Acromioclavicular, Clavicle, and Sternoclavicular Injuries in Athletes

Editor

KATHERINE J. COYNER

CLINICS IN SPORTS MEDICINE

www.sportsmed.theclinics.com

Consulting Editor
MARK D. MILLER

October 2023 • Volume 42 • Number 4

ELSEVIER

1600 John F. Kennedy Boulevard • Suite 1800 • Philadelphia, Pennsylvania, 19103-2899

http://www.theclinics.com

CLINICS IN SPORTS MEDICINE Volume 42, Number 4
October 2023 ISSN 0278-5919, ISBN-13: 978-0-443-18386-7

Editor: Megan Ashdown
Developmental Editor: Malvika Shah

Clinics in Sports Medicine (ISSN 0278-5919) is published quarterly by Elsevier Inc., 360 Park Avenue South, New York, NY 10010-1710. Months of issue are January, April, July, and October. Business and Editorial Offices: 1600 John F. Kennedy Blvd., Ste. 1800, Philadelphia, PA 19103-2899. Customer Service Office: 3251 Riverport Lane, Maryland Heights, MO 63043. Periodicals postage paid at New York, NY and additional mailing offices. Subscription prices are $379.00 per year (US individuals), $773.00 per year (US institutions), $100.00 per year (US students), $421.00 per year (Canadian individuals), $953.00 per year (Canadian institutions), $100.00 (Canadian students), $494.00 per year (foreign individuals), $953.00 per year (foreign institutions), and $235.00 per year (foreign students). Foreign air speed delivery is included in all *Clinics* subscription prices. All prices are subject to change without notice. **POSTMASTER:** Send address changes to *Clinics in Sports Medicine*, Elsevier Health Sciences Division, Subscription Customer Service, 3251 Riverport Lane, Maryland Heights, MO 63043. Customer Service (orders, claims, online, change of address): Elsevier Health Sciences Division, Subscription Customer Service, 3251 Riverport Lane, Maryland Heights, MO 63043. **Tel: 1-800-654-2452 (U.S. and Canada); 314-447-8871 (outside U.S. and Canada). Fax: 314-447-8029. E-mail: journalscustomerservice-usa@elsevier.com (for print support); journalsonlinesupport-usa@ elsevier.com (for online support).**

Reprints. For copies of 100 or more of articles in this publication, please contact the Commercial Reprints Department, Elsevier Inc., 360 Park Avenue South, New York, NY 10010-1710. Tel.: 212-633-3874; Fax: 212-633-3820; E-mail: reprints@elsevier.com.

Clinics in Sports Medicine is covered in *MEDLINE/PubMed (Index Medicus) Current Contents/Clinical Medicine, Excerpta Medica,* and *ISI/Biomed.*

Contributors

CONSULTING EDITOR

MARK D. MILLER, MD
S. Ward Casscells Professor, Head, Department of Orthopaedic Surgery, Division of Sports Medicine, University of Virginia, Charlottesville, Virginia, USA; Team Physician, Miller Review Course, Harrisonburg, Virginia, USA

EDITOR

KATHERINE J. COYNER, MD, MBA
UConn Health Sports Medicine Fellowship Director, Orthopaedic Team Physician UConn Athletics, University of Connecticut Health Center; Associate Professor, Department of Orthopeadic Surgery, University of Connecticut School of Medicine, Associate Sports Medicine Fellowship Director, Farmington, Connecticut, USA

AUTHORS

RAMESSES A. AKAMEFULA, BS
Tulane University School of Medicine, New Orleans, Louisiana, USA

JOHN M. APOSTOLAKOS, MD, MPH
Steadman Philippon Research Institute, Vail, Colorado, USA

BLAKE M. BACEVICH, BS
Sports Medicine, Mass General Hospital, Harvard Medical School, Boston, Massachusetts, USA

KNUT BEITZEL, PhD
Professor, Orthoparc Klinik, Cologne, Germany

LEAH BROWN, MD, FAAOS
Associate Clinical Professor, Banner Orthopaedic Sports Medicine, University of Arizona College of Medicine - Phoenix, Scottsdale, Arizona, USA

E. LYLE CAIN, Jr, MD
Fellowship Director, ASMI, American Sports Medicine Institute, Andrews Sports Medicine and Orthopaedic Center, Birmingham, Alabama, USA

FERDINAND J. CHAN, MD
Montefiore Einstein, Department of Orthopaedic Surgery, Bronx, New York, USA

PETER S. CHANG, MD
The Steadman Clinic, Steadman Philippon Research Institute, Vail, Colorado, USA

KATHERINE J. COYNER, MD, MBA
UConn Health Sports Medicine Fellowship Director, Orthopaedic Team Physician UConn Athletics, University of Connecticut Health Center; Associate Professor, Department of Orthopeadic Surgery, University of Connecticut School of Medicine, Associate Sports Medicine Fellowship Director, Farmington, Connecticut, USA

TYLER R. CRAM, DO
Department of Orthopedic Surgery, University of Colorado School of Medicine, Aurora, Colorado, USA

NATALIA CZERWONKA, MD
Resident Physician, Department of Orthopedic Surgery, Columbia University Irving Medical Center, NewYork-Presbyterian Hospital, New York, New York, USA

ALIRIO J. DEMEIRELES, MD, MBA
Resident Physician, Department of Orthopedic Surgery, Columbia University Irving Medical Center, NewYork-Presbyterian Hospital, New York, New York, USA

CORY EDGAR, MD, PhD
Assistant Professor, Co-Director, UConn Institute for Sports Medicine, Director of Biomechanical Research, Department of Orthopaedic Surgery, University of Connecticut, Head, Team Physician: US Coast Guard Academy, Farmington, Connecticut, USA

CHRISTOPHER M. EDWARDS, BS
Department of Orthopedic Surgery, University of Connecticut School of Medicine, Farmington, Connecticut, USA

SAMUEL R. ENGEL, MA
Department of Orthopedic Surgery, University of Connecticut School of Medicine, Farmington, Connecticut, USA

RACHEL M. FRANK, MD
Department of Orthopedic Surgery, University of Colorado School of Medicine, Aurora, Colorado, USA

WADE GOBBELL, MD
Department of Orthopedic Surgery, University of Connecticut School of Medicine, Farmington, Connecticut, USA

BONNIE GREGORY, MD
Assistant Professor, Department of Orthopaedic Surgery, The University of Texas Health Science Center at Houston/McGovern Medical School, Houston, Texas, USA

JEFFREY D. HASSEBROCK, MD
Department of Orthopedic Surgery, University of Colorado School of Medicine, Aurora, Colorado, USA

MATTHEW J. KRAEUTLER, MD
Department of Orthopaedic Surgery and Sports Medicine, Houston Methodist Hospital, Houston, Texas, USA

WILLIAM N. LEVINE, MD
Frank E. Stinchfield Professor and Chair, Department of Orthopedic Surgery, Columbia University Irving Medical Center, NewYork-Presbyterian Hospital, New York, New York, USA

BENJAMIN J. LEVY, MD
Montefiore Einstein, Department of Orthopaedic Surgery, Bronx, New York, USA

JAYSON LIAN, MD
Montefiore Einstein, Department of Orthopaedic Surgery, Bronx, New York, USA

BENJAMIN C. MAYO, MD
Department of Orthopaedic Surgery, University of Connecticut, UConn Musculoskeletal
Institute, Farmington, Connecticut, USA

AUGUSTUS D. MAZZOCCA, MS, MD
Chief of Sports Medicine Division of Sports Medicine, Department of Orthopaedic
Surgery, Massachusetts General Hospital, Harvard School of Medicine, Massachusetts
General Brigham, Boston, Massachusetts, USA

MARY K. MULCAHEY, MD
Division director of sports medicine Department of Orthopaedic Surgery and
Rehabilitation, Loyola University Medical Center, Maywood, Illinois, USA

COLIN P. MURPHY, MD
Orthopedic Surgery Resident University of North Dakota Orthopaedic Surgery Residency
Program, Fargo, North Dakota, USA

ROBERT J. NASCIMENTO, MD
Assistant Clinical Professor Division of Sports Medicine, Department of Orthopaedic
Surgery, Massachusetts General Hospital, Harvard School of Medicine, Massachusetts
General Brigham, Boston, Massachusetts, USA

EVAN A. O'DONNELL, MD
Division of Sports Medicine, Department of Orthopaedic Surgery, Massachusetts General
Hospital, Harvard School of Medicine, Massachusetts General Brigham, Boston,
Massachusetts, USA

BRITTANY OLSEN, MD
Department of Orthopaedic Surgery, The University of Texas Health Science Center at
Houston/McGovern Medical School, Houston, Texas, USA

NOZIMAKHON K. OMONULLAEVA, BS
Sports Medicine, Mass General Hospital, Boston, Massachusetts, USA; Nova
Southeastern University, College of Osteopathic Medicine, Fort Lauderdale, Florida, USA

DAVID PARKER, MD
Orthopaedic Fellow, ASMI, American Sports Medicine Institute, Andrews Sports
Medicine and Orthopaedic Center, Birmingham, Alabama, USA

LIAM A. PEEBLES, BA
Tulane University School of Medicine, New Orleans, Louisiana, USA

NICHOLAS P.J. PERRY, MD
Physician Division of Sports Medicine, Department of Orthopaedic Surgery,
Massachusetts General Hospital, Harvard School of Medicine, Massachusetts General
Brigham, Boston, Massachusetts, USA

MARK D. PRICE, MD
Orthopedic Surgeon Division of Sports Medicine, Department of Orthopaedic Surgery,
Massachusetts General Hospital, Harvard School of Medicine, Massachusetts General
Brigham, Boston, Massachusetts, USA

CAPT MATTHEW T. PROVENCHER, MD, MBA, MC, USNR (Ret)
Professor of Surgery & Orthopaedics The Steadman Clinic, Steadman Philippon Research Institute, Vail, Colorado, USA

NIKOLAOS PLATON SACHINIS, PhD
First Orthopaedic Department of Aristotle University of Thessaloniki, "Georgios Papanikolaou" Hospital, Greece

MIHIR M. SHETH, MD
Southern California Orthopedic Institute, Van Nuys, California, USA

THEODORE B. SHYBUT, MD
Associate Professor Baylor College of Medicine, Houston, Texas, USA

DANIEL J. STOKES, MD
Research Fellow Department of Orthopedic Surgery, University of Colorado School of Medicine, Aurora, Colorado, USA

LISA M. TAMBURINI, MD
Orthopeadic Surgery Resident Department of Orthopaedic Surgery, University of Connecticut, UConn Musculoskeletal Institute, Farmington, Connecticut, USA

MYRA TRIVELLAS, MD
Department of Orthopaedic Surgery, Duke University School of Medicine, Durham, North Carolina, USA

RYAN J. WHALEN, BS, CSCS
Research Coordinator Steadman Philippon Research Institute, Vail, Colorado, USA

JOCELYN WITTSTEIN, MD
Associate Professor, Department of Orthopaedic Surgery, Duke University School of Medicine, Durham, North Carolina, USA

Contents

Foreword: Acromioclavicular–Clavicle–Sternoclavicular: Strutting Horizontally   xiii

Mark D. Miller

Preface: Acromioclavicular, Clavicle, and Sternoclavicular Injuries in Athletes   xv

Katherine J. Coyner

Management of Acromioclavicular Joint Injuries: A Historic Account   539

Liam A. Peebles, Ramesses A. Akamefula, Matthew J. Kraeutler, and
Mary K. Mulcahey

There has been a rapid evolution in best practice management of acromio-clavicular (AC) joint injuries. AP, Zanca, scapular Y, and dynamic axillary radiographic views provide optimal visualization of the joint and may assess for the presence of horizontal AC instability. Severity of AC joint pathology is classified according to the 6-tier Rockwood scoring system. Over 160 surgical techniques have been described for AC joint repair and reconstruction in the last decade; as a result, determining the optimal treatment algorithm has become increasingly challenging secondary to the lack of consistently excellent clinical outcomes.

Acromioclavicular Joint Anatomy and Biomechanics: The Significance of Posterior Rotational and Translational Stability   557

Nicholas P.J. Perry, Nozimakhon K. Omonullaeva, Blake M. Bacevich,
Robert J. Nascimento, Evan A. O'Donnell, Mark D. Price, and
Augustus D. Mazzocca

The shoulder girdle extends from the sternoclavicular joint to the scapular stabilizing muscles posteriorly. It consists of 3 joints and 2 mobile regions. The shoulder girdle is statically stabilized by the acromioclavicular and coracoclavicular capsuloligamentous structures and dynamically stabilized by the trapezius, deltoid, and deltotrapezial fascia. During humerothoracic elevation, the clavicle elevates, protracts, and rotates posteriorly through the sternoclavicular joint while the scapula tilts posteriorly and rotates upward. The purpose of this article is to review the anatomy and biomechanics of the acromioclavicular joint and the shoulder girdle.

Diagnosis and Nonoperative Treatment of Acromioclavicular Joint Injuries in Athletes and Guide for Return to Play   573

Brittany Olsen and Bonnie Gregory

Injury to the acromioclavicular (AC) joint accounts for approximately 40% to 50% of all shoulder injuries. In contact sports, the prevalence of AC joint injury increases. This injury is frequently encountered and treated by fellowship-trained as well as general orthopedic surgeons. As such, it is important to understand the diagnostic and treatment pathways for AC joint disruption. The treatment pathways in athletes may be different from those in the general population. This article will focus on the diagnosis and non-operative treatment of AC joint injuries in athletes. We will also comment on return-to-play guidelines after this nonoperative treatment.

Open Anatomic Coracoclavicular Ligament Reconstruction for Acromioclavicular Joint Injuries   589

E. Lyle Cain Jr. and David Parker

Open reconstruction of the coracoclavicular (CC) and acromioclavicular (AC) ligaments results in excellent reduction of severely displaced AC dislocations, most commonly Grades III and V. Anatomic CC reconstruction through clavicular bone tunnels can prevent vertical instability, whereas the addition of an acromial limb of the graft can increase horizontal stability. Autograft tendon is preferred in the young athletic group of collision sports participants, although allograft has had acceptable results. Accessory fixation may be placed to protect the graft during healing, or for severe instability, especially for athletes involved in contact sports.

Arthroscopic Repair and Reconstruction of Coracoclavicular Ligament   599

Jeffrey D. Hassebrock, Daniel J. Stokes, Tyler R. Cram, and Rachel M. Frank

Acromioclavicular joint separations are common shoulder injuries that require prompt recognition, diagnosis, and treatment. Deciding on a treatment algorithm relies on a detailed knowledge of anatomy and a thorough understanding of the specific functional demands of the patient in question. When a repair or reconstruction is indicated, arthroscopic assistance can be a helpful tool to ensure a safe, anatomic reconstruction that minimizes morbidity and maximizes the potential return to high-level function.

Risk for Fracture with Acromioclavicular Joint Reconstruction and Strategies for Mitigation   613

Nikolaos Platon Sachinis and Knut Beitzel

Acromioclavicular (AC) joint injuries are a common cause of shoulder pain, especially among athletes. Surgical reconstruction of the AC joint can lead to complications such as fracture of the coracoid process, clavicle or acromion, which can negatively affect the patient's outcome. The purpose of this review is to discuss the risk factors for fractures associated with AC joint reconstruction, as well as the strategies that can be used to mitigate this risk. Risk factors for fractures include low mineral density, coracoid/clavicle drilling, larger holes in the coracoid, and the number of tunnels used for reconstruction.

Surgical Pearls and Pitfalls for Anatomic Acromioclavicular/Coracoclavicular Ligament Reconstruction   621

Peter S. Chang, Colin P. Murphy, Ryan J. Whalen, John M. Apostolakos, and Matthew T. Provencher

Injuries to the acromioclavicular (AC) joint are common shoulder injuries in contact/collision athletes. There are a number of different surgical options that can be used to treat these injuries. The majority of these injuries can be treated nonoperatively with an early return to play for type I and II injuries. Surgical intervention and AC/CC (coracoclavicular) ligament reconstruction have excellent postoperative outcomes if complications can be avoided. This review will focus on the pearls and pitfalls for anatomic AC and CC ligament reconstruction for high-grade AC joint injuries.

Midshaft Clavicle Fractures: When Is Surgical Management Indicated and Which Fixation Method Should Be Used?   633

Myra Trivellas and Jocelyn Wittstein

For displaced midshaft clavicle fractures, operative treatment either with open reduction and plate fixation or with intramedullary fixation has been shown to provide earlier return to work and sport, improved functional outcomes, greater patient-reported satisfaction with appearance, and significantly decreased incidence of nonunion and malunion when compared with conservative treatment. Operative intervention is not without risks associated with surgery. Shared decision-making with the patient and understanding patient goals allows surgeons to recommend a management option that the patient will be comfortable with and will follow to achieve a satisfactory outcome.

Getting Athletes Back on the Field: Management of Clavicle Fractures and Return to Play   649

Wade Gobbell, Christopher M. Edwards, Samuel R. Engel, and Katherine J. Coyner

This chapter provides an overview of the prevalence of clavicle fractures in athletes. The evaluation and management of clavicle fractures in athletes is summarized, including surgical considerations, rehabilitation protocols, and return to sport guidelines. In this population, high rates of union are observed, but careful timing of return to sport is paramount to optimize performance and prevent reinjury.

Clavicle Nonunion and Malunion: Surgical Interventions for Functional Improvement   663

Alirio J. deMeireles, Natalia Czerwonka, and William N. Levine

Clavicle nonunion and malunion are relatively uncommon but, when symptomatic, can result in pain and dysfunction that requires surgical intervention. Various reconstructive and grafting techniques are available to achieve stable fixation and union. In the setting of persistent nonunion, vascularized bone grafting may be necessary. A thorough understanding of the patient's type of nonunion and potential for healing is crucial for achieving satisfactory results because is thoughtful preoperative planning and surgical fixation.

Dual- Versus Single-Plate Fixation of Clavicle Fractures: Understanding the Rationale Behind both Approaches   677

Lisa M. Tamburini, Benjamin C. Mayo, and Cory Edgar

Clavicle fractures are a common injury resulting from a high-energy force, such as a fall onto the shoulder, motor vehicle accident, or sporting activity. Although some clavicle fractures may be treated nonoperatively, operative treatment results in higher union rates and faster return to activity. Here we discuss the operative treatment options for plating of clavicle fractures; specifically, a single plate placed either superiorly or anteriorly or two plates placed orthogonally. Because both techniques provide adequate stability, fracture and patient characteristics should guide the surgical decision making regarding single versus dual plating of clavicle fractures.

Classification of Distal Clavicle Fractures and Indications for Conservative Treatment

685

Jayson Lian, Ferdinand J. Chan, and Benjamin J. Levy

Management of distal clavicle fractures depends on a clear understanding of the injury's proximity to the ligamentous attachments joining the clavicle and scapula. Various classification systems have been proposed to guide treatment. Despite this, controversy between operative and nonoperative management remains for certain fracture patterns. Patient-specific factors, concomitant injuries, fracture characteristics (displacement, shortening, and rotation) should all be considered when deciding on treatment. When nonoperative management is indicated, patients should be immobilized in a sling for 2 weeks, followed by gradual range of motion, and strengthening exercises.

Operative Management for Displaced Distal Clavicle Fractures

695

Mihir M. Sheth and Theodore B. Shybut

This article reviews techniques and outcomes of surgical fixation for distal clavicle fractures. Near 100% union has been reported for several techniques. The most common are locked plating, coracoclavicular fixation and a combination of plating with CC fixation. Hook plates are useful for particular fracture patterns, but there can be complications specific to this implant. Low-profile constructs are favored due to the high rates of symptomatic hardware. Fixation of subacute and chronic injuries can provide reliable functional improvements, but is inferior to acute fixation. Surgery is generally the treatment of choice for displaced fractures in athletes.

Traumatic Sternoclavicular Dislocations in Athletes: Diagnosis, Indications for Surgical Reconstruction, and Guide for Return to Play

713

Leah Brown and Lisa M. Tamburini

Injuries to the sternoclavicular (SC) joint are rare, however, when they occur prompt recognition, evaluation, and treatment are crucial. SC joint injuries can occur following high-energy mechanisms such as motor vehicle collisions and contact sports. Injury to the SC joint can be evaluated with the use of plain radiographs as well as computed tomography. If an injury to the SC joint is suspected, injury to vital mediastinal structures must be evaluated. SC joint dislocations can be treated by either closed reduction or open reduction and stabilization. Many stabilization methods have been described including plate stabilization and ligament reconstruction.

Atraumatic Sternoclavicular Joint Instability: Prevalence, Etiology, and Management   723

Wade Gobbell, Christopher M. Edwards, Samuel R. Engel, and
Katherine J. Coyner

Sternoclavicular joint instability is a rare complaint in the orthopedic clinic, but patients can experience chronic pain and functional impacts. Causes of instability may be posttraumatic, infectious, autoimmune, degenerative, or secondary to generalized laxity. Conservative treatment is the initial approach to management and involves activity modification, physical therapy, oral nonsteroidal anti-inflammatory drugs, and corticosteroid injections. Surgery is indicated when conservative treatment does not manage symptoms. Figure-of-eight reconstruction techniques provide greatest biomechanical strength but are associated with risk of neurovascular injury. Other reconstruction methods have been shown to mitigate these risks with favorable short-term outcomes.

CLINICS IN SPORTS MEDICINE

FORTHCOMING ISSUES

January 2024
Mental Health Considerations in the Athlete
Siobhán M. Statuta, *Editor*

April 2024
Equality, Diversity, and Inclusion in Sports Medicine
Joel Boyd, Constance Chu and Erica Taylor, *Editors*

July 2024
Precision ACL Reconstruction
Volker Musahl, and Alan Getgood, *Editors*

RECENT ISSUES

July 2023
On-the-Field Emergencies
Eric McCarty, Sourav Poddar, and Alex Ebinger, *Editors*

April 2023
Coaching, Mentorship and Leadership in Medicine: Empowering the Development of Patient-Centered Care
Dean C. Taylor, Joe Doty, Jonathan F. Dickens, and Carolyn M. Hettrich, *Editors*

January 2023
Advances in the Treatment of Rotator Cuff Tears
Brian C. Werner, *Editor*

SERIES OF RELATED INTERESTED

Orthopedic Clinics
https://www.orthopedic.theclinics.com/
Foot and Ankle Clinics
https://www.foot.theclinics.com/
Hand Clinics
https://www.hand.theclinics.com/
Physical Medicine and Rehabilitation Clinics
https://www.pmr.theclinics.com/

THE CLINICS ARE AVAILABLE ONLINE!
Access your subscription at:
www.theclinics.com

Foreword

Acromioclavicular–Clavicle–Sternoclavicular: Strutting Horizontally

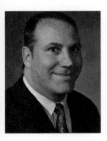

Mark D. Miller, MD
Consulting Editor

The clavicle is the only long horizontal bone in the body and plays a vital role in stabilizing the upper extremities. Because of its vulnerable location and subcutaneous nature, it is prone to injury, especially in athletes. The clavicle's attachments to the acromion via the acromioclavicular (AC) joint and sternum via the sternoclavicular (SC) joint are robust, but are also not uncommonly injured Treatment of these injuries is often challenging, and even the most secure fixation can fail. That makes this topic an ideal subject for an issue in *Clinics in Sports Medicine*.

I invited Dr Katherine Coyner, an expert in the treatment of these injuries, to put together a treatise on the diagnosis and treatment of injuries of these vital components of the shoulder girdle. As expected, she has done an excellent job. The issue focuses on the AC joint, offering a historical, anatomic, and biomechanical review as well as discussing diagnosis and treatment options. We have all heard the premise that if there are multiple ways to fix something, then we haven't figured out the best way to do it — well, that is certainly apropos for treatment of AC injuries. Several good articles on clavicle fractures and their treatment follow, and the issue concludes with two well-written articles on SC injuries and their treatment.

So, there you have it — a complete guide to the diagnosis and treatment of this vital horizontal strut. Thank you to Dr Coyner and all contributing authors — now let's get to

Clin Sports Med 42 (2023) xiii–xiv
https://doi.org/10.1016/j.csm.2023.06.015
0278-5919/23/© 2023 Published by Elsevier Inc.

sportsmed.theclinics.com

work and find the best operations with the least amount of complications and shoulder the responsibility of treating these often challenging problems.

Mark D. Miller, MD
Department of Orthopaedic Surgery
University of Virginia
James Madison University
400 Ray C. Hunt Drive, Suite 330
Charlottesville, VA 22908-0159, USA

E-mail address:
MDM3P@hscmail.mcc.virginia.edu

Preface

Acromioclavicular, Clavicle, and Sternoclavicular Injuries in Athletes

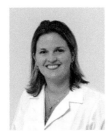

Katherine J. Coyner, MD, MBA
Editor

As the guest editor for this issue on acromioclavicular, clavicle, and sternoclavicular injuries in athletes, I am thrilled to present a comprehensive guide on the diagnosis, management, and treatment of these complex injuries. As an orthopedic sports surgeon with experience treating athletes at all levels of competition, I have seen firsthand the impact that these types of injuries can have on an athlete's performance, career, and quality of life.

The acromioclavicular, clavicle, and sternoclavicular joints are essential components of the shoulder girdle, and injuries to these structures can present significant management challenges. This issue includes a comprehensive review of the anatomy, biomechanics, and pathophysiology of the shoulder complex, along with a comprehensive approach to diagnosis, imaging, and treatment. By providing the latest advances in surgical techniques, readers will have access to the most up-to-date information on managing these injuries in athletes.

This issue brings together leading experts in the field of orthopedic surgery and sports medicine to provide a comprehensive overview of these injuries. Our contributors represent a diverse range of backgrounds, experiences, and perspectives, ensuring that readers have access to a wide range of perspectives of acromioclavicular, clavicle, and sternoclavicular injuries in athletes from various populations. Each article is written

Clin Sports Med 42 (2023) xv–xvi
https://doi.org/10.1016/j.csm.2023.06.014
0278-5919/23/© 2023 Published by Elsevier Inc.

sportsmed.theclinics.com

by an expert in the field with a focus on evidence-based medicine and practical guidance for the clinician.

Katherine J. Coyner, MD, MBA
University of Connecticut Health Center
Department of Orthopeadic Surgery
UConn Athletics
263 Farmington Avenue
Farmington, CT 06030, USA

Management of Acromioclavicular Joint Injuries: A Historic Account

Liam A. Peebles, BA[a], Ramesses A. Akamefula, BS[a],
Matthew J. Kraeutler, MD[b], Mary K. Mulcahey, MD[c],*

KEYWORDS

- Acromioclavicular joint • Acromioclavicular reconstruction
- Coracoclavicular ligaments

KEY POINTS

- Treatment strategies for acromioclavicular (AC) joint injuries date back to the first century, and since then, major advancements in surgical and nonsurgical interventions to restore AC joint anatomy and biomechanics have been discovered.
- The original classification systems introduced and modified by Tossy (1963), Allman (1964), and Rockwood (1984) have stood the test of time and are still used in daily practice for the assessment and treatment of AC joint injuries.
- Although there is a historical consensus on treating Rockwood type I and II AC joint injuries nonoperatively, debate regarding the optimal management of type III injuries persists today.
- Early operative techniques for treating AC joint separation fall under several general classifications: (1) AC joint fixation or ligamentous repair; (2) CC ligament transfer involving transfer of the CA ligament to the distal clavicle; (3) CC ligament reinforcement with sutures, cerclage, sling, or screw fixation; and (4) free graft augmentation or reconstruction of the CC ligament complex.

INTRODUCTION
Acromioclavicular Joint Anatomy

The shoulder girdle consists of the scapula and the clavicle, giving rise to 5 major articulating regions that help with upper extremity movements.[1] One of these regions is the acromioclavicular (AC) joint, which is an articulation that helps attach the upper limb to the axial skeleton.[2] The AC joint can be described as a freely moving, diarthrodial joint

[a] Tulane University School of Medicine, 1430 Tulane Avenue, #2070, New Orleans, LA, USA;
[b] Department of Orthopedics & Sports Medicine, Houston Methodist Hospital, 6445 Main Street, #2300, Houston, TX, USA; [c] Department of Orthopaedic Surgery and Rehabilitation, Loyola University Medical Center, Maywood, IL, USA
* Corresponding author. 2160 South 1st Avenue #3328, Maywood, IL 60153.
E-mail address: mary.mulcahey.md@gmail.com

Clin Sports Med 42 (2023) 539–556
https://doi.org/10.1016/j.csm.2023.05.001
0278-5919/23/© 2023 Elsevier Inc. All rights reserved.

sportsmed.theclinics.com

that is formed via the articulation between the medial border of the anterior side of the acromion and the distal end of the clavicle.[3] More specifically, this relationship consists of the medial facet of the clavicle, oriented posterior-laterally, that articulates with the acromion, which is oriented anterior-medially.[3] The overall shapes of these facets have been described in the literature as variable, but a concave or flattened-shaped acromial facet articulating with a convex clavicular facet seems to be the most common anatomy described.[4]

Current quantitative studies illustrate that the AC joint is about 9 mm in height in the superior-to-inferior direction, and 19 mm in depth in the anterior-to-posterior direction.[5] The width of the AC joint has also been quantified and appears to decline with age. On average, females have an AC joint space width between 1 mm and 6 mm, while males have a joint space width between 1 mm and 7 mm.[6] Finally, the plane of the AC joint formally slants between 20° and 30° relative to the anterior-medial and superior-lateral aspects of the joint.[7] However, variations exist in which the clavicle overrides the acromion, giving an almost horizontal orientation, or even a completely flush orientation leading to a vertical alignment.[7]

Acromioclavicular Ligament and Capsular Anatomy

The AC ligaments stabilize the AC joint, primarily functioning as a restraint to horizontal joint translation.[8,9] This stabilizing effect is about 3 times more prominent in the anterior-posterior direction when compared with the restraint it provides vertically.[8,9] In addition, the AC ligaments also function as clavicular restraints, keeping the clavicle from rotating posteriorly.

The AC ligament complex can be described as thickenings of the AC joint capsule itself, subsequently giving rise to multiple structures.[10] This complex of ligaments may further be divided into 2 major bundles, one oriented superiorly and posteriorly about the joint, and one bundle oriented anteriorly and inferiorly.[11,12] Running in an oblique manner, the superior-posterior (SP) bundle of the AC ligament complex reinforces the AC joint capsule and has been noted to be the stronger of the 2 bundles.[13] More specifically, the SP bundle reinforces the AC joint between the posterior aspect of the distal clavicle and the anterior aspect of the acromion.[14] Grossly, the superior portion of the AC capsule itself has been described as thicker when compared with the inferior capsule. This added thickness also comes with an acromial attachment that is wider compared with the inferior AC joint capsule.[14] The inferior-anterior (IA) bundle originates at the anterior aspect of the acromion or the AC joint capsule, with multiple insertions across the anterior and inferior portions of the joint capsule, and the distal clavicle along its anterior margin.[13] The IA bundle has greater variability in morphology and presence, with variations in origins and insertion points along the joint capsule, acromion, and clavicle.[15] Additionally, the IA bundle is typically smaller and contributes less to AC joint capsule stability when compared with the SP bundle.[16] Finally, compared with the superior portion, the inferior portion of the AC joint capsule consists of much thinner ligamentous tissues, thereby providing minimal reinforcement of the AC joint.[16]

Coracoclavicular Ligament Anatomy

The coracoclavicular (CC) ligaments are the primary stabilizers of the AC joint, predominantly working in the vertical plane when the shoulder girdle is in an uncompromised state.[8] In instances where the AC joint capsule is disrupted, the CC ligaments may also function secondarily as a primary AC joint stabilizer in the horizontal plane.[12] The larger of the 2 ligaments, the trapezoid ligament (TL) has a quadrilateral structure and inserts on the distal end of the clavicle adjacent to the trapezoidal ridge.[17,18] Quantitative analysis illustrates that this insertion ranges between 1.5 cm and 3.0 cm from the AC joint.[17,18] Functionally, the TL resists clavicular displacement in the posterior direction, while additionally preventing AC joint compression.[1] Conical in shape, the conoid ligament traverses in a more vertical fashion and is positioned posterior-medially compared with the trapezoid ligament.[19] The conoid ligament fibers have been described as twisting as they ascend, eventually attaching to the conoid tubercle located on the inferior surface of the clavicle.[17] Functionally, the conoid ligament restrains the clavicle from translating superiorly.[17] Thus, the conoid ligament is a primary stabilizer of the AC joint in the vertical plane.[10,13–16]

Pathophysiology of Acromioclavicular Joint Injury

AC joint injuries can be divided into 2 distinct categories, those that are direct and those that are nondirect. The more common of the two, direct AC joint injuries result from an external force acting on the AC joint itself.[20] A common example of a direct AC joint injury may include an individual falling on the shoulder while the arm is adducted. This typically results in the scapula being forced inferiorly relative to the clavicle and at first disrupts the AC ligament, but can also cause injury to the CC ligaments following a more severe injury and greater displacement of the acromion.[9] Indirect AC joint injuries may also occur during a fall, but commonly arise while the individual tries to brace the fall with an extended, or outstretched arm and hand.[21] This mechanism forces the humerus superiorly and toward the acromion, thus disrupting the AC joint and its components. Indirect injuries often affect the AC ligaments, but commonly spare the CC ligaments, typically leading to a lower-grade injury (via Rockwood grading system).[22] Regardless of the mechanism of injury, AC joint injuries are often diagnosed based on patient history, physical examination, and imaging.[23]

Early Accounts of Acromioclavicular Joint Injury

Records of AC joint injuries can be traced as far back as 400 BC.[24] Historic accounts of Hippocrates (460–370 BC) have illustrated his commentary on the misdiagnosis of AC joint injuries for glenohumeral joint injuries.[24] Treatment strategies for AC joint injuries also date back to the first century and include tight bandaging. Since then, major advancements in surgical and nonsurgical interventions to restore AC joint anatomy and biomechanics have been discovered.

Incidence, Etiology, and Epidemiology

Most AC joint injuries occur in young adults between the ages of 20 and 40 years.[25,26] Males sustain AC joint injuries at a rate 5 times higher than females.[25,26] Especially within athletic populations, AC joint injuries can be extremely common, and depending on the individual sport, may comprise up to 40% to 50% of shoulder injuries.[27] As illustrated previously, the most common etiology of AC joint pathology is a direct external force to the shoulder with the arm in an adducted position. This mechanism of injury frequently occurs in individuals participating in contact sports such as football, lacrosse, hockey, and rugby.[28]

Much of the current literature states that up to 9% of all shoulder injuries involve damage to the AC joint also.[29] However, some authors speculate that this statistic evolved from a book chapter that dates to 1958 and may overestimate the incidence of overall AC joint pathology when compared with more recent data that suggest AC joint injuries occur in only 4% of shoulder injuries.[30] Despite current suggestions, hospital data pertaining to the incidence of AC joint injuries may be inaccurate and underestimated, because of those patients with less severe (ie, Rockwood Type I and II injuries) AC joint injuries who do not pursue evaluation and treatment.[26]

ASSESSMENT OF ACROMIOCLAVICULAR INJURIES
Radiographic Evaluation

Typically, a standard shoulder trauma series of plain radiographs are used to evaluate AC joint injures.[31] The anterior-posterior (AP) and Zanca views are frequently used to evaluate the AC joint and distal clavicle, with the Zanca view accepted as the more accurate by many surgeons (**Fig. 1**).[32] Although the standard AP view illustrates the AC joint, oftentimes an angulated AP view must be applied for optimal visualization to avoid possible overpenetration as a result of increased radiolucency from overlapping structures.[33] For example, the Zanca view utilizes a 10° to 15° cephalad tilt to achieve a better view of the clavicle by decreasing the amount of scapula and clavicle superimposed on one another.[32,34] Additional views such as the lateral (or scapular Y) (**Fig. 2**) and dynamic axillary views (**Fig. 3**) may also be utilized, especially in the case of evaluating horizontal instability and differentiating between Type III and Type IV injuries.[35,36] Standard bilateral AP and bilateral Alexander views may also be used to increase diagnostic accuracy by using the contralateral AC joint to better determine native anatomy. Moreover, as opposed to solely using visual inspection, specific measurements of the contralateral noninjured AC and CC ligaments via radiographic imaging may also increase sensitivity and evaluation of pathology.[37]

Stress radiographs may also be used to assess AC joint injuries and can be performed while the patient is holding a weight in the hand of the affected side; however, many shoulder surgeons have noted that weightbearing radiographs are unnecessary in the evaluation of AC joint pathologies.[38–40] Standard motivations to use stress radiographs include increased sensitivity and detection of possible underlying joint pathology such as unmasking higher-grade AC joint injuries.[41] Despite this, in some studies, paradoxical CC joint narrowing has been seen while using weightbearing radiographs in 33% of healthy volunteers and up to 10% in those diagnosed with an AC joint injury.[42] A 1999 study by Yap and colleagues[39] surveyed 105 members of the American Shoulder and Elbow Society and found that most (85/105, 81%) respondents recommended against the use of weighted stress views, questioning the utility and practicality of the radiographs in the acute setting. The authors also reported that of the respondents who did use stress radiographs in their practice, most indicated that the results did not impact their treatment decision making. These trends are supported in more recent studies, as Shaw and colleagues[43] reported in a 2018 survey of 37 orthopedic surgeons that only 13% used weighted stress radiographs, and even fewer (10%) felt that their treatment plan would vary based on stress radiograph findings. In the senior author's practice, weightbearing radiographs are not typically ordered for the assessment of acute AC joint injuries. Finally, advanced diagnostic imaging modalities such as CT and MRI are not routinely employed when assessing the AC joint.[41,44] Although this is primarily because of their higher costs and poor

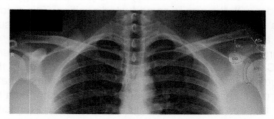

Fig. 1. Bilateral AP radiograph demonstrating Rockwood Type V AC joint injury. AC$_D$, AC distance; CC$_D$, coracoclavicular distance; CL, clavicle; CO, coracoid; G, glenoid; HH, humeral head.

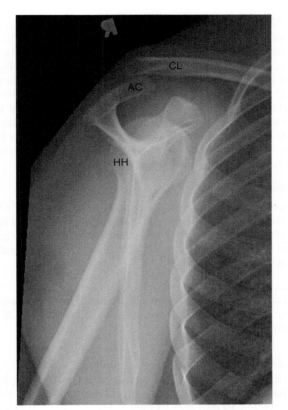

Fig. 2. Right shoulder in the scapular Y view demonstrating a Rockwood Type III A joint injury. AC, acromion; CL, clavicle; HH, humeral head.

availability, CT and MRI are thought to be of low diagnostic value in surgical planning for acute AC joint injuries, as there is normally no need to observe osseous or neurovascular structures in detail.[41,44]

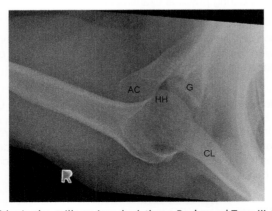

Fig. 3. Right shoulder in the axillary view depicting a Rockwood Type III AC joint injury. AC, acromion; CL, clavicle; HH, humeral head; G, glenoid.

Tossy and Allman Classification

Tossy and colleagues[45] first described a classification system for AC joint injuries in 1963. This characterized AC joint injuries into 3 types. Type I injuries included those in which there is sprain of the AC ligaments, but both the AC and CC ligaments are still intact. Type II injuries are those where the AC ligaments are ruptured, with partial tearing of the CC ligaments. Type III injuries demonstrate complete disruption of both the AC and CC ligaments, leading to vertical AC joint instability. In 1967, Allman further described a similar AC joint injury classification system as Tossy that included a 3-type classification system with virtually the same Type I and Type III class injuries. However, Allman described Type II injuries being characterized by rupturing of the AC ligaments with sprain of the CC ligaments.[46]

Rockwood Classification

Allman's classification system was modified and expanded in 1984, when Rockwood proposed a new 6-tier system to classify AC joint injuries.[45,47,48] The Rockwood classification allows clinicians to determine the severity of AC joint injury based on the ligament complexes involved, the degree of injury, and direction of displacement when evaluated using radiographic imaging.[47–49]

Type I
Low-grade injury caused by AC joint strain with no apparent displacement of the distal clavicle on radiographic imaging. AC ligaments are sprained, but CC ligaments and deltotrapezial complex are intact.[5]

Type II
Disruption of the AC ligaments and AC capsule is evident, resulting in horizontal instability and ability to displace the clavicle during palpation.[21] CC ligaments may be sprained, but remain functional and within range of normal anatomy (ie, CC ligaments maintain length between 10 mm and 13 mm).[48] Radiographic imaging may demonstrate AC joint widening of greater than 7 mm and inferior translation of the acromion relative to the clavicle.[33]

Type III
Evidence of disruption to the AC and CC ligaments. Radiographic imaging may demonstrate up to 100% displacement of the distal clavicle.[33,48] These injuries can be reduced passively during physical examination.

Type IV
Complete disruption of AC and CC ligament complexes with displacement of the distal clavicle posteriorly in the horizontal plane.[50] This injury commonly presents with AP instability and a punctured trapezial fascia.[48]

Type V
Complete disruption of the AC and CC ligament complexes with the CC joint distance more than 100%, but less than 300% compared with the uninjured, contralateral CC ligament length. Unlike Type III injuries, Type V injuries may not be reduced, typically because of buttonholing of the distal clavicle through the deltotrapezial fascia. This leads to another hallmark of Type V injuries, which includes significant disruption of the trapezius and deltoid muscles and fascia.[48,51,52]

Type VI
Complete disruption of the AC and CC ligament complexes with inferior translation of the distal clavicle. This type of injury is extremely rare and requires surgical intervention.[1,22,53]

Grade VI injuries may also be further divided depending on specific location of inferior clavicular displacement, which can either be subacromial (Type VIA), or subcoracoid (Type VIB).[20,48,54]

MANAGEMENT OF ACROMIOCLAVICULAR JOINT INJURIES
Nonoperative Management

Literature prior to the 1960s advocated for more aggressive nonoperative protocols focused on immobilization and reduction of the deformity for all AC joint injuries.[55] This is demonstrated in a 1946 study by Urist[55] and colleagues of 41 patients that reported on the conservative management of complete AC joint dislocations, which generally refers to Type III, IV, V, and VI injuries according to the Rockwood system. The authors noted that a key to successful conservative management was using splints capable of overcorrecting the joint deformity. Using this technique, Urist and colleagues[55] reported successful correction of the deformity and symptomatic relief in approximately 80% of patients treated nonoperatively. In the 20% of patients failing conservative management, deformity, pain, and range of motion (ROM) limitations were common indications for surgical intervention. Palpable posterior displacement and abnormal mobility of the distal clavicle after 3 weeks of nonoperative treatment in these patients were highly suggestive of failure and recurrence of the dislocation.[55]

As management trends evolved in the 1980s and 1990s, surgeons emphasized minimal intervention, treating patients with a sling and immobilization for shorter periods of time.[46,56] Anatomic reduction became a nonessential feature of management, and greater focus was placed on early ROM, strengthening, and return to activity. This was demonstrated in a 1992 survey by Cox and colleagues[57] that reported most surgeons (including 96% of team physicians) preferred to manage Type III injuries nonoperatively. A randomized controlled trial by Larsen and colleagues[58] in 1986 supported this updated approach to nonoperative management by comparing outcomes following conservative or operative treatment of AC joint dislocations. In 84 patients, it was found that most did as well, if not better, with nonoperative management and had significantly shorter rehabilitation periods.[58]

Optimal treatment for AC joint pathology has been heavily debated. Currently, the consensus among most surgeons is that treatment is generally type dependent, with Type IV, V, and VI injuries treated surgically.[59] Although the optimal management of Rockwood Type III AC joint injuries remains controversial, nonoperative treatment is recommended for Type I and II injuries and has yielded reliable outcomes historically.[46,56,60] Sling immobilization and analgesics have thus become mainstays in the nonoperative management of Type I and II injuries. With pain being the primary complaint of patients with these injuries, early treatment should prioritize rest and pain control prior to returning to activity. Rest and application of ice for 1 to 2 weeks or until resolution of symptoms are generally sufficient for Type I injuries, and athletes may be able to return to sport in as soon as 1 to 2 weeks or once they are asymptomatic. Type II AC joint injuries are similarly managed with ice and sling immobilization for 2 weeks; however, the period for return to full activity may take up to 6 to 8 weeks. Because of the increased sagittal plane translation associated with Type II injuries, patients are prone to developing more degenerative changes than those with Type I injuries and thus may require oral nonsteroidal anti-inflammatory drugs or steroid injections later in their treatment course.[9,60–62]

Evolution of Surgical Techniques

In Type IV, V, and VI injuries and some Type III AC joint injuries, surgical management is typically indicated. Techniques for AC joint reconstruction vary and involve different approaches to restoring AC joint stability (**Table 1**). Early operative techniques for treating AC joint separation fall under several general classifications: (1) AC joint fixation or ligamentous repair; (2) CC ligament transfer involving transfer of the CA ligament to the distal clavicle; (3) CC ligament reinforcement with sutures, cerclage, sling, or screw fixation; and (4) free graft augmentation or reconstruction of the CC ligament complex.

Repair of the AC ligaments and reinforcement of the superior AC ligament with the joint meniscus was advocated for in a 1963 study by Sage and Salvatore,[63] and many authors have supplemented this technique with transarticular pins to support the repair.[36,64–66] This approach was popularized early on because of its ease of application and may be performed percutaneously or in an open manner with either smooth or threaded pins. Rigid fixation of the AC joint with a Kirschner wire (K-wire) allows healing of the disrupted CA ligaments by restoring the distance between the clavicle and the coracoid, although this approach has lost popularity because of a high incidence of pin migration, loss of reduction, and degenerative arthritis postoperatively.[67–69] Other authors have supported AC joint plating for management of AC joint separations to reduce the deformity and allow for soft tissue healing.[70–72] Although good-to-excellent results have been reported in up to 90% of cases, hook plating of the AC joint may be associated with impingement on subacromial structures and the development of rotator cuff lesions.[20,73,74]

A 1968 study by Neviaser[75] provided one of the earliest accounts of CA ligament transfer to the distal clavicle to restore AC joint stability without repair of the CC ligaments, and multiple variations of this technique have since been proposed.[64,76] CA ligament transfer with CC ligament screw fixation has also demonstrated reliable outcomes, although some authors have viewed this approach as inadequate for more severe AC joint injuries.[77–79] In the landmark study by Weaver and Dunn in 1972, the authors treated 15 patients with Type III injuries with distal clavicle resection and CC ligament reconstruction using the CA ligament.[80] The original technique has been shown to provide adequate stabilization of the AC joint and pain reduction in most patients.[81,82] Multiple variations of the Weaver-Dunn procedure have since been proposed, including augmentation of the transferred CA ligament with cerclage suture, wire, metal fixation, bone block transfer, or soft tissue autografts and allografts.[82–84] These techniques aim to address persistent pain and recurrent subluxation that has been associated with the traditional Weaver-Dunn procedure.

The native distance between the coracoid and clavicle may also be restored with rigid screw fixation or by using nonrigid synthetic materials. CC ligament repair with percutaneous screws was first described by Bosworth and colleagues[85] in 1941, although this approach has since been shown to be associated with a relatively high technical failure rate.[86] Kennedy and colleagues[87] reported on the use of CC screws with AC joint debridement and trapeziodeltoid repair in 1968, and subsequent studies documented outcomes following CC ligament repair with Bosworth screw fixation.[88–90] Numerous other studies have also advocated for CC ligament repair with cerclage techniques using absorbable and nonabsorbable synthetic devices.[91–96] CC ligament repair with a suture sling has been shown to provide inadequate joint reduction, and the efficacy of polydioxanone (PDS) cerclage has been investigated in multiple comparative studies.[93–95] A 1993 study by Gohring and colleagues[94] reported on 64 complete AC joint dislocations treated with either tension band, hook plate, or braided PDS cord and found the incidence of early postoperative complications to be 43%, 58%, and 17%, respectively. At a mean follow-up time of 35 months, the authors reported recurrent AC joint instability in 32% of patients in the tension band group, 50% in those treated with hook plates, and 24% in the PDS cord group.[94]

Table 1
Classification of original surgical techniques for acromioclavicular joint stabilization

Treatment Classification	Technique	Original Authors, Year
AC joint fixation or ligamentous repair	AC ligament repair and superior AC ligament reinforcement with meniscus	Sage and Salvatore,[63] 1963
	AC ligament repair with transarticular pins	Ahstrom,[64] 1971; Bearden et al,[36] 1973; Augereau et al,[65] 1981; Bartonicek et al,[66] 1988
	AC joint fixation with Wolter, Crook, or Hook plating	Broos et al,[70] 1997; Habernek et al,[71] 1993; Henkel et al,[72] 1997
CC ligament repair with coracoacromial ligament (CAL) transfer to distal clavicle	CAL transfer without CC ligament repair	Neviaser et al,[75] 1968
	CAL transfer with CC ligament screw fixation	Verhaven et al,[79] 1993; Kumar et al,[78] 1995; Guy et al,[77] 1998;
	Distal clavicle resection with CC ligament reconstruction using the CAL	Weaver and Dunn,[80] 1972
	Modified Weaver-Dunn procedure	Kawabe et al,[83] 1984; Shoji et al,[84] 1986; LaPrade et al,[82] 2005
CC ligament repair with sutures, cerclage, sling, screw fixation	CC ligament repair with percutaneous screws	Bosworth et al,[85] 1941
	CC ligament screws with AC joint debridement	Kennedy et al,[87] 1968
	CC ligament repair with cerclage	Gohring et al,[94] 1993; Gollwitzer[95] 1993; Hessman et al,[92] 1995; Colosimo et al,[91] 1996; Clayer et al,[93] 1997
	CC ligament repair with suture sling	Gohring et al,[94] 1993; Gollwitzer[95] 1993; Clayer et al,[93] 1997
CC ligament graft augmentation or reconstruction	Anatomic AC and CC reconstruction with semitendinosus allograft	Jones et al,[97] 2001; Tauber et al,[101] 2009
	Arthroscopic AC and CC reconstruction with gracilis autograft and suture-button tapes	Martetschläger et al,[110] 2016
	Arthroscopic AC reconstruction with double TightRope system	Scheibel et al, 2011
	Arthroscopic CC and AC reconstruction with semitendinosus allograft and clavicular screws	Tauber et al,[111] 2016
	Open all-suture anchor AC reconstruction closing the circle technique	Ângelo et al,[114] 2022
	Open AC reconstruction with semitendinosus or gracilis allograft and interference screws	Aliberti et al,[113] 2020
	Open AC reconstruction with 2 holes in the clavicle all suture technique	Mardani-Kivi et al,[112] 2022

Lastly, anatomic reconstruction of the CC ligamentous complex with soft tissue grafts has risen in popularity over the last 2 decades. Jones and colleagues[97] were the first to describe this technique in 2001 to anatomically recreate the AC and CC ligament complexes. This approach involves drilling 2 clavicular tunnels at the conoid and trapezoid footprints, passing the graft through each tunnel and through the base of coracoid and using the remaining graft limb to reconstruct the AC ligaments. Several in vitro studies have provided biomechanical evidence to support this approach, and it has been shown to be superior to the traditional Weaver-Dunn technique with arthroscopic suture fixation.[98–100] By using a semitendinosus allograft to reconstruct the CC ligament complex, Tauber and colleagues[101] reported significantly better clinical and radiographic outcomes of this approach compared with a modified Weaver-Dunn technique in a series of 24 patients with complete AC joint dislocations.

Emerging Techniques to Address Horizontal Acromioclavicular Joint Instability

The presence of horizontal AC joint instability has been identified as a predictor of inferior clinical outcomes, regardless of operative technique, and thus greater emphasis has been placed on addressing the injured ligamentous anatomy.[50] Although multiple techniques have been proposed to restore vertical joint integrity with CC ligament reconstruction, recent studies have recognized the AC capsule as a contributor to horizontal and rotational stability.[50,102–105] More specifically, the superior aspect of the AC ligament complex has been identified in cadaveric and biomechanical studies as the primary resistor to vertical and rotational translation.[61,103,106,107] Furthermore, there is new biomechanical evidence that suggests anatomic reconstruction of the CC ligaments results in a significantly higher stability of the AC joint in the horizontal plane than reconstruction of the CC ligaments in a nonanatomic configuration.[108] Emerging techniques for open and arthroscopic reconstruction of the AC and CC ligaments have also demonstrated improved clinical and radiographic outcomes and the ability to restore native horizontal stability.[109–114]

In the setting of chronic AC separation, Martetschläger and colleagues[110] proposed an arthroscopically assisted AC and CC ligament reconstruction technique that employs gracilis autograft protected by suture-button tapes (Dog Bone and FiberTape, Arthrex, Naples, FL, USA) to improve horizontal and vertical stability. By looping the graft in front of the clavicle and using fewer, smaller drill holes in the clavicle and coracoid, this technique reduces the risk of weakening the native bony architecture. In theory, this approach mitigates the potential for complications associated with previous graft augmentation techniques such as rupture of the graft, hardware failure, and fracture of the clavicle or coracoid through bone tunnels caused by decreased bone strength.[115–117] Scheibel and colleagues[118] described an arthroscopically assisted AC joint reconstruction technique using a double TightRope (Arthrex) system, consisting of a round clavicular and an oblong coracoid titanium button connected by nonabsorbable Number 5 Fiberwire suture (Arthrex) to augment the torn conoid and trapezoid ligaments in acute AC joint injuries. This technique yielded good-to-excellent outcomes in 28 patients at a mean follow-up of 26.5 months (range, 20.1–32.8 months), although patients with failed correction of horizontal instability were found to have inferior clinical outcomes.[118] In contrast, Tauber and colleagues[111] found that combined anatomic arthroscopic CC ligament reconstruction plus AC ligament reconstruction with a semitendinosus tendon and clavicular interference screw fixation better restored horizontal stability and provided superior clinical and radiographic outcomes when compared with isolated CC reconstruction using the AC Graf-tRope system (Arthrex) with a gracilis tendon.

Multiple open techniques for AC joint reconstruction to correct horizontal instability have also been described in the literature.[112–114] Ângelo and colleagues[114] recently published an all-suture anchor technique that stabilizes the AC joint vertically, horizontally, and rotationally. Using 2 vertical tunnels in the coracoid and clavicle and anterior-to-posterior horizontal tunnels in the acromion and clavicle, this technique reconstructed a circle of stability brought together by the lateral clavicle, the acromion, the coracoid process and the CC, AC, and coracoacromial (CA) ligaments. Aliberti and colleagues[113] also described a novel open reconstruction technique that utilizes a semitendinosus or gracilis allograft with interference screw fixation to restore horizontal stability of the AC joint. The graft is passed across the AC joint in a Figure-8 fashion and fixed to the acromion and clavicle posteriorly to reconstruct the posterior AC capsule, and the native capsule and ligaments are repaired with an additional figure-eight suture over the top of the allograft reconstruction. In a 2022 randomized controlled trial, Mardani-Kivi and colleagues[112] examined acute AC joint horizontal instability following complete dislocation and repair in 104 patients using 1 of 2 Ethibond suture techniques, the loop technique, or the 2 holes in the clavicle technique.

The 2-hole technique involves 2 vertical tunnels in the distal clavicle 1 cm apart, passing a Number 5 Ethibond suture through the first tunnel and looping it around the coracoid to exit through the second tunnel with subsequent flat pinning of the acromion to the clavicle and AC joint capsular repair. The loop technique loops the anchor suture around the clavicle and coracoid instead of passing through a drilled tunnel, and the AC joint is again stabilized with a similar flat pin and capsular repair.

Although both techniques provide significant improvements in Constant Score and Taft Scores at 3, 9, and 12 months, the 2-hole technique resulted in better horizontal stabilization radiographically at all follow-up periods up to 1 year.[112]

SUMMARY

The current and historic literature indicate a rapid and multifaced evolution in best practice management of AC joint injuries. AP, Zanca, scapular Y, and dynamic axillary radiographic views provide optimal visualization of the joint and may reliably assess for the presence of horizontal AC instability. The severity of AC joint pathology is typically classified according to the 6-tier Rockwood scoring system, which was previously adapted from the Tossy and Allman classifications and includes the degree of injury and direction of displacement on radiographs. Over 160 surgical techniques have been described for AC joint repair and reconstruction in the last decade; thus determining the optimal treatment algorithm has become increasingly challenging secondary to the lack of consistently excellent clinical outcomes. Future clinical studies should aim to assess patient outcomes and residual horizontal instability following open AC and CC ligament reconstruction with soft tissue allografts.

CLINICS CARE POINTS

- Careful clinical evaluation with a thorough clinical examination is crucial in determining the severity of AC joint injuries and guides treatment decision making. Imaging studies such as radiographs (AP, Zanca, scapular Y, and dynamic axillary views) and MRI may be useful in further characterizing the injury.
- Optimal management of AC joint injuries should be further guided by the Rockwood classification system, which considers ligament complexes involved, the degree of injury, and direction of displacement when evaluated using radiographic imaging.

- Nonoperative management is generally appropriate for Type I and II AC joint injuries, which involves rest, ice, and physical therapy. This approach typically involves a period of sling immobilization followed by physical therapy to restore ROM and strength.

- Physical therapy for AC joint injuries may include exercises to strengthen the rotator cuff, scapular stabilizers, and other muscles surrounding the shoulder joint. In some cases, corticosteroid injections may be used in the management of persistent pain and inflammation.

- Surgical management may be necessary for more severe AC joint injuries, including Type III, IV, V, and VI injuries. Surgical stabilization options include AC joint fixation or ligamentous repair; CC ligament transfer involving transfer of the CA ligament to the distal clavicle; CC ligament reinforcement with sutures, cerclage, sling, or screw fixation; and free graft augmentation or reconstruction of the CC ligament complex.

- Postoperative management should include adequate pain control, monitoring for signs of infection or hardware failure, and physical therapy to restore ROM, strength, and dynamic stability. Rehabilitation should be tailored to the severity of the injury and the specific surgical technique used, with a gradual progression of activities and return to play to minimize the risk of postoperative complications.

- Long-term outcomes of AC joint injuries typically vary depending on injury severity and the treatment modality used, with surgical management generally resulting in better outcomes for more severe injuries (Type IV to VI).

DISCLOSURES

M.K. Mulcahey is a paid speaker/presenter for Arthrex, Inc. All other authors (L.A. Peebles, R.A. Akamefula, M.J. Kraeutler) have no disclosures to report.

REFERENCES

1. Lee KW, Debski RE, Chen CH, et al. Functional evaluation of the ligaments at the acromioclavicular joint during anteroposterior and superoinferior translation. Am J Sports Med 1997;25(6):858–62.
2. Ludewig PM, Phadke V, Braman JP, et al. Motion of the shoulder complex during multiplanar humeral elevation. J Bone Joint Surg Am 2009;91(2):378–89.
3. Depalma AF. Surgical anatomy of acromioclavicular and sternoclavicular joints. Surg Clin North Am 1963;43:1541–50.
4. Yoo Y. Acromioclavicular joint. In: Bain GI, Itoi E, diGiacomo G, et al, editors. Normal and Pathological anatomy of the shoulder. Heidelberg, Germany: Springer Berlin; 2015. p. 159–69.
5. Frank RM, Cotter EJ, Leroux TS, et al. Acromioclavicular joint injuries: evidence-based treatment. J Am Acad Orthop Surg 2019;27(17):e775–88.
6. Petersson CJ, Redlund-Johnell I. Radiographic joint space in normal acromio-clavicular joints. Acta Orthop Scand 1983;54(3):431–3.
7. Renfree KJ, Wright TW. Anatomy and biomechanics of the acromioclavicular and sternoclavicular joints. Clin Sports Med 2003;22(2):219–37.
8. Fukuda K, Craig EV, An KN, et al. Biomechanical study of the ligamentous system of the acromioclavicular joint. J Bone Joint Surg Am 1986;68(3):434–40.
9. Debski RE, Parsons IM 3rd, Fenwick J, et al. Ligament mechanics during three degree-of-freedom motion at the acromioclavicular joint. Ann Biomed Eng 2000; 28(6):612–8.
10. Stine IA, Vangsness CT Jr. Analysis of the capsule and ligament insertions about the acromioclavicular joint: a cadaveric study. Arthroscopy 2009;25(9):968–74.

11. Nakazawa M, Nimura A, Mochizuki T, et al. The orientation and variation of the acromioclavicular ligament: an anatomic study. Am J Sports Med 2016;44(10): 2690–5.

12. Provencher MT, LeClere L, Romeo AA, et al. Avoiding and managing complications of surgery of the acromioclavicular joint. In: Meislin R, Halbrecht J, editors. Complications in knee and shoulder surgery: management and treatment options for the sports medicine orthopedist. England: Springer London; 2009. p. 245–64.

13. Nolte PC, Ruzbarsky JJ, Midtgaard KS, et al. Quantitative and qualitative surgical anatomy of the acromioclavicular joint capsule and ligament: a cadaveric study. Am J Sports Med 2021;49(5):1183–91.

14. Peebles LA, Aman ZS, Kraeutler MJ, et al. Qualitative and quantitative anatomic descriptions of the coracoclavicular and acromioclavicular ligaments: a systematic review. Arthrosc Sports Med Rehabil 2022;4(4):e1545–55.

15. Boehm TD, Kirschner S, Fischer A, et al. The relation of the coracoclavicular ligament insertion to the acromioclavicular joint: a cadaver study of relevance to lateral clavicle resection. Acta Orthop Scand 2003;74(6):718–21.

16. Chahla J, Marchetti DC, Moatshe G, et al. Quantitative assessment of the coracoacromial and the coracoclavicular ligaments with 3-dimensional mapping of the coracoid process anatomy: a cadaveric study of surgically relevant structures. Arthroscopy 2018;34(5):1403–11.

17. Renfree KJ, Riley MK, Wheeler D, et al. Ligamentous anatomy of the distal clavicle. J Shoulder Elbow Surg 2003;12(4):355–9.

18. Harris RI, Vu DH, Sonnabend DH, et al. Anatomic variance of the coracoclavicular ligaments. J Shoulder Elbow Surg 2001;10(6):585–8.

19. Flores DV, Goes PK, Gomez CM, et al. Imaging of the acromioclavicular joint: anatomy, function, pathologic features, and treatment. Radiographics 2020; 40(5):1355–82.

20. Mazzocca AD, Arciero RA, Bicos J. Evaluation and treatment of acromioclavicular joint injuries. Am J Sports Med 2007;35(2):316–29.

21. Bontempo NA, Mazzocca AD. Biomechanics and treatment of acromioclavicular and sternoclavicular joint injuries. Br J Sports Med 2010;44(5):361–9.

22. Li X, Ma R, Bedi A, et al. Management of acromioclavicular joint injuries. J Bone Joint Surg Am 2014;96(1):73–84.

23. Saccomanno MF, Ieso DE, Milano G. Acromioclavicular joint instability: anatomy, biomechanics and evaluation. Joints 2014;2(2):87–92.

24. Rockwood CA, Young DC. Disorders of the acromioclavicular joint. In: Rockwood CA, Matsen FAI, editors. The shoulder. Philadelphia, PA, USA: WB Saunders; 1990. p. 413–76.

25. Pallis M, Cameron KL, Svoboda SJ, et al. Epidemiology of acromioclavicular joint injury in young athletes. Am J Sports Med 2012;40(9):2072–7.

26. Fraser-Moodie JA, Shortt NL, Robinson CM. Injuries to the acromioclavicular joint. J Bone Joint Surg Br 2008;90(6):697–707.

27. Sirin E, Aydin N, Mert Topkar O. Acromioclavicular joint injuries: diagnosis, classification and ligamentoplasty procedures. EFORT Open Rev 2018;3(7):426–33.

28. Millett PJ, Braun S, Gobezie R, et al. Acromioclavicular joint reconstruction with coracoacromial ligament transfer using the docking technique. BMC Musculoskelet Disord 2009;10:6.

29. Chillemi C, Franceschini V, Dei Giudici L, et al. Epidemiology of isolated acromioclavicular joint dislocation. Emerg Med Int 2013;2013:171609.

30. Beitzel K, Cote MP, Apostolakos J, et al. Current concepts in the treatment of acromioclavicular joint dislocations. Arthroscopy 2013;29(2):387–97.
31. Petri M, Warth RJ, Greenspoon JA, et al. Clinical results after conservative management for Grade III acromioclavicular joint injuries: does eventual surgery affect overall outcomes? Arthroscopy 2016;32(5):740–6.
32. Zanca P. Shoulder pain: involvement of the acromioclavicular joint. (Analysis of 1,000 cases). Am J Roentgenol Radium Ther Nucl Med 1971;112(3):493–506.
33. Vaatainen U, Pirinen A, Makela A. Radiological evaluation of the acromioclavicular joint. Skeletal Radiol 1991;20(2):115–6.
34. Waldrop JI, Norwood LA, Alvarez RG. Lateral roentgenographic projections of the acromioclavicular joint. Am J Sports Med 1981;9(5):337–41.
35. Tauber M, Koller H, Hitzl W, et al. Dynamic radiologic evaluation of horizontal instability in acute acromioclavicular joint dislocations. Am J Sports Med 2010;38(6):1188–95.
36. Bearden JM, Hughston JC, Whatley GS. Acromioclavicular dislocation: method of treatment. J Sports Med 1973;1(4):5–17.
37. Schneider MM, Balke M, Koenen P, et al. Inter- and intraobserver reliability of the Rockwood classification in acute acromioclavicular joint dislocations. Knee Surg Sports Traumatol Arthrosc 2016;24(7):2192–6.
38. Sluming VA. A comparison of the methods of distraction for stress examination of the acromioclavicular joint. Br J Radiol 1995;68(815):1181–4.
39. Yap JJ, Curl LA, Kvitne RS, et al. The value of weighted views of the acromioclavicular joint. Results of a survey. Am J Sports Med 1999;27(6):806–9.
40. Beitzel K, Mazzocca AD, Bak K, et al. ISAKOS upper extremity committee consensus statement on the need for diversification of the Rockwood classification for acromioclavicular joint injuries. Arthroscopy 2014;30(2):271–8.
41. Pogorzelski J, Beitzel K, Ranuccio F, et al. The acutely injured acromioclavicular joint - which imaging modalities should be used for accurate diagnosis? A systematic review. BMC Musculoskelet Disord 2017;18(1):515.
42. Bossart PJ, Joyce SM, Manaster BJ, et al. Lack of efficacy of 'weighted' radiographs in diagnosing acute acromioclavicular separation. Annals of Emergency Medicine 1988;17(1):20–4.
43. Shaw KA, Synovec J, Eichinger J, et al. Stress radiographs for evaluating acromioclavicular joint separations in an active-duty patient population: What have we learned? J Orthop 2018;15(1):159–63.
44. Berthold DP, Muench LN, Dyrna F, et al. Current concepts in acromioclavicular joint (AC) instability - a proposed treatment algorithm for acute and chronic AC-joint surgery. BMC Musculoskelet Disord 2022;23(1):1078.
45. Tossy JD, Mead NC, Sigmond HM. Acromioclavicular separations: useful and practical classification for treatment. Clin Orthop Relat Res 1963;28:111–9.
46. Allman FL Jr. Fractures and ligamentous injuries of the clavicle and its articulation. J Bone Joint Surg Am 1967;49(4):774–84.
47. Gorbaty JD, Hsu JE, Gee AO. Classifications in brief: Rockwood classification of acromioclavicular joint separations. Clin Orthop Relat Res 2017;475(1):283–7.
48. Rockwood C. 2nd edition. Injuries to the acromioclavicular joint, vol. 1. Philadelphia, PA, USA: JB Lippincott; 1984. Fractures in adults.
49. Kraeutler MJ, Williams GR Jr, Cohen SB, et al. Inter- and intraobserver reliability of the radiographic diagnosis and treatment of acromioclavicular joint separations. Orthopedics 2012;35(10):e1483–7.
50. Aliberti GM, Kraeutler MJ, Trojan JD, et al. Horizontal instability of the acromioclavicular joint: a systematic review. Am J Sports Med 2020;48(2):504–10.

51. Simovitch R, Sanders B, Ozbaydar M, et al. Acromioclavicular joint injuries: diagnosis and management. J Am Acad Orthop Surg 2009;17(4):207–19.
52. Willimon SC, Gaskill TR, Millett PJ. Acromioclavicular joint injuries: anatomy, diagnosis, and treatment. Phys Sportsmed 2011;39(1):116–22.
53. Strobel K, Pfirrmann CW, Zanetti M, et al. MRI features of the acromioclavicular joint that predict pain relief from intraarticular injection. AJR Am J Roentgenol 2003;181(3):755–60.
54. Gerber C, Galantay RV, Hersche O. The pattern of pain produced by irritation of the acromioclavicular joint and the subacromial space. J Shoulder Elbow Surg 1998;7(4):352–5.
55. Urist MR. Complete dislocations of the acromiclavicular joint; the nature of the traumatic lesion and effective methods of treatment with an analysis of forty-one cases. J Bone Joint Surg Am 1946;28(4):813–37.
56. Lemos MJ. The evaluation and treatment of the injured acromioclavicular joint in athletes. Am J Sports Med 1998;26(1):137–44.
57. Cox JS. Current method of treatment of acromioclavicular joint dislocations. Orthopedics 1992;15(9):1041–4.
58. Larsen E, Bjerg-Nielsen A, Christensen P. Conservative or surgical treatment of acromioclavicular dislocation. A prospective, controlled, randomized study. J Bone Joint Surg Am 1986;68(4):552–5.
59. Bergfeld JA, Andrish JT, Clancy WG. Evaluation of the acromioclavicular joint following first- and second-degree sprains. Am J Sports Med 1978;6(4):153–9.
60. Bradley JP, Elkousy H. Decision making: operative versus nonoperative treatment of acromioclavicular joint injuries. Clin Sports Med 2003;22(2):277–90.
61. Debski RE, Parsons IMt, Woo SL, et al. Effect of capsular injury on acromioclavicular joint mechanics. J Bone Joint Surg Am 2001;83(9):1344–51.
62. Nuber GW, Bowen MK. Acromioclavicular Joint Injuries and Distal Clavicle Fractures. J Am Acad Orthop Surg 1997;5(1):11–8.
63. Sage FP, Salvatore JE. Injuries of the acromioclavicular joint: a study of results in 96 patients. South Med J 1963;56:486–95.
64. Ahstrom JP Jr. Surgical repair of complete acromioclavicular separation. JAMA 1971;217(6):785–9.
65. Augereau B, Robert H, Apoil A. [Treatment of severe acromio-clavicular dislocations. A coraco-clavicular ligamentoplasty technique derived from Cadenat's procedure (author's transl)]. Ann Chir 1981;35(9 Pt 1):720–2. Traitement des luxations acromio-claviculaires de stade III. Ligamentoplastie a partir du ligament acromio-coracoidien selon une technique derivee de celle de Cadenat.
66. Bartonicek J, Jehlicka D, Bezvoda Z. [Surgical treatment of acromioclavicular luxation]. Acta Chir Orthop Traumatol Cech 1988;55(4):289–309. Operacni lecba akromioklavikularni luxace.
67. Leidel BA, Braunstein V, Kirchhoff C, et al. Consistency of long-term outcome of acute Rockwood Grade III acromioclavicular joint separations after K-wire transfixation. J Trauma 2009;66(6):1666–71.
68. Lizaur A, Sanz-Reig J, Gonzalez-Parreno S. Long-term results of the surgical treatment of type III acromioclavicular dislocations: an update of a previous report. J Bone Joint Surg Br 2011;93(8):1088–92.
69. Norrell H Jr, Llewellyn RC. Migration of a threaded Steinmann pin from an acromioclavicular joint into the spinal canal. A case report. J Bone Joint Surg Am 1965;47:1024–6.
70. Broos P, Stoffelen D, Van de Sijpe K, et al. [Surgical management of complete Tossy III acromioclavicular joint dislocation with the Bosworth screw or the

Wolter plate. A critical evaluation]. Unfallchirurgie 1997;23(4):153–9 ; discussion 160. Operative Versorgung der vollstandigen AC-Luxation Tossy III mit der Bosworth-Schraube oder der Wolter-Platte. Eine Kritische Betrachtung.

71. Habernek H, Weinstabl R, Schmid L, et al. A crook plate for treatment of acromioclavicular joint separation: indication, technique, and results after one year. J Trauma 1993;35(6):893–901.

72. Henkel T, Oetiker R, Hackenbruch W. [Treatment of fresh Tossy III acromioclavicular joint dislocation by ligament suture and temporary fixation with the clavicular hooked plate]. Swiss Surg 1997;3(4):160–6. Die Behandlung der frischen AC-Luxation Tossy III durch Bandnaht und temporare Fixation mit Klavikula-Hakenplatte.

73. Lin HY, Wong PK, Ho WP, et al. Clavicular hook plate may induce subacromial shoulder impingement and rotator cuff lesion–dynamic sonographic evaluation. J Orthop Surg Res 2014;9:6.

74. Phadke A, Bakti N, Bawale R, et al. Current concepts in management of ACJ injuries. J Clin Orthop Trauma 2019;10(3):480–5.

75. Neviaser JS. Acromioclavicular dislocation treated by transference of the coraco-acromial ligament. A long-term follow-up in a series of 112 cases. Clin Orthop Relat Res 1968;58:57–68.

76. Auge WK 2nd, Fischer RA. Arthroscopic distal clavicle resection for isolated atraumatic osteolysis in weight lifters. Am J Sports Med 1998;26(2):189–92.

77. Guy DK, Wirth MA, Griffin JL, et al. Reconstruction of chronic and complete dislocations of the acromioclavicular joint. Clin Orthop Relat Res 1998;(347):138–49.

78. Kumar S, Sethi A, Jain AK. Surgical treatment of complete acromioclavicular dislocation using the coracoacromial ligament and coracoclavicular fixation: report of a technique in 14 patients. J Orthop Trauma 1995;9(6):507–10.

79. Verhaven E, DeBoeck H, Haentjens P, et al. Surgical treatment of acute type-V acromioclavicular injuries in athletes. Arch Orthop Trauma Surg 1993;112(4):189–92.

80. Weaver JK, Dunn HK. Treatment of acromioclavicular injuries, especially complete acromioclavicular separation. J Bone Joint Surg Am 1972;54(6):1187–94.

81. Rauschning W, Nordesjo LO, Nordgren B, et al. Resection arthroplasty for repair of complete acromioclavicular separations. Arch Orthop Trauma Surg 1980;97(3):161–4.

82. LaPrade RF, Hilger B. Coracoclavicular ligament reconstruction using a semi-tendinosus graft for failed acromioclavicular separation surgery. Arthroscopy 2005;21(10):1277.

83. Kawabe N, Watanabe R, Sato M. Treatment of complete acromioclavicular separation by coracoacromial ligament transfer. Clin Orthop Relat Res 1984;185:222–7.

84. Shoji H, Roth C, Chuinard R. Bone block transfer of coracoacromial ligament in acromioclavicular injury. Clin Orthop Relat Res 1986;208:272–7.

85. Bosworth B. Acromioclavicular separation: a new method of repair. Surg Gynecol Obstet 1941;73:866–71.

86. Tsou PM. Percutaneous cannulated screw coracoclavicular fixation for acute acromioclavicular dislocations. Clin Orthop Relat Res 1989;243:112–21.

87. Kennedy JC. Complete dislocation of the acromioclavicular joint: 14 years later. J Trauma 1968;8(3):311–8.

88. Lowe GP, Fogarty MJ. Acute acromioclavicular joint dislocation: results of operative treatment with the Bosworth screw. Aust N Z J Surg 1977;47(5):664–7.

89. Tiefenboeck TM, Popp D, Boesmueller S, et al. Acromioclavicular joint disloca-tion treated with Bosworth screw and additional K-wiring: results after 7.8 years - still an adequate procedure? BMC Musculoskelet Disord 2017;18(1):339.

90. Esenyel CZ, Ozturk K, Bulbul M, et al. Coracoclavicular ligament repair and screw fixation in acromioclavicular dislocations. Acta Orthop Traumatol Turc 2010;44(3):194–8.

91. Colosimo AJ, Hummer CD 3rd, Heidt RS Jr. Aseptic foreign body reaction to Dacron graft material used for coracoclavicular ligament reconstruction after type III acromioclavicular dislocation. Am J Sports Med 1996;24(4):561–3.

92. Hessmann M, Gotzen L, Gehling H. Acromioclavicular reconstruction augmented with polydioxanonsulphate bands. Surgical technique and results. Am J Sports Med 1995;23(5):552–6.

93. Clayer M, Slavotinek J, Krishnan J. The results of coraco-clavicular slings for acromio-clavicular dislocation. Aust N Z J Surg 1997;67(6):343–6.

94. Gohring U, Matusewicz A, Friedl W, et al. [Results of treatment after different sur-gical procedures for management of acromioclavicular joint dislocation]. Chir-urg 1993;64(7):565–71. Behandlungsergebnisse nach unterschiedlichen Operationsverfahren zur Versorgung einer Schultereckgelenksprengung.

95. Gollwitzer M. [Surgical management of complete acromioclavicular joint dislo-cation (Tossy III) with PDS cord cerclage]. Aktuelle Traumatol 1993;23(8): 366–70. Operative Versorgung der kompletten Schultereckgelenkluxation (Tossy III) mit PDS-Kordel.

96. Kiefer H, Claes L, Burri C, et al. The stabilizing effect of various implants on the torn acromioclavicular joint. A biomechanical study. Arch Orthop Trauma Surg 1986;106(1):42–6.

97. Jones HP, Lemos MJ, Schepsis AA. Salvage of failed acromioclavicular joint reconstruction using autogenous semitendinosus tendon from the knee. Surgi-cal technique and case report. Am J Sports Med 2001;29(2):234–7.

98. Costic RS, Labriola JE, Rodosky MW, et al. Biomechanical rationale for develop-ment of anatomical reconstructions of coracoclavicular ligaments after complete acromioclavicular joint dislocations. Am J Sports Med 2004;32(8):1929–36.

99. Grutter PW, Petersen SA. Anatomical acromioclavicular ligament reconstruction: a biomechanical comparison of reconstructive techniques of the acromioclavic-ular joint. Am J Sports Med 2005;33(11):1723–8.

100. Mazzocca AD, Santangelo SA, Johnson ST, et al. A biomechanical evaluation of an anatomical coracoclavicular ligament reconstruction. Am J Sports Med 2006; 34(2):236–46.

101. Tauber M, Gordon K, Koller H, et al. Semitendinosus tendon graft versus a modi-fied Weaver-Dunn procedure for acromioclavicular joint reconstruction in chronic cases: a prospective comparative study. Am J Sports Med 2009; 37(1):181–90.

102. Voss A, Imhoff AB. Editorial commentary: why we have to respect the anatomy in acromioclavicular joint surgery and why clinical shoulder scores might not give us the information we need. Arthroscopy 2019;35(5):1336–8.

103. Dawson PA, Adamson GJ, Pink MM, et al. Relative contribution of acromiocla-vicular joint capsule and coracoclavicular ligaments to acromioclavicular stabil-ity. J Shoulder Elbow Surg 2009;18(2):237–44.

104. Dyrna F, Imhoff FB, Haller B, et al. Primary stability of an acromioclavicular joint repair is affected by the type of additional reconstruction of the acromioclavic-ular capsule. Am J Sports Med 2018;46(14):3471–9.

105. Dyrna FGE, Imhoff FB, Voss A, et al. The integrity of the acromioclavicular capsule ensures physiological centering of the acromioclavicular joint under rotational loading. Am J Sports Med 2018;46(6):1432–40.

106. Morikawa D, Dyrna F, Cote MP, et al. Repair of the entire superior acromioclavicular ligament complex best restores posterior translation and rotational stability. Knee Surg Sports Traumatol Arthrosc 2019;27(12):3764–70.

107. Klimkiewicz JJ, Williams GR, Sher JS, et al. The acromioclavicular capsule as a restraint to posterior translation of the clavicle: a biomechanical analysis. J Shoulder Elbow Surg 1999;8(2):119–24.

108. Schobel T, Theopold J, Fischer JP, et al. Anatomical versus non-anatomical configuration of double coraco-clavicular tunnel technique in acromioclavicular joint reconstruction. Arch Orthop Trauma Surg 2022;142(4):641–8.

109. Teixeira Ramos J, Silva Gomes D, Quinaz Neto P, et al. Arthroscopic-assisted acromioclavicular joint dislocation repair: a modified technique for horizontal stabilization using suture anchors. Arthrosc Tech 2021;10(2):e283–8.

110. Martetschlager F, Tauber M, Habermeyer P, et al. Arthroscopically assisted acromioclavicular and coracoclavicular ligament reconstruction for chronic acromioclavicular joint instability. Arthrosc Tech 2016;5(6):e1239–46.

111. Tauber M, Valler D, Lichtenberg S, et al. Arthroscopic stabilization of chronic acromioclavicular joint dislocations: triple- versus single-bundle reconstruction. Am J Sports Med 2016;44(2):482–9.

112. Mardani-Kivi M, Asadi K, Leili EK, et al. Horizontal instability after acromioclavicular joint reduction using the two-hole technique is preferred over the loop technique: a single-blind randomized clinical trial. Clin Shoulder Elb 2022;25(3):224–9.

113. Aliberti GM, Mulcahey MK, Brown SM, et al. Restoring horizontal stability of the acromioclavicular joint: open acromioclavicular ligament reconstruction and repair with semitendinosus allograft. Arthrosc Tech 2020;9(10):e1619–26.

114. Angelo AC, Maia Dias C, de Campos Azevedo C. Combined vertical, horizontal, and rotational acromioclavicular joint stabilization: "closing the circle" technique. Arthrosc Tech 2022;11(8):e1479–86.

115. Spiegl UJ, Smith SD, Euler SA, et al. Biomechanical consequences of coracoclavicular reconstruction techniques on clavicle strength. Am J Sports Med 2014;42(7):1724–30.

116. Martetschlager F, Saier T, Weigert A, et al. Effect of coracoid drilling for acromioclavicular joint reconstruction techniques on coracoid fracture risk: a biomechanical study. Arthroscopy 2016;32(6):982–7.

117. Martetschlager F, Horan MP, Warth RJ, et al. Complications after anatomic fixation and reconstruction of the coracoclavicular ligaments. Am J Sports Med 2013;41(12):2896–903.

118. Scheibel M, Droschel S, Gerhardt C, et al. Arthroscopically assisted stabilization of acute high-grade acromioclavicular joint separations. Am J Sports Med 2011;39(7):1507–16.

Acromioclavicular Joint Anatomy and Biomechanics
The Significance of Posterior Rotational and Translational Stability

Check for updates

Nicholas P.J. Perry, MD[a,b,*], Nozimakhon K. Omonullaeva, BS[b,c],
Blake M. Bacevich, BS[b,d], Robert J. Nascimento, MD[a,b],
Evan A. O'Donnell, MD[a,b], Mark D. Price, MD[a,b],
Augustus D. Mazzocca, MS, MD[a,b]

KEYWORDS

- Acromioclavicular joint • Coracoclavicular ligaments • Conoid • Trapezoid
- Biomechanics • Posterior rotation

KEY POINTS

- Acromioclavicular (AC) joint dislocations are often reflective of a larger soft tissue injury to the multiple static (AC and coracoclavicular capsuloligamentous structures) and dynamic (trapezius, deltoid, and deltotrapezial fascia) stabilizers of shoulder girdle.
- Clavicular motion during humerothoracic elevation is reliant on strong capsuloligamentous connections between the distal clavicle and scapula.
- After an injury to the capsuloligamentous structures, the kinetic chain between the clavicle and scapula is disrupted causing increased scapular internal rotation and downward rotation.
- Refined understanding of the biomechanics of the shoulder girdle should help inform advances in surgical techniques with the ultimate goal of restoring injured anatomy and resolving pathomechanic adaptations.

INTRODUCTION

AC joint injuries and dislocations, which are associated with varying degrees of damage to nearby ligamentous, fascial, and muscular tissue, are a common source of pain

[a] Division of Sports Medicine, Department of Orthopaedic Surgery, Massachusetts General Hospital, Harvard School of Medicine, Massachusetts General Brigham, Boston, MA 02115, USA; [b] Sports Medicine, Mass General Hospital, 175 Cambridge Street, 4th Floor, Boston, MA 02114, USA; [c] Nova Southeastern University, College of Osteopathic Medicine, 3301 College Avenue, Fort Lauderdale, FL 33314, USA; [d] Harvard Medical School, Boston, MA 02115, USA
* Corresponding author. Sports Medicine, Mass General Hospital, 175 Cambridge Street, 4th Floor, Boston, MA 02114.
E-mail address: npperry@mgh.harvard.edu

Clin Sports Med 42 (2023) 557–571
https://doi.org/10.1016/j.csm.2023.05.002
0278-5919/23/© 2023 Elsevier Inc. All rights reserved.

and dysfunction of the shoulder girdle.[1,2] Despite significant research efforts, there remains an opaque understanding of the precise anatomy and biomechanics of the shoulder girdle. This knowledge gap has contributed to the inability to develop a gold standard surgical solution to injuries of the AC joint and surrounding tissues. Recently, more detailed anatomic and biomechanical investigations have begun providing a clearer vision while suggesting new treatment options. The purpose of this article is to provide an in-depth review of the anatomy and biomechanics of the AC joint and related structures of the shoulder girdle.

ANATOMY

The shoulder girdle is an anatomic region, which extends anteriorly from the sternoclavicular (SC) joint to the broad scapular stabilizing muscles posteriorly. It consists of 3 joints and 2 gliding regions.[3] The joints include the SC joint, the AC joint, and the glenohumeral (GH) joint, while the gliding regions are the subacromial space and the scapulothoracic (ST) space (**Fig. 1**). Humerothoraciac motion, such as arm abduction, requires circumferentially coordinated movement from the SC joint to the ST space with its large stabilizing muscles.[4,5] The AC joint and supporting structures act as an important link in this kinetic chain and contribute to fluid shoulder motion. Given the large anatomic area of the shoulder girdle, it is important to understand and inspect the entire shoulder girdle during evaluation of an AC joint injury.

Osteology

Clavicle
The clavicle is a curvilinear bone with a medial convexity and a lateral concavity. It is the only horizontal long bone in the body and is one of the first bones to ossify during fetal development.[3] The medial clavicular epiphysis does not ossify until 18 to 20 years old, and it does not fuse to the diaphysis until 23 to 25 years old.[6] The clavicle's length is approximately 14.1 cm $\pm$ 0.9 cm and is proportional to patient height.[7,8] The medial aspect of the clavicle features a large and broad facet that articulates with the synovial-lined SC joint.[9] It is stabilized by the large costoclavicular ligament, in addition to the anterior and posterior SC ligaments.[10] The sternocleidomastoid provides

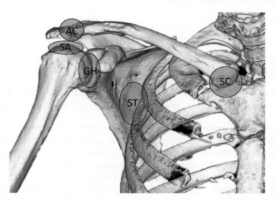

Fig. 1. Three-dimensional CT demonstrates the 3 joints and 2 gliding regions of the shoulder girdle. The SC joint connects the clavicle to the sternum. The acromioclavicular (AC) joint connects the clavicle to the scapula. The GH connects the scapula to the humerus. The ST and subacromial (SA) spaces are nonarticular gliding regions. (CT Scan courtesy of Marc Succi, MD from Department of Radiology, Massachusetts General Hospital, Boston, MA, USA.)

dynamic stability. The SC joint is the only direct skeletal connection between the axial skeleton and the upper extremity. The SC joint is the only direct skeletal connection between the axial skeleton and the upper extremity. In contrast, the lateral aspect of the clavicle is relatively narrow and rectangular in shape, measuring approximately 2 cm in width and 1 cm in height.[7] The conoid and trapezoid tuberosities represent the insertion site of the conoid and trapezoid ligaments, which are the lateral coracoclavicular (CC) ligaments. These insertion sites are proportional to the length of the clavicle. Specifically, when measuring from the lateral edge of the clavicle, the trapezoid and conoid tuberosities are located approximately 17% and 31%, respectively, along the length of the clavicle.[7,8] Given the average clavicle length of 15 cm, the trapezoid and conoid ligaments insert approximately 2.5 cm and 4.6 cm from the lateral edge of the clavicle.[3,7]

While protecting vital neurovascular structures medially, the clavicle also serves several important biomechanical functions. Statically, it provides suspensory support to the arm through the lateral CC ligaments and AC capsuloligamentous structures.[11,12] Dynamically, it is thought to provide 2 main functions. First, with its medial edge anchored at the SC joint, the clavicle provides a pivot point and guides the shoulder girdle during shoulder motion. Second, the "strut" function of the clavicle helps lateralize the glenoid face and prevents the shoulder girdle from collapsing medially, especially during overhead activities.[13] In an interesting comparative anatomy study, Veegar and colleagues claim the clavicle is a key component in the success of human bipedalism and upper extremity dexterity.[12]

Scapula

The scapula is a broad, flat bone with complex geometry and includes the glenoid, coracoid, and acromion. The scapula is approximately 15 cm $\pm$ 1 cm in length and 13 cm $\pm$ 1 cm in width.[14] It is important to consider the length of the scapula, which provides a long moment arm and high torque-generating capability to the scapular stabilizing muscles (especially in the context of a ligament reconstructive construct, which may have a small [3 cm] or nonexistent moment arm). The scapular body is surrounded by musculature and serves as the origin of the rotator cuff muscles. The acromion process is the lateral extension of the scapular spine and articulates with the clavicle to form the AC joint. The coracoid process is a bony projection with an apex to base length of 41 mm and width of 25 mm.[7,8,15]

Acromioclavicular joint

The AC joint is a diarthrodial, synovial joint formed by the articulation of the lateral clavicle with the medial facet of the acromion. The joint is approximately 1 cm superior-to-inferior and 2 cm anterior-to-posterior.[3] The plane of the AC joint is inclined 20° to 30° inferiorly and 20° to 40° posteriorly.[3,16] However, the AC joint does have significant morphologic variations, and these numbers may vary widely. The articulating geometry may also vary from flat, oblique, and curved.[17,18] Given the bony geometry, the only motion with significant bony constraint is medialization of the acromion, which is blocked by the clavicle. The remaining 5° of motion are restrained and controlled by capsular, ligamentous, and muscular structures. Static stabilizers include the AC capsuloligamentous structures, lateral CC ligaments (trapezoid and conoid), and, perhaps, the medial CC ligament. Dynamic stabilizers include the deltoid, trapezius, and the deltotrapezial fascia.

Static Stabilizers

Acromioclavicular joint and ligaments

Classically, the AC capsuloligamentous structures have been conceptualized as homogenous fibers perpendicular to the joint line.[19] However, recent detailed anatomic studies have begun elucidating the more nuanced structure.[16,20,21] Nakazawa and colleagues described the AC capsuloligamentous system as being composed of 2 main structures: the superoposterior (SP) bundle and the anteroinferior (AI) bundle.[16] The SP bundle is a distinct, consistent ligamentous structure approximately 3.0 mm ± 0.5 mm thick.[16] Several authors have demonstrated that it is not perpendicular to the AC joint line, but rather, an oblique structure originating on the posterior aspect of the distal clavicle and inserting on the anterosuperior acromion.[16,20] The angle of obliquity with respect to the distal third of the clavicle is approximately 30° to 40°.[16,20] In contrast, the AI bundle is thin (1.6 ± 0.5 mm) with an inconsistent location.[16,20] Evaluating the insertional anatomy of the AC capsuloligamentous structures, Nolte and colleagues demonstrated that the superior capsuloligamentous structures had a broader insertional footprint compared with the inferior capsuloligamentous structures on both the clavicle (superior 6.4 mm [5.8–6.9] vs inferior 4.4 mm [3.9–4.8]) and the acromion (superior 4.6 mm [4.2–4.9] vs inferior 4.0 mm [3.6–4.4]).[20] Furthermore, their study carefully mapped out the distance from the AC joint line to the insertional footprints, which showed the superior capsuloligamentous on the clavicle had the furthest footprint from the AC joint cartilage (4.6 mm; 95% CI 4.2–4.9) and the inferior capsuloligamentous structures on the acromion had the shortest distance from the AC joint cartilage (2.5 mm; 95% CI 2.2–2.7).

Coracoclavicular ligaments: the conoid and trapezoid

The conoid and trapezoid form an inverted triangle connecting the base of the coracoid and the distal third of the clavicle (**Fig. 2**). The trapezoid ligament has a quadrilateral shape and forms the more anterior, lateral limb of the inverted triangle, whereas the conoid has a conical shape and forms the nearly vertical posteromedial limb.[7,8,22] On the coracoid, the trapezoid is the more anterior structure, with a minimal distance from the coracoid apex to the trapezoid center of 27.0 mm (95% CI 23.7–30.3).[8] The distance between the center of the conoid and trapezoid was 8.8 mm (95% CI 7.4–10.3). Additionally, the trapezoid has a slightly larger coracoid insertional footprint compared with the conoid (44.3 mm^2 vs 37.0 mm^2).[8] The conoid's insertion on the coracoid is in close proximity to the suprascapular nerve (13.8 ± 4.0 mm) and the suprascapular artery (7.1 ± 3.3 mm).[22]

On the clavicle, the conoid inserts posteriorly and medially compared with the trapezoid (**Fig. 3**). The center of the attachment site for these ligaments is 16.2 mm (95% CI 14.1–18.4) apart.[8] The total span of the footprint, measured from the lateral fibers of the trapezoid to the medial fibers of the conoid, is 25.6 mm (95% CI 22.3–28.9), representing approximately 20% of the total clavicular length.[8] This span may be an important biomechanical feature, which provides a moment arm to help resist torque. When measuring the distance from the lateral edge to the center of the ligaments, the distance is roughly 25 mm for the trapezoid and 45 mm for the conoid.[7] Shibata and colleagues found these distances varied depending on the overall length of the clavicle; however, the ratio of the distance from the lateral edge of the clavicle to ligament insertion site compared with total clavicular length was relatively constant at 17% for the trapezoid and 30% for the conoid.[8,22]

The "more" medial coracoclavicular ligament

In juxtaposition to the well-defined conoid and trapezoid ligaments, some authors have described a "more" medial CC ligament, which is not well understood. Its existence and clinical relevance are highly debated, with some authors reporting they were

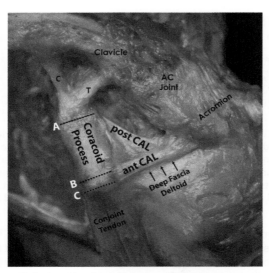

Fig. 2. Finely dissected left shoulder displaying the conoid (C) and trapezoid (T) CC ligament and coracoacromial ligament (CAL) bundles. The deep fascia of the deltoid is shown attaching to the anterior CAL bundle. Note that overlap was observed between the conjoint tendon and the anterior CAL bundle. The distances measured from the most distal attachment of the trapezoid (A) to the superior tip of the coracoid process (B) and the tip of the coracoid (C). AC, acromioclavicular; ant CAL, anterior coracoacromial ligament; post CAL, posterior coracoacromial ligament. (Reprint with permission Chahla et al. Quantitative Assessment of the Coracoacromial and the Coracoclavicular Ligaments With 3-Dimensional Mapping of the Coracoid Process Anatomy: A Cadaveric Study of Surgically Relevant Structures. *Arthroscopy* 2018;34(5):1403-1411.)

unable to identify the ligament or isolate it from the clavipectoral fascia.[23,24] However, this variation may be a result of different cadaveric preservation techniques.[25] In detailed anatomic dissections, several authors describe a consistent "more" medial CC ligament, which spans from the base of the medial coracoid to the inferior medial third of the clavicle with a lower expansion to the first rib (**Fig. 4**).[23,24] The "more"

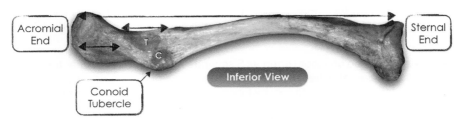

Fig. 3. Inferior view of a cadaveric left clavicle showing the attachment shapes of the trapezoid (T) and conoid (C) ligaments. The mean clavicle length was 14.1 cm [13.4, 14.8], and the mean distance between the most lateral insertions of the CC ligaments from the lateral aspect of the clavicle at the AC joint was 15.7 mm. (Reprint with permission Chahla et al. Quantitative Assessment of the Coracoacromial and the Coracoclavicular Ligaments With 3-Dimensional Mapping of the Coracoid Process Anatomy: A Cadaveric Study of Surgically Relevant Structures. *Arthroscopy.* 2018;34(5):1403-1411.)

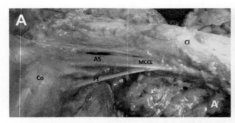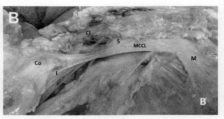

Fig. 4. (*A*) Coracoid origin: anterosuperior and posteroinferior bundles (right shoulder). AS, anterosuperior bundle; Cl, clavicle; Co, coracoid process; MCCL, medial coracoclavicular ligament; PI, posteroinferior bundle. (*B*) Fascial expansions (right shoulder). Cl, clavicle; Co, coracoid process; I, inferior; M, medial; MCCL, medial coracoclavicular ligament; S, superior. (Reprint with permission Moya et al. The medial coracoclavicular ligament: anatomy, biomechanics, and clinical relevance—a research study. *JSES Open Access*. 2018;2(4):183-189.)

medial CC ligament is 48.9 ± 2.4 mm long and 18.3 ± 0.9 mm wide.[24] It is anterior to the subclavius muscle at a 20° angle compared with the long axis of the clavicle. Histologic evaluation of this tissue suggests it is ligamentous in nature with organized and densely packed collagen fibers.[26] Please note, "more" medial CC ligament is our naming convention to avoid confusion with the conoid ligament, which could also be described as the medial CC ligament.

Dynamic Stabilizers

Similar to other anatomic regions, the shoulder girdle and the AC joint are supported by dynamic stabilizers, in addition to static stabilizers. However, unlike the GH joint, the synergistic effect of dynamic and static stabilizers for the shoulder girdle and AC joint is not well understood or cemented in the collective consciousness of the orthopedic community.

Deltoid

The deltoid muscle is composed of 3 distinct functional units, often separated by a tendinous raphe: the anterior deltoid on the lateral clavicle, the lateral deltoid on the acromion, and the posterior deltoid on the lateral aspect of the scapular spine (**Fig. 5**).[3,27,28] The anterior deltoid originates on the superior, anterior, and inferior aspects of the lateral 37% of the clavicle.[28] The fibers of the anterior deltoid continue laterally and cover 90.9 ± 7.3% of the anterior AC capsuloligamentous structures without extension to the superior portion.[28] In close proximity to the AC joint, there is typically a tendinous raphe, which separates the anterior and middle deltoid.[27,28]

Trapezius

The trapezius may be conceptualized as 3 separate motor units: the upper trapezius, the middle trapezius, and the lower trapezius. This concept is supported by the recent advances in tendon transfer surgery by Elhassan and colleagues, who have successfully isolated the lower trapezius for transfer.[29] A similar distinction between the upper trapezius and middle trapezius may be relevant for shoulder girdle function. Levasseur and colleagues have identified a consistent fat stripe that separates the upper trapezius, inserting on the lateral clavicle, from the middle trapezius, inserting on the acromion.[28] This suggests a different force vector generated by each of these muscles. Interestingly, the upper trapezius inserts on the lateral 37% of the posterior clavicle, mirroring the anterior deltoid on the anterior clavicle.[28] The muscular fibers of the upper trapezius also cover 15% to 20% of the superior portion of the lateral clavicle.[28]

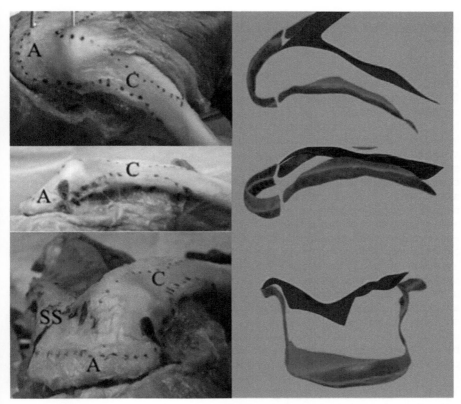

Fig. 5. Anatomical footprints of the deltoid (*red*) and trapezius (*blue*) muscles to the clavicle, acromion, and scapular spine with corresponding digitized surface footprint meshes of a right shoulder. Top, superior view. Middle, anterior view. Bottom, lateral view. (A, acromion; C, clavicle; SS, scapular spine.) (Reprint with permission LeVasseur et al. Three-Dimensional Footprint Mapping of the Deltoid and Trapezius: Anatomic Pearls for Acromioclavicular Joint Reconstruction. *Arthroscopy.* 2022;38(3):701-708.)

However, this leaves approximately 80% of the superior portion of the lateral clavicle and AC capsuloligamentous structures as a bare area devoid of direct muscular attachments.

Deltotrapezial fascia

The deltotrapezial fascia is the aponeurotic extension of the superficial fascia of the upper trapezius, which traverses the bare area of the lateral clavicle and AC capsuloligamentous structures, merging with the superficial fascia of the anterior and middle deltoid.[25,28,30] It exists between the insertion of the upper trapezius and origin of the anterior deltoid. Although the deltotrapezial fascia is adherent to the underlying clavicular periosteum and AC capsuloligamentous tissues, careful dissection and histologic evaluation has shown it to be a distinct structure.[25] It is 1 to 2 mm thick with a mean thickness of 1.7 mm.[25] The deltotrapezial fascia seems to have characteristics of both dynamic and static stabilizers. Its adherence to the underlying structures may provide static, mechanical reinforcement to the AC capsuloligamentous tissues. However, by bridging the bare area between the upper trapezius and anterior deltoid and connecting the fascia of these muscles, it may have a dynamic sling effect to stabilize the shoulder girdle and dampen force transmission (similar to a dashpot in mechanical modeling).

Biomechanics

Description of motion

Given the complex, three-dimensional motion of the shoulder girdle and the surrounding individual joints (ST, SC, AC, GH), it is paramount to clearly define the shoulder motion for data reproducibility and homogeneity.[31,32] To aid this endeavor, the International Society of Biomechanics has published suggested standard coordinate systems for the description of clavicular and scapular motion, similar to the coordinate system shown in **Fig. 6**.[33] Clavicular motion is centered at the SC joint. The lateral clavicular axis is parallel to the longitudinal axis of the clavicle. The superior clavicular axis is parallel to the longitudinal axis of the thorax. The anterior clavicular axis is perpendicular to the plane of the previous 2 axes. Rotations about the clavicular axes are termed: anterior/posterior axial rotation for the lateral clavicular axis; protraction/retraction for the superior clavicular axis; and elevation/depression for the anterior clavicular axis. Scapular motion is centered at the AC joint. The lateral scapular axis is a line from the root of the scapular spine to the AC joint. The superior scapular axis is parallel to the longitudinal axis of the thorax. The anterior scapular axis is perpendicular to the plane of the previous 2 axes and parallel to the scapular body. Rotation about the scapular axes are termed as follows: anterior/posterior tilting for the lateral scapular axis, internal/external scapular rotation for the superior scapular axis, and upward/downward rotation for the anterior scapular axis. GH motion terms should be used to describe relative motion between the humeral head and the glenoid. Composite motion of the shoulder girdle and the change in position between the humeral

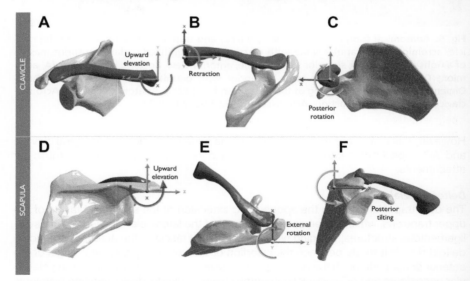

Fig. 6. Local coordinate system of clavicle (*A–C*) and scapula (*E, F*). Definition of SC (*A–C*) and ST (*D–F*) motion. Using a 3D coordinate system and Cardan or Euler angles, following International Society of Biomechanics recommendation. (Reprint with permission Velasquez Garcia et al Anteroinferior bundle of the acromioclavicular ligament plays a substantial role in the joint function during shoulder elevation and horizontal adduction: a finite element model. *J Orthop Surg.* 2022;17(1):73.)

shaft and the thorax can be described as humerothoracic motion. When precision of language is required for clinical or research purposes, consideration should be given to preferential use of these well-defined terms rather than other ill-defined terms.

Physiologic motion

Humerothoracic motion is the result of coordinated motion between the GH and ST joints, with about 30% to 40% of motion originating from the ST joint. The ratio of one-third ST motion to two-thirds GH motion is termed scapulohumeral rhythm.[32] During humerothoracic elevation in the healthy shoulder, the general motion of the clavicle is elevation, retraction, and posterior rotation, which is reciprocated by the scapula's upward rotation and posterior tilting.[12,31,32] Scapular internal rotation seems to be more dependent on the plane of humerothoracic elevation (forward flexion vs abduction).[12] Because the long axis of the clavicular is nearly perpendicular to the plane of scapular upward rotation, rotation of the clavicle around its longitudinal axis and scapular upward rotation are well matched and require minimal adjustment through the AC joint.[12] The AC and CC capsuloligamentous structures are strong, but not stiff, creating a deformable link between the clavicle and the scapula, which allows a maximum of 20° rotation through the AC joint.[12,34] Biomechanical studies by Harris and Koh demonstrated that the CC ligaments allow for 8 to 14 mm elongation.[35,36]

In order to overcome the limitations of cadaveric studies and cutaneous-based position transducers, Ludewig and colleagues conducted an invasive study with transcortical fixation of motion trackers in patients with normal shoulder function to better describe physiologic motion.[31] With cortically based transducers in the humeral shaft, clavicle, scapular spine, and a cutaneous-based transducer on the sternum, the subjects performed humerothoracic elevation in several planes of motion during data collection. Through the SC joint, the clavicle's motion relative to the sternum was 16° of retraction, 6° of elevation, and 31° of posterior axial rotation. Through the AC joint, the scapula's motion relative to the clavicle was 11° of upward rotation, 19° of posterior tilting, and 8° of internal rotation. Finally, through the ST space, the scapula's motion relative to the thorax was 21° of posterior tilting, 40° of upward rotation, and 2° of external rotation. The authors concluded there is a significant amount of posterior rotation that occurs through the SC joint, whereas the AC joint has less relative motion, as the scapula rotates upward. They conceptualized the clavicle as an intercalated segment that is passively moved through the various capsuloligamentous attachments because there is no muscle attaching to the clavicle capable of producing posterior rotation. This suggests the importance of the static and dynamic stabilizers' ability to resist rotational and posterior translational forces while maintaining the physiologic position of the distal clavicle and the acromion.

Pathomechanics After Injury

Isolated acromioclavicular capsuloligamentous injuries

Several authors have investigated the kinematic effects of an isolated injury to the AC capsuloligamentous structures, which seems to occur most frequently at the clavicular insertion.[37] Complete disruption of AC capsuloligamentous structures with uninjured CC ligaments in a cadaveric model resulted in increased AP translation of the distal clavicle compared with the native state (8.0 vs 15.4 mm).[34] Interestingly, increased axial compression of the AC joint decreased the magnitude of translation, which may suggest the contribution of dynamic stabilizing structures. Similarly, Kurata and colleagues demonstrated increased posterior and superior translation of the distal clavicle after selectively transecting the AI bundle and SP ligament at the AC joint.[38]

Their data suggest the SP ligament contributes significantly more of the stabilizing forces compared with the AI bundle.

More recently, authors have also begun to examine the rotational stability of the AC capsuloligamentous structures in addition to translational stability. This is likely reflective of our greater understanding of normal shoulder girdle kinematics and the significant amount of clavicular posterior rotation during thoracohumeral elevation. Using a distal clavicle-scapula cadaveric model, Dyrna and colleagues measured the resistive forces to 10 mm of posterior translation and 20° of posterior rotation in an uninjured model and complete AC capsuloligamentous injury model (CC ligaments intact).[39] After complete dissection of the AC capsuloligamentous structures, the resistive forces to posterior translation were reduced by 75% compared with the intact state, and resistive forces to posterior rotation were reduced by 94% compared with the intact state. Morikawa and colleagues demonstrated a similar reduction in resistive forces and the ability to partially restore the resistance to posterior translation and posterior rotation after surgical repair of the AC capsuloligamentous structures.[40]

These studies represent a growing body of literature, which suggest the importance of AC capsuloligamentous structures for shoulder girdle stability and physiologic kinematics. Surgeons should carefully consider the contribution of these structures and the need to potentially include AC capsuloligamentous structure repair or reconstruction when treating this patient population.

Isolated coracoclavicular injuries

Clinically, an isolated CC disruption with intact AC capsuloligamentous structures and intact deltotrapezial fascia does not seem to be an entity. However, several authors have used this as an investigational model to understand the mechanical properties of these structures. Dawson and colleagues showed that complete disruption of conoid and trapezoid with the AC capsuloligamentous structures intact yields increased superior−inferior translation (5 vs 12 mm).[34] As previously discussed, axial compression of the AC joint seems to stabilize the joint.

Combined acromioclavicular and coracoclavicular injuries

Rupture of the AC capsuloligamentous structures, the CC ligaments, and the deltotrapezial fascia disrupts the kinematic chain between the clavicle and the scapula with several pathomechanical consequences. In a whole body cadaver biomechanical study, Oki and colleagues showed the resting position of the scapula has more internal rotation and downward rotation compared with the intact state.[41] During passive thoracohumeral coronal plane elevation, there was decreased scapular upward rotation and increased clavicular retraction after ligamentous disruption.[41]

In another interesting whole body cadaveric study, Matsumura and colleagues evaluated the biomechanical consequences of midshaft clavicular discontinuity.[11] This model is pertinent to the discussion of pathomechanical effects of AC-CC disruption because it provides another perspective on the kinetic chain between the clavicle and scapula. Similar to AC-CC disruption models, the clavicle discontinuity model demonstrated decreased upward rotation, posterior tilting, and external rotation of the scapula with thoracohumeral elevation.

These cadaveric studies seem to correlate with the observed clinical manifestation of chronic disruptions of the shoulder girdle, specifically increased downward rotation of the scapula with a reciprocal upward rotation of the inferior pole of the scapula. This prominent inferior pole of the scapula seems to be a consistent clinical finding in patients with chronic high-grade AC-CC injuries, which is apparent on physical examination.[42]

The downward rotation and anterior tilting of the scapula away from the clavicle may also affect the anterior deltoid by changing the length–tension relationship. Due to the anterior deltoid originating on the distal clavicle, it may experience a unique change in working-length when compared with the lateral and posterior deltoid, which originate on the acromion and scapular spine, respectively. This increased length may result in decreased strength and increased fatigability of the anterior deltoid during humero-thoracic forward flexion.

Trapezial and deltotrapezial fascia injury

Dynamic stabilization of the shoulder girdle and the individual contribution of the trapezius, deltoid, and deltotrapezial fascia is a relatively new concept. However, there are a few studies, which have attempted to investigate the biomechanical function of these structures. Synchronization of the upper trapezius, which retracts and elevates the distal clavicle, and the middle trapezius, which retracts the scapula, may decrease the forces exerted on the static AC capsuloligamentous structures and CC ligaments during thoracohumeral motion. If this dynamic off-loading occurs in the healthy shoulder, it may have significant implications to protect the reconstructed ligaments and suggest the importance of surgically addressing these structures at the time of reconstruction.

In order to investigate the stabilization provided by the trapezius to the AC joint during scapular movement, Trudeau and colleagues performed a cadaveric biomechanical study with sequential sectioning of the trapezoidal insertion on the scapular and clavicle.[43] Their model did not have any injuries to the CC ligamentous or AC capsuloligamentous structures. To simulate muscular resistance to movement, the origins of the upper trapezius and middle trapezius were loaded with weights on a pulley system, which exerted approximately 10% of the estimated contraction force. After complete injury to the trapezoidal clavicular and scapular insertion, there was a 12.3% decrease in rotary torque for 12° of scapular internal rotation. Resistance to external rotation did not significantly change. The authors suggest unaddressed trapezoidal injury may contribute to loss of reduction after CC reconstruction due to loss of the dynamic stabilizing effect of the upper and middle trapezius and overreliance on the purely static stability of the ligamentous reconstruction.

Using a whole cadaveric model, Pastor and colleagues attempted to isolate the contribution of the deltotrapezial fascia to shoulder girdle stability after injury to the AC capsuloligamentous structures.[30] Using passive thoracohumeral motion, the authors investigated clavicular and scapular kinematic differences after complete AC capsuloligamentous injury followed by stripping of the deltotrapezial fascia off the clavicle. The authors did demonstrate a small but statically significant increase in anterior rotation of the clavicle (1.11). It should be noted that the experimental design did not simulate muscle forces, which may be a confounding factor if the deltotrapezial fascia acts more as a dynamic stabilizer rather than a static stabilizer.

IMPLICATIONS FOR SURGICAL TECHNIQUE: AUTHOR'S OPINION

Given the increased understanding of the shoulder girdle's anatomy and biomechanics, there are several implications for surgical technique. First, there are a multiple anatomic structures injured during an AC dislocation injury. Surgeons should strive to understand what specific anatomic structures are injured in their patients and attempt to restore native anatomy. Physical examination can help give clues. For example, posteriorly displaced clavicles often violate the trapezoid fascia and can result in painful spasm of the muscle. Additionally, irreducible AC joint injuries may represent higher degree of tissue damage, with interposing tissue. These 2 findings on physical examination, posterior displacement and irreducible dislocation, seem to correlate with increased difficulty with nonoperative management, and these patients may benefit from surgical intervention. Second, these injuries have complex three-dimensional pathomechanics, far more than the simple vertical displacement, which is often used as an inadequate surrogate. Third, the clavicle is an intercalated segment, which relates on capsuloligamentous attachments to the scapula in order to move in space and continue to perform its strut function (preventing excessing protraction of the scapula). Posterior rotation of the clavicle is a key component of this motion. For these reasons, an isolated CC reconstruction wrapped around the coracoid and clavicle is probably inadequate. The senior author has several key points to help mitigate these issues during surgical reconstruction. First, it is important to attempt to repair any deltoid or deltotrapezial fasica injuries by reattaching these structures to the anterior and posterior aspect of the distal clavicle with bone anchors. This fixation to bone will help reconstitute rotational control. Often, the origin of the deltoid is primarily muscle and may be reinforced with running suture to increase holding strength of the anchor's suture. Second, given the strut function of the clavicle and primary issue of instability, distal clavicle excisions should be avoided if possible. Maintaining a congruent, articulated AC joint will allow for the clavicle to keep the scapula is proper position. Allow the clavicle to provide compressive resistance forces will off load some of these forces from the reconstructed ligaments. Finally, if there is adequate native capsular tissue or graft tissue, repair or reconstruction of the posterosuperior AC capsuloligamentous tissues with direct suturing or use of long graft limb will likely help reconstitute the connection between clavicle and scapula.

FUTURE DIRECTION

Future studies should continue to evolve our understanding of physiologic motion of the shoulder girdle; the specific contribution of newly described structures, such as the "more" medial CC ligament and AC posterosuperior ligament; and the role of dynamic stabilizers, such as the upper trapezius and anterior deltoid. Detailed understanding of the pathologic and compensatory kinematics after injury will help further inform the development of new surgical techniques. Studies capturing the complex ST kinematics using whole-body cadaveric models (vs isolated distal clavicle-acromion models) will be important. Investigators should also push the limitations of our current conceptual framework. For example, AC/CC injuries are often represented as a one-dimensional diastasis between the coracoid and the clavicle; however, clinicians and researchers should be mindful of the complex anatomy, interdependence of the 5 mobile regions, and the multiplanar kinematics of the shoulder girdle.

SUMMARY

The shoulder girdle anatomically extends anteriorly from the SC joint to the broad scapular stabilizing muscles posteriorly. There are 3 joints and 2 mobile regions that form a kinetic chain, which allows for the complex kinematics required to accurately position the arm in space. The shoulder girdle is statically stabilized by the AC and CC capsuloligamentous structures and dynamically stabilized by the trapezius and deltoid muscles. During humerothoracic elevation, the clavicle elevates, protracts, and posteriorly rotates through the SC joint while the scapula increases posterior tilting and upward rotation. Clavicular motion, particularly posterior axial rotation, is reliant on strong capsuloligamentous attachments and should be conceptualized as an intercalated segment. After injury to the AC and CC capsuloligamentous structures, the kinetic chain between the clavicle and scapula is disrupted resulting in various pathomechanical consequences, such as increased scapular internal rotation and downward rotation. A detailed understanding of the biomechanical characteristics of the shoulder girdle and the contributions of various structures can help guide the development of the next generation of reconstructive procedures.

CLINICS CARE POINTS

- The trapezoid and conoid ligaments insert approximately 2.5 cm and 4.6 cm from the lateral edge of the clavicle, which are important landmarks for the anatomic CC reconstruction.
- Proper reconstruction of the AC joint's newly described posterosuperior ligament, with its 30° obliquity, may be an important consideration in surgical designs to improve posterior translational stability of clavicle.
- During arm elevation, the general motion of the clavicle is elevation, retraction, and posterior rotation, which is reciprocated by the scapula's upward rotation, posterior tilt, and external rotation.
- Disruption of the AC and CC capsuloligamentous structures causes increased internal and downward rotation of the scapula during rest and decreased scapular upward rotation, posterior tilt, and external rotation during arm elevation.

DISCLOSURES

A.D. Mazzocca reports research grants and is a consultant for Arthrex. Remaining authors have no disclosures.

REFERENCES

1. Gumina S, Carbone S, Postacchini F. Scapular Dyskinesis and SICK Scapula Syndrome in Patients With Chronic Type III Acromioclavicular Dislocation. Arthrosc J Arthrosc Relat Surg 2009;25(1):40–5.
2. Dunphy TR, Damodar D, Heckmann ND, et al. Functional Outcomes of Type V Acromioclavicular Injuries With Nonsurgical Treatment. J Am Acad Orthop Surg 2016;24(10):728–34.
3. Flores DV, Goes PK, Gómez CM, et al. Imaging of the Acromioclavicular Joint: Anatomy, Function, Pathologic Features, and Treatment. Radiographics 2020; 40(5):1355–82.
4. Lawrence RL, Braman JP, Keefe DF, et al. The Coupled Kinematics of Scapulothoracic Upward Rotation. Phys Ther 2020;100(2):283–94.
5. Flores-Hernandez C, Eskinazi I, Hoenecke HR, et al. Scapulothoracic rhythm affects glenohumeral joint force. JSES Open Access 2019;3(2):77–82.
6. Bishop JY, Flatow EL. Pediatric Shoulder Trauma. Clin Orthop 2005;432:41–8.
7. Rios CG, Arciero RA, Mazzocca AD. Anatomy of the Clavicle and Coracoid Process for Reconstruction of the Coracoclavicular Ligaments. Am J Sports Med 2007;35(5):811–7.
8. Chahla J, Marchetti DC, Moatshe G, et al. Quantitative Assessment of the Coracoacromial and the Coracoclavicular Ligaments With 3-Dimensional Mapping of the Coracoid Process Anatomy: A Cadaveric Study of Surgically Relevant Structures. Arthrosc J Arthrosc Relat Surg 2018;34(5):1403–11.
9. Dhawan R, Singh RA, Tins B, et al. Sternoclavicular joint. Shoulder Elb 2018; 10(4):296–305.

10. Lee JT, Campbell KJ, Michalski MP, et al. Surgical Anatomy of the Sternoclavicular Joint: A Qualitative and Quantitative Anatomical Study. J Bone Jt Surg 2014; 96(19):e166.

11. Matsumura N, Nakamichi N, Ikegami H, et al. The function of the clavicle on scapular motion: a cadaveric study. J Shoulder Elbow Surg 2013;22(3):333–9.

12. Veeger HEJ, van der Helm FCT. Shoulder function: The perfect compromise between mobility and stability. J Biomech 2007;40(10):2119–29.

13. Voss A, Imhoff AB. Editorial Commentary: Why We Have To Respect The Anatomy In Acromioclavicular Joint Surgery And Why Clinical Shoulder Scores Might Not Give Us The Information We Need. Arthrosc J Arthrosc Relat Surg 2019;35(5):1336–8.

14. von Schroeder HP, Kuiper SD, Botte MJ. Osseous anatomy of the scapula. Clin Orthop 2001;383:131–9.

15. Xin L, Luo J, Chen M, et al. Anatomy and Correlation of the Coracoid Process and Coracoclavicular Ligament Based on Three-Dimensional Computed Tomography Reconstruction and Magnetic Resonance Imaging. Med Sci Monit 2021;27. https://doi.org/10.12659/MSM.930435.

16. Nakazawa M, Nimura A, Mochizuki T, et al. The Orientation and Variation of the Acromioclavicular Ligament: An Anatomic Study. Am J Sports Med 2016; 44(10):2690–5.

17. DePalma AF. Surgical Anatomy of Acromioclavicular and Sternoclavicular Joints. Surg Clin North Am 1963;43(6):1541–50.

18. Colegate-Stone T, Allom R, Singh R, et al. Classification of the morphology of the acromioclavicular joint using cadaveric and radiological analysis. J Bone Joint Surg Br 2010;92-B(5):743–6.

19. Thompson JC. Netter's concise orthopaedic anatomy. 2nd edition, updated edition. Amsterdam, The Netherlands: Saunders Elsevier; 2016.

20. Nolte PC, Ruzbarsky JJ, Midtgaard KS, et al. Quantitative and Qualitative Surgical Anatomy of the Acromioclavicular Joint Capsule and Ligament: A Cadaveric Study. Am J Sports Med 2021;49(5):1183–91.

21. Velasquez Garcia A, Salamé Castillo F, Ekdahl Giordani M, et al. Anteroinferior bundle of the acromioclavicular ligament plays a substantial role in the joint function during shoulder elevation and horizontal adduction: a finite element model. J Orthop Surg 2022;17(1):73.

22. Shibata T, Izaki T, Miyake S, et al. Anatomical study of the position and orientation of the coracoclavicular ligaments: Differences in bone tunnel position by gender. Orthop Traumatol Surg Res 2019;105(2):275–80.

23. Moya D, Poitevin LA, Postan D, et al. The medial coracoclavicular ligament: anatomy, biomechanics,and clinical relevance—a research study. JSES Open Access 2018;2(4):183–9.

24. Filho RB, Freitas MM de, Nunes RHR, et al. Acromioclavicular, Coracoclavicular and Medial Coracoclavicular Ligaments Assessment in Acromioclavicular Dislocation. Rev Bras Ortop 2021;56(6):777–83.

25. Czerwonatis S, Steinke H, Hepp P, et al. Nameless in anatomy, but famous among surgeons: The so called "deltotrapezoid fascia". Ann Anat Anat Anz Off Organ Anat Ges 2020;231:151488.

26. Stimec BV, Lädermann A, Wohlwend A, et al. Medial coracoclavicular ligament revisited: an anatomic study and review of the literature. Arch Orthop Trauma Surg 2012;132(8):1071–5.

27. Rispoli DM, Athwal GS, Sperling JW, et al. The anatomy of the deltoid insertion. J Shoulder Elbow Surg 2009;18(3):386–90.

28. LeVasseur MR, Mancini MR, Kakazu R, et al. Three-Dimensional Footprint Mapping of the Deltoid and Trapezius: Anatomic Pearls for Acromioclavicular Joint Reconstruction. Arthrosc J Arthrosc Relat Surg 2022;38(3):701–8.
29. Elhassan BT, Sanchez-Sotelo J, Wagner ER. Outcome of arthroscopically assisted lower trapezius transfer to reconstruct massive irreparable posterior-superior rotator cuff tears. J Shoulder Elbow Surg 2020;29(10):2135–42.
30. Pastor MF, Averbeck AK, Welke B, et al. The biomechanical influence of the deltotrapezoid fascia on horizontal and vertical acromioclavicular joint stability. Arch Orthop Trauma Surg 2016;136(4):513–9.
31. Ludewig PM, Phadke V, Braman JP, et al. Motion of the Shoulder Complex During Multiplanar Humeral Elevation. J Bone Jt Surg-Am 2009;91(2):378–89.
32. Lefèvre-Colau MM, Nguyen C, Palazzo C, et al. Recent advances in kinematics of the shoulder complex in healthy people. Ann Phys Rehabil Med 2018;61(1):56–9.
33. Wu G, van der Helm FCT, DirkJan, et al. ISB recommendation on definitions of joint coordinate systems of various joints for the reporting of human joint motion—Part II: shoulder, elbow, wrist and hand. J Biomech 2005;38(5):981–92.
34. Dawson PA, Adamson GJ, Pink MM, et al. Relative contribution of acromioclavicular joint capsule and coracoclavicular ligaments to acromioclavicular stability. J Shoulder Elbow Surg 2009;18(2):237–44.
35. Harris RI, Wallace AL, Harper GD, et al. Structural properties of the intact and the reconstructed coracoclavicular ligament complex. Am J Sports Med 2000;28(1):103–8.
36. Koh SW, Cavanaugh JM, Leach JP, et al. Mechanical Properties of the Shoulder Ligaments under Dynamic Loading. Stapp Car Crash J 2004;48:125–53.
37. DiCosmo MB, Rumpf N, Mancini MR, et al. Clavicular-Sided Tears Were the Most Frequent Mode of Failure During Biomechanical Analysis of Acromioclavicular Ligament Complex Failure During Adduction of the Scapula. Arthrosc Sports Med Rehabil 2021;3(6):e1723–8.
38. Kurata S, Inoue K, Hasegawa H, et al. The Role of the Acromioclavicular Ligament in Acromioclavicular Joint Stability: A Cadaveric Biomechanical Study. Orthop J Sports Med 2021;9(2). 232596712098294.
39. Dyrna FGE, Imhoff FB, Voss A, et al. The Integrity of the Acromioclavicular Capsule Ensures Physiological Centering of the Acromioclavicular Joint Under Rotational Loading. Am J Sports Med 2018;46(6):1432–40.
40. Morikawa D, Dyrna F, Cote MP, et al. Repair of the entire superior acromioclavicular ligament complex best restores posterior translation and rotational stability. Knee Surg Sports Traumatol Arthrosc 2019;27(12):3764–70.
41. Oki S, Matsumura N, Iwamoto W, et al. The Function of the Acromioclavicular and Coracoclavicular Ligaments in Shoulder Motion: A Whole-Cadaver Study. Am J Sports Med 2012;40(11):2617–26.
42. Peeters I, Braeckevelt T, Herregodts S, et al. Kinematic Alterations in the Shoulder Complex in Rockwood V Acromioclavicular Injuries During Humerothoracic and Scapulothoracic Movements: A Whole-Cadaver Study. Am J Sports Med 2021;49(14):3988–4000.
43. Trudeau MT, Peters JJ, Hawthorne BC, et al. The Role of the Trapezius in Stabilization of the Acromioclavicular Joint: A Biomechanical Evaluation. Orthop J Sports Med 2022;10(9). 232596712211189.

Diagnosis and Nonoperative Treatment of Acromioclavicular Joint Injuries in Athletes and Guide for Return to Play

Brittany Olsen, MD, Bonnie Gregory, MD*

KEYWORDS

- Acromioclavicular joint • AC sprain • Shoulder separation • AC joint

KEY POINTS

- Acromioclavicular (AC) joint injuries are common in contact athletes.
- Many AC joint injuries can be managed nonoperatively but it is important to understand to diagnosis and treatment options in the athletic population.
- This article reviews the role for nonoperative treatment and outlines return-to-play considerations.

INTRODUCTION

In 2005 to 2006, the US Center for Disease Control and Prevention (CDC) conducted a study, which estimated that roughly 4.2 million students in the United States participated in high school sports. Within these 4.2 million athletes, there were 1.2 million injuries that occurred, 80% being new injuries.[1,2] Contact sports such as football, wrestling, and men's and women's soccer accounted for the highest number of injuries.[1] The CDC also released more current information. They demonstrated that, in 2019, 57.4% of all high school students was a part of at least one sports team compared with 56% in 2005 when the first study was performed. It can be extrapolated that there was an even higher number of injuries in 2019 given that more students were involved in sports competitions.[3]

When evaluating an athlete on the field, the trainer, coach, or physician should follow the order of "ABCDE," which stands for airway, breathing, circulation, disability, and extremity. After ruling out any immediate danger to the athlete, the attention can be

Department of Orthopaedic Surgery, University of Texas Health Science Center at Houston/McGovern Medical School, 6400 Fannin Street, Suite 1700, Houston, TX 77030, USA
* Corresponding author.
E-mail address: bonnie.p.gregory@uth.tmc.edu

Clin Sports Med 42 (2023) 573–587
https://doi.org/10.1016/j.csm.2023.05.003
0278-5919/23/© 2023 Elsevier Inc. All rights reserved.

directed toward that limb that is injured.[1] The most pressing injuries include ones that involve the brain, spine, or neurovascular injury, and those should take precedent over other injuries. Usually, if the injury involves only the upper extremity, the athlete should be able to walk themselves off of the field or court with the assistance of the trainer, coach, or physician. In this case, the evaluation should be done on the sidelines or somewhere that limits possible distractions. This helps to create an environment for a more thorough evaluation as you try to determine the mechanism, severity of injury, any concurrent injuries, and whether the athlete is safe to return to game play.

Injuries involving the shoulder consist of roughly 80% of injuries sustained in contact sports,[4] whereas injuries to the acromioclavicular (AC) joint account for 3% to 12% of all injuries.[5] The incidence of these injuries increases to roughly 40% to 50% when evaluating only those athletes involved in contact sports.[6] AC joint injuries have been found to be the third most common injury seen in college hockey players.[7] In elite college football players, AC joint injuries consist of 41% of all shoulder injuries, making these injuries the fourth most common injury sustained.[6] When looking at gender, men sustain anywhere from 2.2 to 8.5 more AC joint injuries than women.[8] Additionally, low-grade AC joint separations (Rockwood grade I and II) occur more frequently than high-grade injuries (Rockwood grade III, IV, V, and VI)[9] (**Fig. 1**).

DEFINITIONS AND INJURY CLASSIFICATION

The classification of AC joint injuries has been described by Rockwood based on the severity of injury to both the AC and coracoclavicular (CC) ligaments. A breakdown of this classification was previously described in the article, "Management of acromioclavicular joint injuries: a historical account" and can be reviewed in **Fig. 1** and **Table 1**.

DIAGNOSIS

The key to diagnosis of an AC joint injury is the history and physical examination. The first step is to discuss the mechanism of injury with the athlete and ensure that the

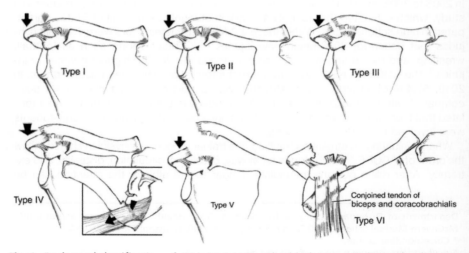

Fig. 1. Rockwood classification of AC joint injuries. The *black arrows* indicate the direction of pull on the extremity. The red arrows demonstrate structures that are injured or sprained without frank tearing. Picture representation of the spectrum of injury and the injured structures.[10]

Table 1
Verbal breakdown of injured structures and associated imaging based on the Rockwood classification of acromioclavicular joint injuries[11]

Type	AC Ligaments	CC Ligaments	Deltopectoral Fascia	X-Ray CC Distance	X-Ray AC Appearance
I	Sprained	Intact	Intact	Normal	Normal
II	Disrupted	Sprained	Intact	<25%	Widened
III	Disrupted	Disrupted	Disrupted	25%–100%	Widened
IV	Disrupted	Disrupted	Disrupted	Increased	Clavicle posteriorly displaced (axillary)
V	Disrupted	Disrupted	Disrupted	100%–300%	N/A
VI	Disrupted	Disrupted	Disrupted	Decreased	Clavicle displaced inferior to coracoid

mechanism fits the pathologic condition. The next step is to examine them preferably without any obstruction to the area. Whether in clinic or on the sidelines, this includes the removal of any pads, equipment, or even a shirt so that the area of the AC joint is well visible. Additionally, the contralateral should be exposed to allow visual inspection of bilateral shoulders with the arms hanging at the sides. Doing this will allow you to inspect the skin over the AC joint in order to determine if there are any open or impending open wounds, road rash, or abrasions over the deformity. This is important because it may change your management to include early surgical intervention or the administration of antibiotics. The physical examination should also be done in the standing or seated position to allow gravity to help exaggerate any deformity that is present.[12,13] Often, there is an obvious deformity of the AC joint compared with the contralateral side; however, in low-grade injuries, this is not always the case. Palpatory examination is also helpful in making the diagnosis on the sideline. A step-off can often be felt or motion of the distal clavicle can be elicited manually. This gives the examiner an idea about the direction of displacement of the distal clavicle with respect to the acromion. Alternatively, the athlete may only have tenderness directly over the AC joint if it a low-grade injury.

Regardless, the athlete will likely have increased pain in the area with range of motion of the shoulder. Specific tests such as the cross-arm abduction test and the active compression test (O'Brien test) can exacerbate the athlete's symptoms.[14] The cross-arm abduction test is done by elevating the arm to 90° and then adducting the arm. The O'Brien test is done by bringing the patient's arm to 90° of forward flexion with the elbow in full extension and then adducting the arm 10° to 15° medial to the sagittal plane of the body and internally rotating the am so that the thumb points downward. The examiner stands behind the patient and provides a downward force to the arm. Then the arm is fully supinated so that the palm is pointing upward and the pressure is reapplied.[12] If pain is elicited superficially over the AC joint during the first maneuver and relieved with the second maneuver, then it is considered a positive test (**Fig. 2**). This test has a sensitivity of 41% with a specificity of 94% for AC joint pathologic condition.[12] Additionally, the initial evaluation should include a simple shoulder shrug maneuver. This will help to evaluate the integrity of the deltotrapezial fascia. If the shoulder shrug reduces the AC joint, it can be assumed that the deltotrapezial fascia is intact.[15] If it does not reduce the AC joint, it would be concerning for detachment of this fascia, which may be indicated a more severe injury. This would be associated with a Rockwood grade III, IV, V, and possibly VI injury.[16] If the athlete is unable to

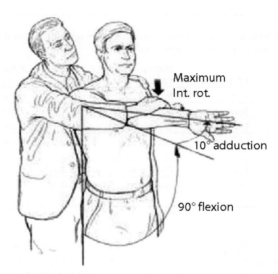

Fig. 2. Demonstrating the O'Brien test.

complete a shoulder shrug on their own due to pain and guarding the provider can help by stabilizing the clavicle and providing upward pressure on the ipsilateral elbow and looking for congruency of the AC joint. The examiner should also assess strength of the injured extremity, any deficits in strength eliminate immediate return to play during that session, regardless of grade of injury. Finally, a thorough neurovascular examination should be conducted of the upper extremity including the cervical spine to rule out any more serious and concomitant injuries.

Other tests should be conducted during the physical examination to look for any associated injuries. Palpation of the clavicle, coracoid, and sternoclavicular joint should be conducted to assess for any point tenderness, which may indicate fracture or further injury.[14] In a study conducted by Tisher and colleagues,[17] they evaluated the intra-articular injuries of 77 patients undergoing surgery for a high-grade AC joint dislocation. They found that 18.2% of these patients had intra-articular injury. Most of these consisted of a superior labrum anterior and posterior (SLAP) tear, whereas 4 patients had a fracture. Another sideline tool that may be useful for evaluation and investigation for an associated clavicle fracture is a tuning fork. This would not rule out a fracture but may give you a higher suspicion for the severity of injury and would push you to evaluate with further imaging.[1]

Another common injury that presents with pain in the neck and shoulder region but is not related to the AC joint includes a stinger. Typically, this presents with a "dead arm." The patient will have unilateral numbness or tingling and weakness in the affected arm. This is usually transient and will resolve on its own within a few minutes. This is important to differentiate from other injuries because it typically resolves quickly and the athlete can return to play without further intervention or precautions.

Regardless of sideline assessment, all presumed AC joint injuries should undergo radiographic examination. A full explanation of the radiographs is described in a previous chapter; however, we will discuss several pertinent considerations regarding selection and interpretation of select radiographic views. The 4 standard radiographic views to assess AC joint injuries include a Grashey anteroposterior (AP) or standard AP view of the shoulder, scapular Y, and axillary and bilateral Zanca views. The AP view helps to evaluate the glenohumeral joint for associated injuries. A Grashey AP will give you a proper AP of the glenohumeral joint and may give subtle clues into a concomitant injury within the glenohumeral joint. A scapular Y view can also be obtained to evaluate the scapula as well as an orthogonal view of both the acromion and the coracoid. An axillary view is used to evaluate the horizontal displacement of the clavicle and is deemed sufficient if there is a full view of the spinoglenoid notch.[18] If an axillary view cannot be obtained due to difficulties with pain and or positioning, a Velpeau axillary lateral view can be obtained. In this situation, the patient is asked to lean backward over the cassette and the beam is directed from superior to inferior.[13] The Zanca view was developed due to the difficulty in evaluating the AC joint on the AP view, as well as the difference in penetration needed to evaluate the glenohumeral joint versus the AC joint.[13] This allows you to quantify the degree of vertical displacement of the AC joint, evaluate for any coexisting fractures of the clavicle or in a younger athlete, a physeal separation, as well as compare it to the contralateral or "normal" side (**Fig. 3**).

The Rockwood classification uses the distance between the superior aspect of the coracoid process and the inferior aspect of the clavicle. The average distance is variable, measuring between 1.1 and 1.3 cm. This variability underscores the importance of comparing to the contralateral side. If this CC distance increases more than 40% to 50% of the contralateral side or 5 mm of difference, there is considered to be a complete tear of the coracoclavicular ligaments[13,19,20] (**Fig. 4**). In terms of the Rockwood classification, if the CC distance in increased but less than 25% of the contralateral side, it is considered a type II injury. If this distance is increased between 25%

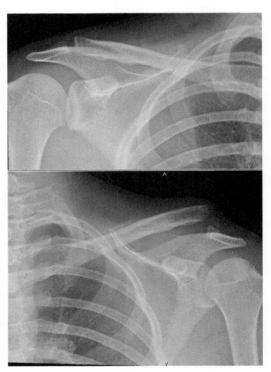

Fig. 3. Bilateral Zanca Views in 17-year-old male patient with left grade III AC joint separation.

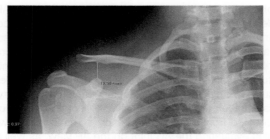

Fig. 4. Increased coracoclavicular ligament distance in a 32F with grade III AC joint separation.

and100% of the contralateral side, it is a type III, and more than 100% increase in the CC distance classifies it as a type V AC joint separation.[12] Of note, if there is an inferior AC joint dislocation, the CC distance would be less than the contralateral side; however, this is exceedingly rare. Additionally, as discussed previously, a stress view may be indicated. However, it is rarely used in clinical setting as this point because it is a painful examination that rarely provides any new information that changes management.[12]

Prompted by the pain associated with and difficulty in obtaining stress views, Vanarthos and colleagues[20] conducted a cadaveric study to determine if an internal rotation view could replace the stress view. They used an AP radiograph of the shoulder with the arm in internal rotation without any weights as seen in **Fig. 5**. They found that sometimes this is helpful to differentiate between a type II and type III AC joint separation and could be used to replace the stress view.[13] However, once again this view adds limited information and typically does not change management.

If an AC joint injury is suspected, however the AC joint seems normal on radiographs and the CC distance is within normal limits to the contralateral side, then a fracture of the coracoid needs to be considered. This is can best viewed with a Stryker notch view. This radiograph is obtained in the supine position with the arm elevated parallel to the long axis of the body and the palm placed behind the head. The x-ray beam is then angled 10° cranially.[12,22]

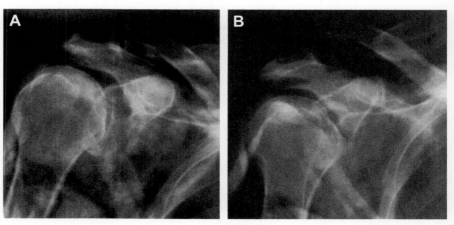

Fig. 5. Picture taken from Vanarthos and colleagues[21] demonstrating the use of internal rotation stress views in the setting of AC joint injury.

Depending on the severity of injury or concern for concomitant injuries, an MRI may be indicated. An MRI can be helpful in differentiating lower grade AC joint dislocation because it allows for the evaluation of the AC joint capsule, the CC ligaments as well as the osseous alignment directly rather than indirectly when using plain radiographs (**Fig. 6**). White and colleagues[22] conducted a study looking at AC joint injuries and evaluation with MRI in the National Hockey League (NHL). They were able to better identify bone bruising and concomitant muscular injury than with plain radiographs or physical examination alone. In this study, 23 out of 24 of their patients were diagnosed with a grade I, II, or III, whereas the last one had a grade V injury. They found that 79% of their cohort sustain a trapezius muscle strain while 50% had a deltoid strain. All of the lower grade injuries were treated nonoperatively in a sling, whereas the grade V injury was treated with surgery. All of the athletes returned to professional NHL competition; however, those with more extensive soft tissue injury, such as muscle strains or higher grade AC joint injury, missed more games.[23] An MRI may also be helpful in cases where there is concern for a rotator cuff tear. Tischer and colleagues[17] found that of 77 patients with AC joint dislocations 11 patients had an SLAP tear and 3 had a rotator cuff tear. They found that these were more likely in traumatic AC dislocations with the rotator cuff tears being more prevalent in the older age group. An MRI would be useful in evaluating these pathologic conditions because it may change your management plan.

Recently, ultrasound has been investigated as a diagnostic imaging tool. One method of assessment of the AC is by conducting a dynamic sonographic evaluation. Peetrons and Bedard[24] discussed the technique of using ultrasound while conducting a crossarm maneuver. In this case, the ultrasound probe is centered over the AC joint and the affected hand is placed on the operative shoulder. When this is done, the ultrasound will show abnormal motion at the AC joint. At rest, the clavicle is raised compared with the AC joint and when the cross-body maneuver is done, the clavicle can be seen to lower to the level of the acromion. The authors describe this examination supplement as being helpful when there are less obvious findings but a mild AC joint sprain is suspected.[24] **Fig. 7** demonstrates their findings. Heers and Hedtmann[25] looked at ultrasound (US) evaluation in relation to radiograph (XR) in the setting of AC

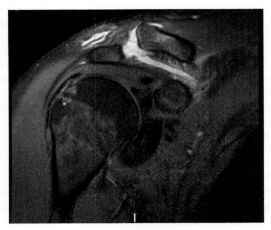

Fig. 6. Coronal MRI of R shoulder demonstrating a complete disruption of the superior and inferior AC joint capsule and coracoclavicular ligaments (type III).

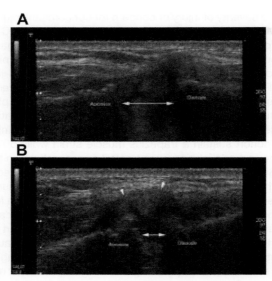

Fig. 7. Picture taken from Peetrons and Bedard[24] demonstrating the ultrasound findings for an AC joint dislocation.

joint dislocations. They determined that ultrasound may overestimate or underestimate the soft tissue injury component not seen on XR. They also stated that US evaluation is most helpful in type III injuries to evaluate the fascial disruption and deltoid or trapezius detachment, which would push the physician toward indicating the athlete for surgery. US evaluation can be helpful because it has become more common to have trained sideline physicians with portable ultrasounds readily available. This is a quick study that can be done at the time of injury on the sidelines or training room to help determine the degree of pathology and next steps quickly.

DISCUSSION

AC joint injuries are consistently treated with either conservative management for the low grade (types I, II) or surgery for the high-grade (types IV, V, VI) injuries. Type III injuries still pose controversy among surgeons. Some surgeons advocate for conservative management, whereas others opt for surgical intervention, and the literature supports both options. The decision to pursue nonoperative versus operative treatment depends on the surgeon's preference and experience, as well as the outcome of discussions with the patient and family. A meta-analysis of 1172 patients with type III AC joint injuries were studied, with 833 of these patients treated with surgery and 339 treated conservatively.[26] The authors found that 88% of those treated surgically and 87% of those treated nonoperatively has satisfactory outcomes. However, the complication rate was much higher after surgery, with infection and need for future surgery being most common. Those undergoing conservative management were more likely to have a cosmetic deformity though. The time required to return to activities, pain level, range of motion, and strength were found to be similar between the 2 cohorts. Therefore, the authors concluded that surgery showed no benefit compared with nonoperative treatment.

Another study evaluating patients treated both operatively and nonoperatively found that both have similar outcomes in terms of rotational strength.[27] However, when compared with the bench press strength, the patients treated conservatively were 17% weaker in their injured arm compared with their contralateral arm. They found that 20% of the patients treated conservatively have suboptimal outcomes. This was mostly encountered during long-term follow-up when increasing demands of strength and endurance caused discomfort. Therefore, athletes that require high loads or collisions may benefit from early operative intervention. This can also be extrapolated to heavy laborers because the demands of their jobs may require similar demands in strength and endurance. There is no consensus in the literature as to which type of treatment is considered the gold standard.

Treatment Options and Rehabilitation

Treatment is typically guided by the Rockwood classification in which types I and II are treated conservatively; types IV, V, and VI are treated surgically; and type III can be treated either conservatively or surgically depending on the physician's preference and discussion with the patient. Surgical treatment options are discussed elsewhere; this article will focus on nonsurgical management with specific consideration regarding the athlete.

The first decision that needs to be made is whether the patient can return to competition immediately. With an AC joint injury, this is mostly dependent on the patient's pain and ability to execute the necessary skills of their position. A quick sideline assessment is needed to inspect the skin over the AC joint and test the athlete's strength. If these are both normal, they should take some time on the sidelines with sport-specific drills to see if they can tolerate those. If the athlete passes these sideline tests, then they could return to competition the same day. If the athlete's skin compromises or their pain inhibits them to being able to compete adequately, they should be held out until they can prove otherwise.

The treatment of an athlete may be different than a normal patient given the need to return them to high level of activities quickly. For athletes with type I AC joint injuries, sling immobilization and OTC medications are only indicated for pain control and usually discontinued within a few days if necessary. For type II AC joint injuries, nonoperative management typically usually includes 1 to 2 weeks of sling immobilization of the affected extremity while working on pain control with anti-inflammatories and/or tylenol as well as ice. Corticosteroid injections (CSIs) can be used immediately to help decrease the pain as well as for all them to return to the game if the injury occurred during competition. In our practice, CSI during competition is limited to athletes with intact strength but significant pain limiting return to game play, after informed consent is provided. If available sideline, this can be done under fluoroscopic or ultrasound guidance for improved accuracy. Caution is warranted for use in throwing or overhead athletes (ie, quarterback) as occasional short-term rotator cuff inhibition can occur due to analgesic potentially entering the subacromial space during injection. Additionally, in higher level athletes, local analgesic without CSIs can be administered each pregame to allow the athlete to continue playing in the subsequent weeks.

Taping may help to decrease the motion of the clavicle on the acromion, which can also help alleviate the athlete's pain. For contact sports, padding can be taped to the shoulder under the uniform to protect them from any blows to the AC joint. This can range from padding found in the training room, to a formal brace to one fitted to the athlete using orthoglass or custom 3D printed brace to protect them from contact (**Figs. 8** and **9**). The physician and trainer would need to check with their league's rules and regulation regarding what is acceptable before fitting the athlete with it. Once the athlete's pain is under control, they can start physical therapy. This usually starts with

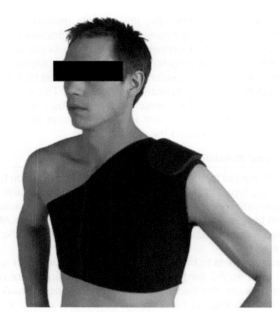

Fig. 8. Padding over the AC joint for protection against contact.

range of motion exercises of the shoulder and scapula and progresses to isometric and then isotonic exercises. They can then work to strengthen their shoulder and scapula and work toward returning to their sport with sport-specific drills and exercises and working back into full game situations. The length of time needed before returning to competition is also dictated by the position of the athlete. In terms of football, a lineman or running back may be able to return quicker than a quarterback or wide receiver. This is because the stress on the AC joint is increased with the arm being overhead. Therefore, overhead athletes may also take longer to recover especially if it is their dominant side. In this case, range of motion and strength need to be as close to normal as possible to allow them to be successful in their position. However, there is no specific return-to-play testing or guidelines based on the different level of injuries in each sport or position.

Few studies regarding treatment of AC joint injuries discuss general rehabilitation protocol. One study reports a rehabilitation protocol focuses on mobility, scapular strengthening, shoulder strengthening, and kinetic chain exercises. It includes 12 supervised exercises done with a physical therapist. They recommend a minimum of 3 hours per week of therapy for the first 6 weeks then 1.5 hours per week until final follow-up.[28] Another study recommended a similar protocol; however, theirs included therapy visits 2 to 3 times per week for 6 weeks and progressed the patient through phases such as acute, recovery, and return-to-sport phases.[9]

Most of the literature on rehabilitation of AC joint injury agrees that protocols should focus on scapular control and kinetic chain exercises. Similarly, many emphasize therapy should only be initiated after a sufficient amount of rest to decrease or even eliminate the pain associated with the initial injury. However, elite in-season athletes with low-grade injuries may wish to initiate rehabilitation with athletic training and physical therapy immediately. Regardless, the first step in rehabilitation and return-to-play

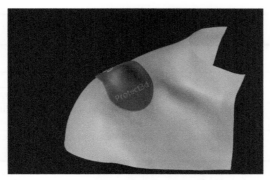

Fig. 9. Custom 3D printed AC joint brace by Protect3D (https://www.nfl.com/playerhealthand safety/equipment-and-innovation/1st-and-future/nfl-2020-1st-and-future-winner-protect3d-using-3d-scanning-and-printing-to-help-).

progression is to work on shoulder and AC joint mobility without excessively loading the AC joint itself.[29] This includes starting with exercises with the arm in an adducted rather than abducted or forward flexed position, which would increase the lever arm and therefore stress across the AC joint. Once achieving short level arm exercises pain-free, the athlete can then progress to a longer level arm. Sciascia and colleagues[9] recommend that the exercises first be performed with the arm in 30° to 40° of abduction before progressing further. They suggest that the patient start their therapy with 1 to 2 sets of 5 to 10 repetitions without any external resistance, using only body weight and gravity. This can be increased as the patient tolerates to a goal of 5 to 6 sets with 10 repetitions in each. Once this step is obtained, resistance can be added starting with lightweights, about 2 to 3 lbs maximum with progression to elastic resistance bands. The longer lever exercises should be implemented later in the rehabilitation protocol ensuring that each step before has been mastered without worsening the patient's symptoms.

1. Exercises with the arm in 30° to 45° of abduction
   a. 1 to 2 sets of 5 to 10 reps → increase to goal of 5 to 6 sets of 10 repetitions each
   b. Body weight and gravity
2. Start adding resistance
   a. 2 to 3 lbs maximum → elastic resistance bands
3. Repeat with arm in 45° to 60° of abduction
4. Repeat with arm in 60° to 90° of abduction

Sciascia and colleagues[29] summarized their approach into 5 succinct steps. The first includes rest and activity modification to control the pain and symptoms of the acute injury. This usually takes about 1 to 2 weeks. The second step is to start exercises that address proximal segment control such as leg, truck, and core strengthening. The third step introduces exercises for scapular, shoulder, and lower extremity mobility. The next step involves short-lever interventions that use trunk and leg mobility to help with scapular positioning and control. Finally, transition through the range of abduction to start working on long lever exercises that start to include unilateral as well as bilateral maneuvers.[29] Typically, if the injury happens during the season, those with type III injuries will follow this pathway as well. Return to play can take anywhere between 1 week and 6 weeks pending the pain tolerance and physical demands of the athlete.

Physical Therapy Progression	
Phase 1	• Rest • Activity modification
Phase 2	• Exercises focusing on proximal segment control (eg, legs, trunk, core)
Phase 3	• Exercises focused on scapular, shoulder, and lower extremity mobility
Phase 4	• Short lever interventions using trunk and leg mobility to help with scapular position and control
Phase 5	• Progress through abduction to work on long lever exercises • Unilateral exercises

Some athletes may benefit from the addition of injections to help get them back to their preinjury level of play.[14] Typically, an initial injection is done within 48 to 72 hours from injury and composed of an analgesic agent such as marcaine or bupivacaine with a corticosteroid. Additional analgesic injections without concomitant corticosteroid may be repeated weekly or as needed before competition, especially for professional or high-level collegiate athletes. Often these injections are successful in allowing the athlete to return to play. Risks of this procedure include residual pain or a slight increased risk for the need of distal clavicle excision.[14] However, these injections have been deemed safe and are not a significant threat to the athlete's career.[12,30] Orchard and colleagues[29] conducted a retrospective study of 100 players in the National Football League who had been injected with local anesthetic on 1023 occasions for 307 injuries. Ninety-eight percent of the athletes stated that they would repeat the procedure again for their injury and only 6% had residual pain. There was no comment of any recurrent injuries the athletes sustained to the AC joint. Their study included more anatomic locations than just the AC joint; however, they found that these injections are both safe and helpful in the context of professional athletes.[30]

Nonoperative management is not without its complications. These can include residual instability, degenerative changes at the AC joint, distal clavicle osteolysis, and continued pain present as early as 6 months after injury.[12,31] Cox and colleagues[31] found that it was not uncommon for an athlete to have residual symptoms, positive examination findings, and radiographic changes after sustaining type I or II AC joint injuries.[32] Not all patients with radiographic changes are symptomatic; however, if they are, this can be successfully treated with an arthroscopic or open distal clavicle excision.

If any athlete fails nonsurgical treatment, surgery should be considered. This time frame for intervention can be as early as 6 weeks after injury if still symptomatic or at the conclusion of the season. As surgical techniques have advanced, delayed reconstruction has equivalent outcomes to acute.[33] Athletes who sustain types IV, V, and VI AC joint injuries have superior outcomes after undergoing surgical intervention as compared with conservative measures.[34,35] This is also true for collision athletes; however, if the athlete can tolerate it, surgery can be considered after the season.

Most studies have looked at the time frame of athletes returning to competition after sustaining an AC joint injury rather than the protocols themselves. One study showed that in a population consisting of Major League Baseball players acute AC joint injuries were more likely to occur in infielders and outfielders, and they typically missed 3 weeks before returning to play.[36] Another study that looked at professional soccer players found that those who sustained an AC joint separation missed roughly 5 to 7 weeks of competition. Eighty-one percent of their cohort was able to return to elite levels of performance similar to preinjured and healthy controls.[37] Neither of these studies reviews their rehab or return-to-play protocols. In the NHL, one study demonstrated that their time frame to return to activity was between 3 and 4 weeks.[23] Their return-to-play criteria included objective measures including manual strength using a handheld dynamometer and Y-balance testing compared with preinjury baseline data. They also underwent functional testing, which includes push-ups, push-pull testing, ability to receive contact during practice, battle with a stick, and shoot confidently. These measures were all compared relative to their own preinjury baseline in the same extremity. Their goal was above 90% of the contralateral side before being cleared to return to professional NHL competition.[23]

Currently, literature has not identified a universal return-to-play protocol after sustaining an AC joint injury. At this point, it is understood that competitive athletes should undergo intense sport-specific movements and exercises before returning to practices and games. The agreed upon pathway thus far includes a period of rest and pain management followed by range of motion exercises and then strengthening of the trunk, scapula, and shoulder musculature. Once this is complete, sports-specific exercises can be introduced. More research needs to be conducted to better characterize sports-specific rehabilitations programs, objective measures for readiness to return to sports and timelines associated with return to play because each sport and each position has different upper extremity demands. Furthermore, once a battery of exercises and objective measures is identified, it can be used as baseline testing at the start of their season and is the marker by which any postinjury rehabilitation can be measured to allow the safest to return to competition.

SUMMARY

Injury to the AC joint is common in the athletic population, in particular in contact sports. Physical examination and imaging are key to assessing extent of injury and as a result nonoperative versus operative treatment. If nonoperative treatment is indicated, bracing/taping, injections, and physical therapy can be used to reliably return athletes to activity within game or within a few weeks depending on severity of injury, level and sport of participation, and position-specific requirements.

CLINICS CARE POINTS

- Sideline assessment of athletic AC joint injuries is key to rule out concomitant injuries such as fracture as well as assess strength and ability to return to play
- Acute corticosteroid or analgesic injections as well as taping/bracing can be used in grade I and II AC sprains to return athletes to play within same game or in subsequent games within first few weeks
- No defined return guideline exists in the literature but full strength and function as well as limited pain can serve as a guideline for athletic return
- Although nonoperative treatment can reliably return athletes to play quickly, degenerative changes at AC and residual pain can be noted even with grade I injuries

DISCLOSURE

B. Gregory is an American Orthopedic Society for Sports Medicine: Board or committee member.

REFERENCES

1. Schupp CM. Sideline evaluation and treatment of bone and joint injury. Curr Sports Med Rep 2009;8(3):119–24.
2. Sports-Related Injuries Among High School Athletes - United States, 2005-2006 School Year. Center for Disease Control and Prevention. Available at: www.cdc.gov/mmwr/preview/mmwrhtml/mm5538a1.htm. Accessed on October 17 2022.
3. Centers for Disease Control and Prevention (CDC). 1991-2019 High School Youth Risk Behavior Survey Data. Available at: http://yrbs-explorer.services.cdc.gov/. Accessed on October 17 2022.
4. Van Lancker HP, Martineau PA. The diagnosis and treatment of shoulder injuries in contact and collision athletes. J Orthop Trauma 2012;26(1):1.
5. Rosso C, Martetschläger F, Saccomanno MF, et al. High degree of consensus achieved regarding diagnosis and treatment of acromioclavicular joint instability among ESA-ESSKA members. Knee Surg Sports Traumatol Arthrosc 2021;29:2325–32.
6. Kaplan LD, Flanigan DC, Norwig J, et al. Prevalence and variance of shoulder injuries in elite collegiate football players. Am J Sports Med 2005;33(8):1142–6.
7. Flik K, Lyman S, Marx RG. American collegiate men's ice hockey: an analysis of injuries. Am J Sports Med 2005;33:183–7.
8. Chillemi C, Franceschini V, Dei Giudici L, et al. Epidemiology of isolated acromioclavicular joint dislocation. Emerg Med Int 2013;2013:171609.
9. Sciascia A, Bois AJ, Kibler WB. Nonoperative management of traumatic acromioclavicular joint injury: a clinical commentary with clinical practice considerations. Int J Sports Phys Ther 2022;17(3):519–40.
10. Tossy JD, Mead MC, Sigmond HM. Acromioclavicular separations: useful and practical classification for treatment. Clin Orthop Relat Res 1963;28:111–9.
11. Williams GR Jr, Nguyen VD, Rockwood CA Jr. Classification and radiographic analysis of acromioclavicular dislocations. Appl Radiol 1989;18:29–34.
12. Epstein D, Day M, Rokito A. Current concepts in the surgical management of acromioclavicular joint injuries. Bull Hosp Joint Dis 2012;70(1):11–24.
13. Arner JW, Provencher MT, Bradley JP, et al. Evaluation and management of the contact athlete's shoulder. J Am Acad Orthop Surg 2022;30:e584–94.
14. Tischer T, Salzmann GM, El-Azab H, et al. Incidence of associated injuries with acute acromioclavicular joint dislocations types III through V. Am J Sports Med 2009;37(1):136–9.
15. Mazzocca AD, Sellards R, Romeo A. Acromioclavicular joint injuries: pediatric and adult. Orthop sports med. Philadelphia: WB Saunders; 2002.
16. Gorbaty JD, Hsu JE, Gee AO. Classifications in brief: rockwood classification of acromioclavicular joint separations. Clin Orthop Relat Res 2017;475(1):283–7.
17. Matsen FA 3rd, Gupta A. Axillary view: arthritic glenohumeral anatomy and changes after ream and run. Clin Orthop Relat Res 2014;472(3):894–902.
18. Bosworth BM. Complete acromioclavicular dislocation. N Engl J Med 1949;241:221–5.
19. Beim GM. Acromioclavicular joint injuries. J Athl Train 2000;35(3):261–7.
20. Vanarthos WJ, Ekman EF, Bohrer SP. Radiographic diagnosis of acromioclavicular joint separation without weight bearing: importance of internal rotation of the arm. AJR Am J Roentgenol 1994;162:120–2.

21. Galatz LM, Williams G. Acromioclavicular joint injuries. In: Bucholz RW, Heckman JD, Court-Brown CM, editors. Rockwood and green's fractures in adults. Philadelphia: Lippincott Williams and Wilkins; 2002. p. 1210–24.

22. White LM, Ehmann J, Bleakney RR, et al. Acromioclavicular joint injuries in professional ice hockey players: epidemiologic and MRI findings and association with return to Play. Orthop J Sports Med 2020;8(11). https://doi.org/10.1177/2325967120964474.

23. Peetrons P, Bédard J. Acromioclavicular joint injury: enhanced technique of examination with dynamic maneuver. J Clin Ultrasound 2007;35:262–7.

24. Heers G, Hedtmann A. Correlation of ultrasonographic findings to Tossy's and Rockwood's classification of acromioclavicular joint injuries. Ultrasound Med Biol 2005 Jun;31(6):725–32.

25. Carbone S, Postacchini R, Gumina S. Scapular dyskinesis and SICK syndrome in patients with a chronic type III acromioclavicular dislocation. Results of rehabilitation. Knee Surg Sports Traumatol Arthrosc 2015;23:1473–80.

26. Schlegel TF, Burks RT, Marcus RL, et al. A prospective evaluation of untreated acute grade III acromioclavicular separations. Am J Sports Med 2001;29(6):699–703.

27. Tamaoki MJ, Lenza M, Matsunaga FT, et al. Surgical versus conservative interventions for treating acromioclavicular dislocation of the shoulder in adults. Cochrane Database Syst Rev 2019;10:Cd007429.

28. Petri M, Warth RJ, Greenspoon JA, et al. Clinical results after conservative management for grade III acromioclavicular joint injuries: does eventual surgery affect overall outcomes? Arthroscopy 2016;32:740–6.

29. Orchard JW. Benefits and risks of using local anaesthetic for pain relief to allow early return to play in professional football. Br J Sports Med 2002;36(3):209–13.

30. White B, Epstein D, Sanders S, et al. Acute acromioclavicular injuries in adults. Orthopedics 2008;31(12). PMID: 19226062.

31. Cox JS. The fate of the acromioclavicular joint in athletic injuries. Am J Sports Med 1981;9(1):50–3.

32. Phillips AM, Smart C, Groom AF. Acromioclavicular dislocation. Conservative or surgical therapy. Clin Orthop Relat Res 1998;353:10–7.

33. Kim SH, Koh KH. Treatment of rockwood type III acromioclavicular joint dislocation. Clin Shoulder Elb 2018;21(1):48–55.

34. Frank RM, Cotter EJ, Leroux TS, et al. Acromioclavicular joint injuries: evidence-based treatment. J Am Acad Orthop Surg 2019;27:e775–88.

35. Frantz T, Ramkumar PN, Frangiamore S, et al. Epidemiology of acromioclavicular joint injuries in professional baseball: analysis from the major league baseball health and injury tracking system. J Shoulder Elbow Surg 2021;30:127–33.

36. Diaz CC, Forlenza EM, Lavoie-Gagne OZ, et al. Acromioclavicular joint separation in UEFA soccer players: a matched-cohort analysis of return to play and player performance from 1999 to 2018. Orthop J Sports Med 2021;9(10). https://doi.org/10.1177/23259671211026262.

37. Ma R, Smith P, Smith M, et al. Managing and recognizing complications after treatment of acromioclavicular joint repair or reconstruction. Curr Rev Musculoskelet Med 2015;8(10):1007.

Open Anatomic Coracoclavicular Ligament Reconstruction for Acromioclavicular Joint Injuries

E. Lyle Cain Jr, MD*, David Parker, MD

KEYWORDS

- Coracoclavicular • Ligament • Reconstruction • Acromioclavicular • Instability

KEY POINTS

- Acromioclavicular (AC) instability is common in sports.
- Several surgical techniques are available to reduce and fix the unstable AC joint.
- Coracoclavicular (CC) ligament reconstruction with autograft or allograft tendon has been successful at maintaining AC reduction.
- Open reconstruction of both the CC and AC joint ligaments provides both coronal and sagittal restraint to motion.
- Our preferred technique for both CC and AC ligament reconstruction is discussed.

INTRODUCTION

Acromioclavicular (AC) joint injuries are one of the most common shoulder injuries. AC joint trauma is responsible for 12% of all shoulder injuries.[1] The AC joint is stabilized by the coracoclavicular (CC) ligaments in the coronal plane and the AC joint ligaments in the sagittal plane. The conoid and trapezoid ligaments comprise the CC ligaments and are located on the undersurface of the clavicle extending to the cephalad portion of the coracoid. The conoid ligament is located 45 mm from the end of the distal clavicle and is more posterior than the trapezoid ligament. The trapezoid ligament is 10 mm more lateral from the conoid and has a more central footprint.[2]

AC joint instability most commonly occurs by falling on an outstretched arm with the direct force acting on the lateral shoulder but can also be caused by direct blow to the top of the AC joint in contact or collision sports (football). AC joint injuries are classified by the Rockwood classification based on the degree and direction of displacement. Type I and II injuries are usually nonsurgical, whereas some type III and most type IV, V, and VI injuries are indicated for surgical intervention.[3]

American Sports Medicine Institute, Andrews Sports Medicine and Orthopaedic Center, 805 Saint, Vincents Drive, Suite 100, Birmingham, AL, 35205, USA
* Corresponding author.
E-mail address: Lyle.Cain@Andrewssm.com

Clin Sports Med 42 (2023) 589–598
https://doi.org/10.1016/j.csm.2023.05.009

sportsmed.theclinics.com

AC joint repair was first described by Cadanet in 1917.[4] Since then, numerous surgical treatment options have been used for achieving adequate AC reduction, including the Bosworth screw, Kirschner wires, or a hook plate.[5,6] These fixation methods have better results when performed in the acute period, but they have increased risks of hardware breakage, wire migration, loss of reduction, and need for later hardware removal.[5-8] Arthroscopic cortical button suspensory fixation techniques are less invasive but do not anatomically reconstruct the AC ligaments and rely on native tissue healing.[9,10] These arthroscopic cortical fixation procedures generally need to be performed acutely unless a graft is used, because the healing response of native tissue is less consistent in chronic injury. The Weaver-Dunn technique involves transfer of the coracoacromial (CA) ligament to the distal clavicle.[5] However, this ligament is not as strong as the native CC ligaments and does not reconstruct the AC ligaments or place the transferred CA ligament tissue in the anatomically correct position.

No gold standard exists for AC joint reconstruction. Most methods used today involve some type of reconstruction of the CC and/or AC ligaments due to increasing knowledge of their biomechanical importance.[11] Many factors must be taken into account when deciding to perform an AC joint reconstruction including sport, arm dominance, age, chronicity, and symptoms. This article describes our technique for open anatomic CC and AC ligament reconstruction for AC joint injuries. The surgical technique has the following goals: (1) both coronal and sagittal AC joint stability; (2) avoidance of graft fraying or bone cut through that may be associated with tenodesis screws or nonabsorbable sutures being passed through bone tunnels; and (3) the addition of braided PDS sutures (Ethicon, Somerville, NJ) around the clavicle to initially unload the forces on the graft.[12]

Indications

Displacement of the AC joint has been classified by Rockwood and colleagues into types I–VI. Generally, types I and II are stable injuries not requiring additional ligamentous reconstruction, where types III–VI often result in chronic instability requiring surgery. The decision to proceed with AC reconstruction depends on several factors including sport, arm dominance, age, chronicity and symptoms. Most patients with grade V AC separation and many with grade III are advised to have surgical reconstruction. The authors generally perform arthroscopic stabilization with dual-button tightrope suspensory fixation through the coracoid and clavicle for acute grade III injuries in lower level athletes, whereas contact or collision athletes indicate the need for additional tissue grafts and fixation, including accessory fixation options described below.

Surgical Technique

Anatomic CC ligament reconstruction has been well described by Mazzocca and colleagues in several publications.[2] Although the authors have used the original Mazzocca technique with good results to restore AC elevation (vertical stability), increased anterior-posterior AC joint/distal clavicle motion is not well-controlled (horizontal stability). Our current technique for unstable AC joint injuries provides reconstruction of both the CC ligaments and AC joint capsule with the same autograft tendon. After passage of the traditional CC ligament graft around the coracoid and through two tunnels in the clavicle, the graft is passed through an oblique acromial tunnel and sutured to the trapezoid graft limb after appropriate elevation and reduction of the shoulder girdle. Tenodesis screws are not placed in the bone tunnels to avoid graft damage, and initial forces on the graft are protected with braided absorbable sutures (nine strands of #0 PDS [Ethicon, Somerville, NJ]) passed around the coracoid and clavicle in a cerclage fashion. In cases of severe instability or concern for high graft forces, especially in collision athletes, a dual-button suspensory construct (AC Tighrope, Arthrex, Naples, FL) may be placed from a coracoid tunnel through the medial clavicle tunnel for accessory fixation. Although several allograft tendon options have been used for CC reconstruction, the authors prefer contralateral gracilis tendon autograft if available.

Approach

The patient is placed supine with slight head elevation and the arm is prepped free to allow shoulder motion during the procedure. A slightly oblique anterior incision is made approximately 5 cm in length beginning just cephalad to the displaced AC joint extending to 2 cm below the coracoid process (**Fig. 1**). The deltotrapezial fascia is incised along the line of the skin incision, and the deltoid muscle is split from the AC joint to the coracoid process. The AC capsule is opened in a T-shaped manner exposing the AC joint, anterior acromion, and distal 5 cm of superior clavicle. Wide clavicle exposure is helpful to allow later graft passage through the bone tunnels. The medial and lateral margins of the coracoid process are exposed using electrocautery to release the CA ligament and pectoralis minor attachments.

Graft Harvest and Preparation

The contralateral lower extremity is prepped and draped for graft harvest. This allows for simultaneous graft harvest and AC joint exposure without compromising the surgical field. An oblique incision 2 cm distal and medial to the tibial tubercle over the pes anserinus tendons leads to the sartorius fascia and easy palpation of the semitendinosus and gracilis tendons. The sartorius fascia is incised in line with the cephalad edge of the gracilis tendon. The superior most gracilis tendon is identified on the undersurface of the fascia with a hemostat clamp, freed of fascial bands, and harvested with a tendon stripper (Stryker, Mahwah, NJ). Care is taken to protect the saphenous nerve

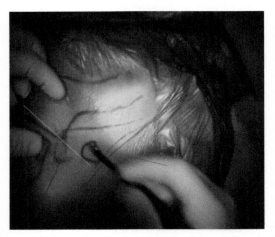

Fig. 1. Right shoulder, with the patient in the supine position. A 6-cm incision is made from the most posterior aspect of the acromioclavicular joint and extends distally to the coracoid process (white *line*). The scalpel is currently over the top of the coracoid (*arrow*). (*From* Scillia AJ, CAIN EL Jr. Acromioclavicular Joint Reconstruction. Arthrosc Tech. 2015 Dec 28;4(6).)

and medial collateral ligament during dissection and harvesting of the gracilis tendon. Both ends of the tendon are prepared by removing muscle fibers and whip stitches are placed with high strength suture (Suture Tape, Arthrex, Naples, FL).

Tunnel Placement

In cases with distal clavicle chondral injury or other significant damage, 8 to 10 mm of distal clavicle is resected before tunnel placement, but the clavicle is not resected in most acute cases. The anatomy of the conoid and trapezoid components of the CC ligament complex determines clavicular tunnel placement. The posteromedial bicortical tunnel is placed with a 3.5-mm drill bit 45 mm from the distal clavicle and slightly posterior to midline to match the native conoid insertion, whereas the second tunnel is 10 mm lateral to the conoid tunnel (35 mm from the distal clavicle) and more central on the clavicle shaft to match the trapezoid footprint (**Fig. 2**). A tunnel is also placed in the anteromedial acromion for AC ligament reconstruction.

Graft Passage and Fixation

Initially, the gracilis and a looped passing suture are passed around the coracoid base using a curved aneurysm hook (Zimmer, Warsaw, IN) from medial to lateral (**Fig. 3**). The lateral limb of gracilis passes through the posteromedial clavicular tunnel, whereas the medial limb passes through the lateral clavicular tunnel, resulting in

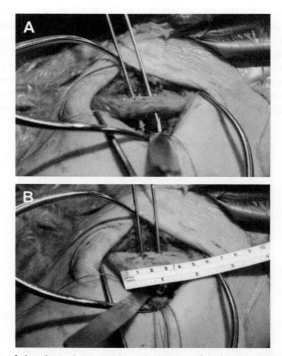

Fig. 2. Placement of the clavicular tunnels with distance for the conoid (medial) and trapezoid (lateral) footprints measured from the distal clavicle. (*From* Berthold DP, Beitzel K, Cerciello S, Mazzocca AD; Anatomic Acromioclavicular Joint Reconstruction, in Surgical Techniques of the Shoulder, Elbow and Knee in Sports Medicine (3rd Edition):2022; pages 327–334. Elsevier.)

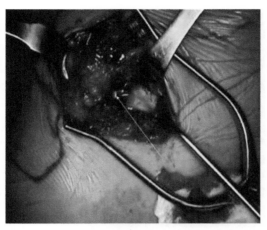

Fig. 3. Aneurysm hook (*arrow*) passes medial to lateral around the exposed coracoid base. (*From* Scillia AJ, CAIN EL Jr. Acromioclavicular Joint Reconstruction. Arthrosc Tech. 2015 Dec 28;4(6).)

crossing of the graft limbs (**Fig. 4**). Excess length is maintained from the medial clavicular limb and is passed through the acromial tunnel from inferior to superior for AC ligament reconstruction (**Fig. 5**). The tails of each limb are then tied end-to-end after AC joint reduction (shoulder girdle cephalad elevation) and is sutured to itself with No 2 nonabsorbable sutures (Arthrex, Naples, FL) (**Fig. 6**). For cases where extra protection is desired, nine strands of #0 PDS absorbable suture are woven together and passed in cerclage fashion around the coracoid (with a looped passing suture) and around the entire clavicle. A square knot is tied anteriorly with the braided PDS sutures (**Fig. 7**). Each end of the knot is sutured with No. 2 nonabsorbable suture to prevent knot prominence associated with the braided PDS sutures (**Fig. 8**). In cases of severe displacement or collision sports athletes, the authors add a dual-button suspensory device (AC tightrope, Arthrex, Naples, FL) through the posteromedial clavicular tunnel and

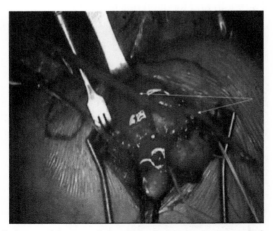

Fig. 4. Gracilis graft (*arrows*) is passed through the clavicular tunnels for reconstruction of the coracoclavicular ligament. (*From* Scillia AJ, CAIN EL Jr. Acromioclavicular Joint Reconstruction. Arthrosc Tech. 2015 Dec 28;4(6).)

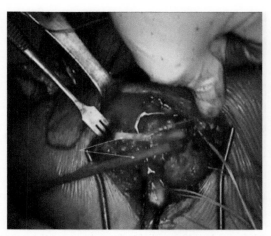

Fig. 5. Gracilis graft (*arrows*) is passed through the acromial tunnel for reconstruction of the acromioclavicular ligament and sutured end to end. (*From* Scillia AJ, CAIN EL Jr. Acromioclavicular Joint Reconstruction. Arthrosc Tech. 2015 Dec 28;4(6).)

coracoid base for additional fixation and protection of the graft during healing. The deltotrapezial fascia is closed with #0 absorbable sutures, and absorbable subcutaneous #3 to 0 Monocryl sutures (Ethicon) and a running subcuticular #3 to 0 Prolene suture (Ethicon) are used to close the skin.

Postoperative Treatment

Sling immobilization is continued for the first 6 weeks postsurgery, and physical therapy begins the day after surgery. Passive motion is allowed unrestricted, but weight-bearing exercises are limited until the 7th week. Gradual strengthening of the upper extremity begins at 7 weeks and is permitted fully at 12 weeks postsurgery. Noncontact sports participation is allowed after completion of the strengthening phase at approximately 4 months, and contact sports are generally unrestricted at 5 to 6 months, when full strength and function has returned.

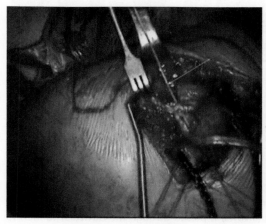

Fig. 6. The graft is sutured to itself using nonabsorbable sutures (*arrow*). (*From* Scillia AJ, CAIN EL Jr. Acromioclavicular Joint Reconstruction. Arthrosc Tech. 2015 Dec 28;4(6).)

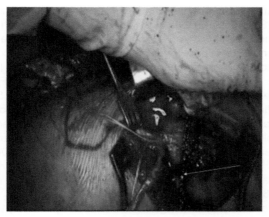

Fig. 7. Braided #0 PDS suture (*arrow*) is being looped around the clavicle and coracoid for cerclage fixation to protect the graft. (*From* Scillia AJ, CAIN EL Jr. Acromioclavicular Joint Reconstruction. Arthrosc Tech. 2015 Dec 28;4(6).)

DISCUSSION

Overall, open anatomic CC ligament reconstruction for AC injuries has had favorable short- to mid-term results with more long-term studies needed. Carofino and colleagues studied 17 patients who had CC ligament reconstruction with semitendinosus allograft with an average 21 month follow-up. They showed that the Amercian Shoulder and Elbow Surgeons Standardized Shoulder Asessment Form (ASES) score increased from 52 preoperatively to 92 postoperatively. The Constant–Murley (CM) score increased from 66.6 to 94.7, and the average Single Assessment Numeric Evaluation (SANE) score was 94.4.[13]

Millett and colleagues studied 2 year outcomes following open AC joint reconstruction. Anatomic CC ligament reconstruction was performed in 31 patients. In seven patients (22.6%), a complication occurred that went on to need a subsequent surgical procedure including graft rupture/attenuation (2), clavicle fractures (2), distal clavicle

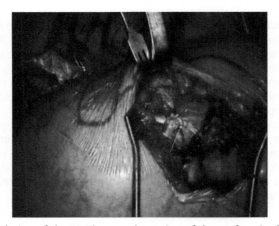

Fig. 8. After completion of the PDS knot and suturing of the graft to itself, the final reconstructed acromioclavicular joint is shown before closure. One should note the nonabsorbable sutures at the end of the square knot (*arrow*) to avoid prominence. (*From* Scillia AJ, CAIN EL Jr. Acromioclavicular Joint Reconstruction. Arthrosc Tech. 2015 Dec 28;4(6).)

hypertrophy (2), and adhesive capsulitis (1). Of the 24 patients who did not have a complication, 20 (83.3%) had subjective outcome data available after a minimum 2-year follow-up period (mean, 3.5 years; range, 2.0–6.2 years). The mean postoperative ASES and 12 item Short Form Physical Score (SF-12 PCS) scores significantly improved when compared with the preoperative baseline values (58.9 vs 93.8 for ASES scores [$P < .001$] and 45.3 vs 54.4 for SF-12 PCS scores [$P = .007$]). At the last follow-up, the SANE and QuickDASH scores were 89.1 and 5.6, respectively, with a median patient satisfaction rating of 9 out of 10. Those who did not need revision surgery had excellent postoperative scores. The mean ASES score was 93.8.[14]

Tauber and colleagues and Hegazy found that semitendinosus autograft was biomechanically and clinically superior to the Modified Weaver-Dunn for AC joint reconstruction.[15,16] Garofalo and colleagues studied open reconstruction of Type V AC injuries with hamstring autograft. They found that ASES scores increased from a median of 38.2 ± 6.2 preoperative to 92.1 ± 4.7 postoperatively ($P \leq .05$). The median VAS score improved from 62 mm (range 45–100 mm) preoperatively to 8 mm (range 0–20 mm) at final follow-up ($P \leq .05$). No patient experienced pain or discomfort with either direct palpation of the AC joint or with cross-body adduction; 30/32 patients (93%) were able to return to their pre-injury level of work and sports activities.[17]

Muench and colleagues reported functional and radiographic outcomes following AC joint reconstruction for Type III and V injuries. They found 92% of patients achieved the minimal clinically important difference in ASES score and 81% achieved substantial clinical benefit. They also found the Rowe score improved from 66.6 ± 15.9 preoperatively to 88.6 ± 12.3 postoperatively, the CM score from 61.6 ± 18.8 to 87.4 ± 15.1, and the Simple Shoulder Test score from 6.2 ± 3.6 to 9.4 ± 3.7 (all $P < .001$). The postoperative side-to-side difference in the CC distance was 3.1 ± 2.7 mm for all degrees of initial displacement, with type III injuries (2.4 ± 1.9 mm) showing significantly lower measurements compared with type V (4.2 ± 3.4 mm) ($P = .02$). Patients maintained this improvement at a minimum of 2-year follow-up.[18]

Recently, Lädermann and colleagues retrospectively studied early versus late anatomic reconstruction of AC joint injuries. They showed that both early and delayed reconstructions provide equivalent clinical scores when both CC and AC ligaments are reconstructed.[19] More long-term studies are needed to determine sustainability of the clinical outcomes for the open anatomic reconstruction technique.

Frank and colleagues evidence-based treatment review article on AC joint surgery discussed the risk of complications after surgical treatment for AC joint injuries including nerve injury, vascular injury, and infection. In addition, the presence of any type of fixation with hardware implants can result in migration and damage to soft tissues including nerves and blood vessels. Failed reconstruction can result from coracoid fracture, graft rupture, and clavicle fracture. Suture granulomas, adhesive capsulitis, and implant pain also may occur.[20]

In summary, open anatomic CC ligament reconstruction for AC joint injuries has good to excellent outcomes in the short- to mid-term follow-up with reported 83% to 100% all-cause survivorship.[12] There is increased stability in the vertical and horizontal plane when both the CC and AC joint tissues are reconstructed; however, there are complications associated with this technique that can include infection, failure of graft, pain, and fractures of the coracoid or clavicle.

SUMMARY

Open reconstruction of the CC and AC ligaments results in excellent reduction of severely displaced AC dislocations, most commonly Grades III and V. Anatomic CC reconstruction through clavicular bone tunnels can prevent vertical instability, whereas the addition of an acromial limb of the graft can increase horizontal stability. Autograft tendon is preferred in the young athletic group of collision sports participants, although allograft has had acceptable results. Accessory fixation may be placed to protect the graft during healing, or for severe instability, especially for athletes involved in contact sports.

CLINICS CARE POINTS

- Open reconstruction of the CC ligaments using either auto- or Allograft has been successful in restoring vertical stability to the injured AC joint.
- Adding a graft limb from the clavicle to acromion to reconstruct the AC ligaments helps control sagittal stability.
- Attention to well-described anatomic relationships will allow the surgeon to correctly place the graft limbs for AC stability.

DISCLOSURE

The authors have nothing to disclose related to this article.

REFERENCES

1. Fraser-Moodie JA, Shortt NL, Robinson CM. Injuries to the acromioclavicular joint. J Bone Joint Surg Br 2008;90(6):697–707.
2. Mazzocca AD, Santangelo SA, Johnson ST, et al. A biomechanical evaluation of an anatomical coracoclavicular ligament reconstruction. Am J Sports Med 2006; 34(2):236–46.
3. Simovitch R, Sanders B, Ozbaydar M, et al. Acromioclavicular joint injuries: diagnosis and management. J Am Acad Orthop Surg 2009;17(4):207–19.
4. Cadenat FM. The treatment of dislocations and fractures of the outer end of the clavicle. Int Clin 1917;27:145–69.
5. Beitzel K, Cote MP, Apostolakos J, et al. Current concepts in the treatment of acromioclavicular joint dislocations. Arthroscopy 2013;29(2):387–97.
6. Wiesel BB, Gartsman GM, Press CM, et al. What went wrong and what was done about it: pitfalls in the treatment of common shoulder surgery. J Bone Joint Surg Am 2013;95(22):2061–70.
7. Sim E, Schwarz N, Höcker K, et al. Repair of complete acromioclavicular separations using the acromioclavicular-hook plate. Clin Orthop Relat Res 1995;314: 134–42.
8. Gerhardt DC, VanDerWerf JD, Rylander LS, et al. Postoperative coracoid fracture after transcoracoid acromioclavicular joint reconstruction. J Shoulder Elbow Surg 2011;20(5):e6–10.
9. Brand JC, Lubowitz JH, Provencher MT, et al. Acromioclavicular joint reconstruction: complications and innovations. Arthroscopy 2015;31(5):795–7.
10. Shin SJ, Kim NK. Complications after arthroscopic coracoclavicular reconstruction using a single adjustable-loop-length suspensory fixation device in acute acromioclavicular joint dislocation. Arthroscopy 2015;31(5):816–24.
11. Dyrna F, Berthold DP, Feucht MJ, et al. The importance of biomechanical properties in revision acromioclavicular joint stabilization: a scoping review. Knee Surg Sports Traumatol Arthrosc 2019;27(12):3844–55.

12. Scillia AJ, Cain EL. Acromioclavicular Joint Reconstruction. Arthrosc Tech 2015; 4(6):e877–83.
13. Carofino BC, Mazzocca AD. The anatomic coracoclavicular ligament reconstruction: surgical technique and indications. J Shoulder Elbow Surg 2010;19(2 Suppl):37–46.
14. Millett PJ, Horan MP, Warth RJ. Two-Year Outcomes After Primary Anatomic Coracoclavicular Ligament Reconstruction. Arthroscopy 2015;31(10):1962–73.
15. Hegazy G, Safwat H, Seddik M, et al. Modified Weaver-Dunn Procedure Versus The Use of Semitendinosus Autogenous Tendon Graft for Acromioclavicular Joint Reconstruction. Open Orthop J 2016;10:166–78.
16. Tauber M, Gordon K, Koller H, et al. Semitendinosus tendon graft versus a modified Weaver-Dunn procedure for acromioclavicular joint reconstruction in chronic cases: a prospective comparative study. Am J Sports Med 2009;37(1):181–90.
17. Garofalo R, Ceccarelli E, Castagna A, et al. Open capsular and ligament reconstruction with semitendinosus hamstring autograft successfully controls superior and posterior translation for type V acromioclavicular joint dislocation. Knee Surg Sports Traumatol Arthrosc 2017;25(7):1989–94.
18. Muench LN, Kia C, Jerliu A, et al. Functional and Radiographic Outcomes After Anatomic Coracoclavicular Ligament Reconstruction for Type III/V Acromioclavicular Joint Injuries. Orthop J Sports Med 2019;7(11). 2325967119884539.
19. Lädermann A, Denard PJ, Collin P, et al. Early and delayed acromioclavicular joint reconstruction provide equivalent outcomes. J Shoulder Elbow Surg 2021;30(3): 635–40.
20. Frank RM, Cotter EJ, Leroux TS, et al. Acromioclavicular Joint Injuries: Evidence-based Treatment. J Am Acad Orthop Surg 2019;27(17):e775–88.

Arthroscopic Repair and Reconstruction of Coracoclavicular Ligament

Jeffrey D. Hassebrock, MD[a], Daniel J. Stokes, MD[a],
Tyler R. Cram, DO[a], Rachel M. Frank, MD[a],*

KEYWORDS

- Coracoclavicular ligaments • Coracoclavicular ligaments anatomy
- Coracoclavicular ligaments reconstruction • Acromial clavicular joint reconstruction

KEY POINTS

- Most acromioclavicular (AC) joint injuries can be treated nonoperatively. However, there is a subset of patients that will require surgical fixation.
- Many surgical techniques have been described, focusing on reconstructing the coracoclavicular ligaments.
- Anatomic reconstruction is superior to nonatomic techniques, but there is an increased risk of fracture.
- Arthroscopic coracoclavicular ligament reconstruction for AC joint injuries can be a safe and reliable surgical technique with promising outcomes.

INTRODUCTION

Injury to the acromioclavicular (AC) ligamentous complex can alter shoulder mechanics and scapular kinematics. Although many AC joint injuries can be treated nonoperatively, a subset of patients will require surgery to reconstruct the coracoclavicular (CC) ligaments. Over 60 techniques have been described for AC joint injuries, including repair and reconstruction. Anatomic reconstructions are superior to nonanatomic reconstructions but come with the potential risk of fracture to the clavicle and coracoid, particularly in a contact athlete. In the discussion, the authors highlight the senior authors preferred technique. An arthroscopically assisted AC joint reconstruction technique using a knotless suture button construct through the clavicle and coracoid base supplemented with an allograft loop tied over the clavicle and around the coracoid to biologically augment healing.

[a] Department of Orthopedic Surgery, University of Colorado School of Medicine, Aurora, CO, USA
* Corresponding author. Department of Orthopedic Surgery, UCHealth CU Sports Medicine – Colorado Center, 2000 South Colorado Boulevard, Tower 1, Suite 4500, Denver, CO 80222.
E-mail address: Rachel.Frank@cuanschutz.edu

Clin Sports Med 42 (2023) 599–611
https://doi.org/10.1016/j.csm.2023.05.004
0278-5919/23/© 2023 Elsevier Inc. All rights reserved.

sportsmed.theclinics.com

BIOMECHANICS

The biomechanics of the AC joint is believed to be more complex than historically suggested, allowing translation and rotation in multiple planes. The clavicle can rotate on average 5° to 8° with concurrent glenohumeral joint (GHJ) and scapulothoracic motion. In addition, loading the AC joint allows translation of 4 to 6 mm in the anterior, posterior, and superior planes.[1] The AC ligaments and joint capsule are the primary restraint to the posterior translation of the distal clavicle. In a cadaveric model, 1 cm of resection has been shown to increase posterior translation up to 32%.[2,3]

The trapezoid ligament primarily functions to resist compression of the AC joint, whereas the conoid is responsible mainly for resisting superior translation of the distal clavicle.[4] Harris and colleagues conducted a cadaveric study and were able to show that the conoid and trapezoid tuberosities provided reliable attachment sites on the clavicle, especially when the length of the clavicle is taken into account.[5] Based on these quantitative studies, the trapezoid center is approximately 2.5 cm from the lateral edge of the clavicle. In contrast, the conoid is approximately 4.6 cm from the distal edge of the clavicle. The average distance between the tuberosities was found to be 9 mm. This allows the conoid and trapezoid ligaments to account for over 50% of the resistance to applied forces. Furthermore, large AC joint displacements increase the resistance capacity of the CC ligaments up to 70%.[4] Maintaining stabilization of the AC and CC ligaments is critical for optimizing shoulder biomechanics.

EVALUATION
History

A detailed history can help guide the clinical evaluation. The interview should address the mechanism of injury, location of pain, restricted range of motion (ROM), deformity, and competition level for an athlete. A patient with an AC joint injury commonly presents after an acute traumatic injury caused by a direct blow to the shoulder with the arm in an adducted position. This results in AC joint pain with restricted active and passive shoulder ROM. In more severe cases, there may be a noticeable deformity.

Physical Examination

Evaluation should include bilateral inspection, palpation, active/passive ROM, strength, and neurovascular testing. It is also important to evaluate the cervical spine and sternoclavicular joint to rule out associated injuries.

- *Visual Inspection*: With the patient sitting upright and arms relaxed to the side, allowing gravity to pull the weight of the arms inferiorly, the examiner will assess for asymmetry of the normal contour, swelling, and deformity accentuated by the maneuver. A prominent distal clavicle is suggestive of AC joint injury.
- *Palpation*: With the patient sitting upright/standing with their arms to the side, the examiner will palpate directly over the AC joint. Reproducible pain/tenderness over the AC joint indicates a positive test and is the most common examination finding with this injury.

Acromioclavicular Joint Special Testing

- *Cross-Body Adduction Test*: With the patient sitting upright and the shoulder flexed to 90°, the examiner will horizontally adduct the arm (**Fig. 1**). Pain about the AC joint indicates a positive test. This test has the highest sensitivity for AC joint injury.[6]
- *Paxinos Sign*: With the patient sitting upright and the arm relaxed to the side, the examiner will support the posterolateral acromion with an anterosuperior force

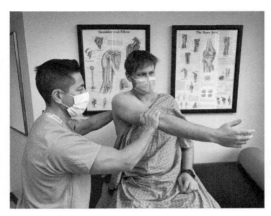

Fig. 1. Cross-body adduction test.

while simultaneously applying an inferiorly directed force to the mid-clavicle (**Fig. 2**). Pain in the AC joint region indicates a positive test.[7]

- *O'Brien's/Active Compression Test*
  - ○ With the patient standing, arms flexed to 90° and fully extended, internally rotated with thumbs facing down, the examiner will apply a resisted downward force (**Fig. 3**A). If the patient reports pain, the test is positive.[7]
  - ○ This test is repeated with the thumb facing upward (**Fig. 3**B). If positive, the patient will report decreased pain compared with the first maneuver. This test has the highest specificity for AC joint injury.[6]
- *Hawkins–Kennedy Test*: With the patient sitting upright and the shoulder and arm at 90° flexion, the examiner will support the scapula while internally rotating the arm. If pain is elicited, this test is positive.[7]

Imaging

Plain film radiographs are obtained for a patient with suspected AC joint injury, including an anteroposterior (AP), a true AP (Grashey), axillary, modified scapular-Y,

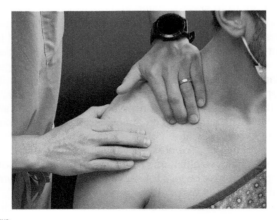

Fig. 2. Paxinos sign.

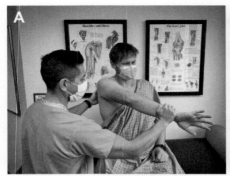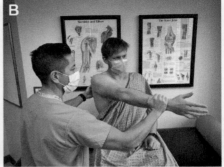

Fig. 3. (*A*) O'Brien's/active compression test (thumb down). (*B*) O'Brien's/active compression test (thumb up).

and Zanca views. MRI should be performed for suspected concomitant intra- or extra-articular GHJ pathology.

Approach/Clinical Evidence

AC joint injuries were initially classified by Tossy and colleagues to include grades I to III. Grade III injuries were later modified and expanded by Rockwood based on the extent and direction of the displacement.[8] The Rockwood classification system (**Table 1**) classifies AC joint injuries from type I to type VI with an increasing severity of soft tissue injury.[9,10]

Treatment

AC joint injuries can be managed operatively or nonoperatively depending on the severity of the injury using the Rockwood classification system. Nonoperative management is often sufficient for Rockwood type I and II AC joint injuries. Discussion continues to surround the management of type III AC dislocation. Evidence has shown positive outcomes in patients treated nonoperatively. Petri and colleagues demonstrated that 71% of patients in the nonoperative cohort were successfully managed without surgery.[11] A prospective study by Schlegel and colleagues revealed that 80% of patients treated nonsurgically had no difference in shoulder ROM or strength.[12] Return to work and return to sport resulted in a quicker recovery for nonoperatively managed patients with comparable clinical outcomes to surgical patients.[13] Nonsurgical treatment has also shown a lower incidence of ossification of the CC ligament with no significant differences in pain, weakness, strength, function, and patient-reported outcome scores between surgical and conservative management.[14]

With the substantial evidence demonstrating good outcomes with nonoperative treatment, the preferred initial treatment of type III injuries is typically nonoperative. However, risk factors associated with conservative management failure need to be identified before eliminating surgery as an option. Risk factors that support consideration for surgical intervention include patients with high physical demands, such as athletes, military personnel, and laborers or individuals who participate in repetitive physical activities, including weightlifters and overhead athletes.[15] Conservative management in this population may be less tolerable due to persistent symptoms and limitations associated with type III dislocation.

Surgical reduction and stabilization are almost always recommended for type IV–VI AC joint separation. Although surgery has historically been indicated for type V

Table 1
Rockwood classification for acromioclavicular joint injury

Rockwood Type	Imaging Findings	Exam Findings
Type I • AC sprain • CC normal	Normal	• Pain over AC joint • No deformity
Type II • AC disruption • CC sprain	• Widened AC joint • CC distance up to 25% > Contralateral side	• Anterior to posterior instability • Pain over AC joint
Type III • AC disruption • CC disruption	• CC distance 25% to 100% > Contralateral side	• Anterior to posterior • Superior to inferior instability • Pain over AC joint • Positive deformity
Type IV • Posterior displacement of clavicle	• Posterior displacement on axillary view	• Irreducible on examination
Type V • AC disruption • CC disruption • Deltopectoral fascia disruption	• CC distance 100% > Contralateral side	• Subcutaneously palpable distal clavicle • Not fully reducible on examination
Type VI • Inferior displacement of clavicle below coracoid	• Widened AC joint • CC distance up to 25% > Contralateral side	• Commonly associated with other shoulder girdle and chest wall pathology

Abbreviations: AC, acromioclavicular; AP, anteroposterior; CC, coracoclavicular.

dislocation, the recent literature proposed a trial of conservative therapy following evidence of successful results.[16] Although a trial of conservative treatment may be indicated and ultimately be effective for type III and V AC joint injury, considerable evidence demonstrates that early surgical intervention leads to more favorable outcomes, specifically regarding type V injuries.[17]

Surgical Technique

Many techniques for AC joint reconstruction have been described. The preferred technique for the senior author is an arthroscopically assisted AC joint reconstruction using a knotless suture button construct quadricortically through the superior and inferior clavicle cortices and bicortically through the base of the coracoid. This is supplemented with an allograft loop tied over the clavicle and around the coracoid to biologically augment healing. Standard beach chair positioning with a wide prep of the involved shoulder is used, as is a sterile arm positioner.

A standard posterior portal is used to access the joint and perform a diagnostic arthroscopy. Under scope visualization, a high anterior working portal is established through the rotator interval. This is used to perform a subcoracoid debridement to remove the rotator interval tissue back to the level of the coracoid. A 70° scope is then used through the same posterior portal, which allows visualized dissection below the coracoid to the level of the scapula and the medial side of the coracoid. This is necessary to visualize proper graft passage. Next, a standard 30° arthroscope can be inserted into the subacromial space, and the same working anterior portal can be used to debride the scar tissue and fibrous tissue of the AC joint to facilitate reduction (distal clavicular excision is not routinely performed for this in our practice). The

70° scope can then be placed back intra-articular from the posterior portal to view the coracoid for the suture button and graft passage.

A small 2 to 2.5 cm incision is made from anterior to posterior over the clavicle in line with the coracoid. Dissection is carried down to the clavicle, ensuring a robust fascial layer is preserved for repair. A guide can then be inserted through the anterior working portal and placed subcoracoid to ensure correct center–center placement at the base of the coracoid while drilling through the clavicle superiorly. A suture button device is then passed and flipped under direct visualization. The senior author prefers to use a passing stitch around the coracoid under direct visualization to shuttle an allograft around the coracoid. Once this has been shuttled around the coracoid and on either side of the clavicle, the arthroscopic portion of the procedure is completed. The suture button construct is assembled and tied down, ensuring the AC joint is appropriately reduced. Fluoroscopy confirms the complete reduction (**Fig. 4**A, B). The two tails of the graft are then tied and sutured over the clavicle. The remaining tails of the allograft are then brought to the acromion and secured with a soft tissue suture anchor. Fascial closure over the graft construct is crucial to minimize soft tissue irritation. Hardware failure is a rare but described phenomenon. The senior author prefers to remove symptomatic hardware arthroscopically using intraoperative fluoroscopy as needed.

DISCUSSION

Various techniques have been described for AC joint injuries, including open repair, Weaver–Dunn, Modified Weaver–Dunn, and arthroscopic or arthroscopic-assisted reconstruction. There is no gold standard for treating AC joint injuries, and the broad technique options make it difficult to compare clinical outcomes. However, evidence indicates that acute AC joint injuries are more amenable to repair, whereas chronic AC joint injuries typically require reconstruction due to the nonviability of the soft tissue.[8] Anatomic reconstructions have also been shown to be superior to nonanatomic reconstructions biomechanically but come with an increased risk of clavicle and coracoid fracture.[13]

Addressing the CC ligaments is critical for optimizing shoulder biomechanics.[18] Physiologic rotation and movement are achieved by restoring horizontal and vertical

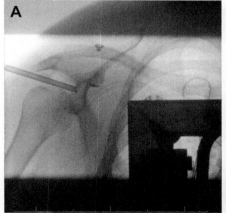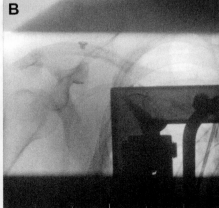

Fig. 4. (*A, B*) Intraoperative fluoroscopy of the right shoulder visualizing the suture button construct is assembled and tied down with appropriate AC joint reduction.

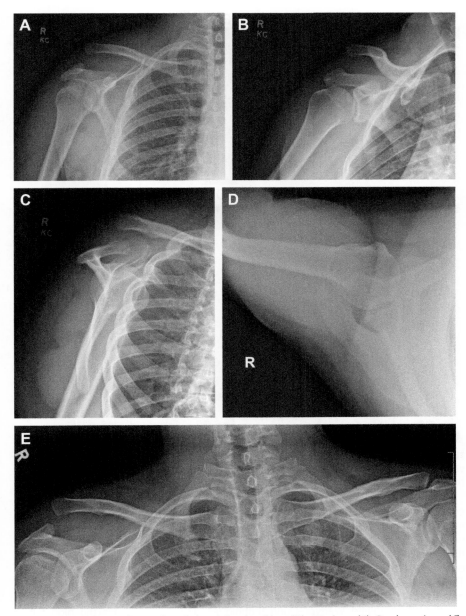

Fig. 5. Preoperative radiographs of the right shoulder: (A) AP view, (B) Grashey view, (C) scapular-Y view, (D) axillary view, and (E) bilateral shoulder Zanca view demonstrating a type V AC joint injury with a significant proximal elevation of the distal clavicle relative to the acromion.

stability.[19] Traditional primary open repair techniques reduce the AC joint, allowing the CC ligaments to heal. Open repair provides good visualization but is highly invasive and requires a larger incision. Primary open repair methods also have an increased

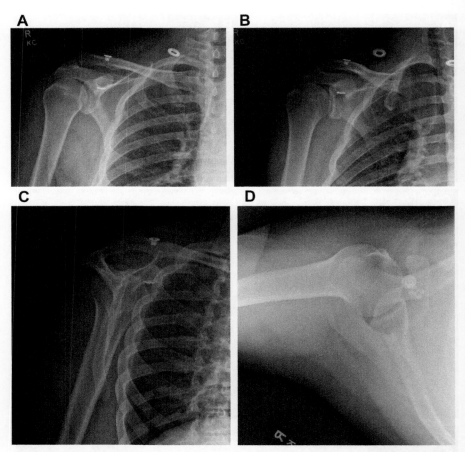

Fig. 6. Radiographs of the right shoulder 10 days postoperative: (*A*) AP view, (*B*) Grashey view, (*C*) scapular-Y view, and (*D*) axillary view demonstrating coracoclavicular ligament reconstruction with an anatomic reduction.

complication and failure rate, typically a result of hardware migration, and have the potential to require additional surgery for hardware removal.[20] The Weaver–Dunn procedure uses the transfer of the coracoacromial ligament to the superior aspect of the excised distal end of the clavicle for an anatomic reduction. This technique is an option for chronic AC joint injuries with low predictability of CC ligament healing.[21] The Weaver–Dunn technique is associated with higher failure rates and retearing of ligaments due to a weaker repair construct without fixation compared with the native CC ligament[22]—modified Weaver–Dunn techniques aimed to address the high failure rates of the coracoacromial ligament transfer technique.[23] Various modifications, such as a suture loop or cerclage, have been presented to increase strength and stability, promote early healing, maintain AC joint reduction, enhance the protection of the CA and CC ligaments, and augment the biological healing.[23] Despite the modified Weaver–Dunn improvements, the force transfer from the medial acromion to the lateral clavicle raises concern for the disruption of physiologic rotation and movement due to the force transfer and a high rate of scapular dyskinesis.[18,19] Problems with failure rates, suboptimal function, and advanced biomechanical studies, the modified

Weaver–Dunn techniques have decreased and shifted in favor of anatomical reconstructions.[24,25] Arthroscopic reconstruction is a minimally invasive option that improves the ability to diagnose and treat concomitant GHJ pathology. However, visualization may be difficult, and many described techniques are nonatomic.

The authors describe an arthroscopically assisted AC joint reconstruction technique using a knotless suture button construct quadricortically through the clavicle and base of the coracoid and supplemented with an allograft loop tied over the clavicle and around the coracoid to biologically augment healing. Arthroscopically assisted AC joint reconstruction is advantageous for diagnosing and treating concomitant GHJ pathology. It also provides an enhanced view of the coracoid base, enabling a more anatomic CC reconstruction.[19] Biomechanically, suture button constructs have demonstrated comparable load strength to the native CC ligament.[26] The allograft loop braces the AC capsule restoring horizontal stability and biologically augments healing while maintaining physiologic motion. The potential disadvantages of this technique include recurrent deformity due to loss of anatomic reduction, cost of the implants, the possibility of abrasion or inflammatory response to the suture material, and the higher learning curve due to the technical demands. Despite these disadvantages, arthroscopic assistance can be a helpful tool to ensure a safe, anatomic reconstruction that minimizes morbidity and maximizes the potential return to high-level function.

Pearls and pitfalls of arthroscopically assisted AC joint reconstruction using a knotless suture button construct

Pearls	Pitfalls
Gain adequate exposure of the coracoid base with either alternative viewing from anterolateral accessory portals or using a 70° arthroscope.	Avoid eccentric placement in either the clavicle or the coracoid base with drill and fixation to minimize the risk of iatrogenic fracture.
Use an intraoperative arm positioner to aid in reducing the AC joint before tightening the button construct.	Avoid under resection of rotator interval and subcoracoid space tissue before starting fixation, as this will make visualization during the case more difficult.
Before starting the surgery, use preoperative fluoroscopic scout shots to assess for adequate visualization.	
Visualize drill placement through coracoid to ensure centered location.	

CASE PRESENTATION

A 31-year-old man, right-hand dominant patient, presented to our clinic with right shoulder pain. He reported an acute snowboarding injury where he had fallen onto an outstretched hand. The patient immediately noted diffuse shoulder pain. He was able to snowboard to the base of the mountain, where he was evaluated at an on-site clinic. At that time, a prominence of the distal clavicle was noted. He was examined, received x-rays, diagnosed with an AC joint separation, provided a sling, and referred to our clinic for follow-up. The patient was further evaluated at our clinic 4-days following the initial injury. His diffuse shoulder pain localized to the anterior aspect of the shoulder with point tenderness about the AC joint and was worse at night when he rolled over onto the affected shoulder. He also endorsed popping in the front of his shoulder, particularly with forward flexion of the arm and pain with overhead movements. He denied any paresthesia. The patient had a prior history of a right shoulder type I AC joint injury that was managed nonoperatively. The patient is an active individual that enjoys playing recreational sports.

On examination, visual inspection revealed ecchymosis and a prominent distal clavicle with an elevation of the distal clavicle relative to the acromion. There was tenderness to palpation over the AC joint. A cross-body adduction test was performed and produced pain. O'Brien's test was also positive, with increased pain with thumbs facing upward.

The standard series shoulder x-rays taken on the date of injury were reviewed. An additional bilateral Zanca view was also captured, demonstrating a Type V AC joint injury with a significant proximal elevation of the distal clavicle relative to the acromion (**Fig. 5**A–E).

After a long discussion with this patient regarding diagnosis and treatment options, the patient opted for early surgical intervention. We proceeded with an arthroscopic-

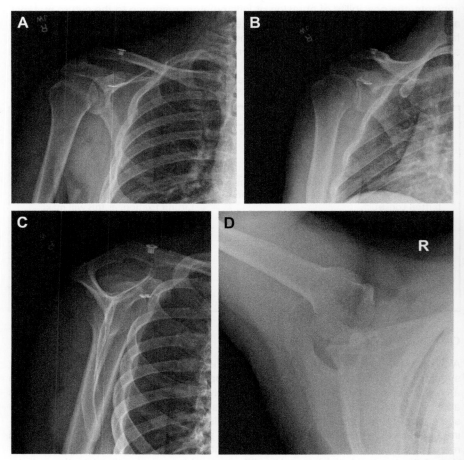

Fig. 7. Radiographs of the right shoulder 6 months postoperative: (*A*) AP view, (*B*) Grashey view, (*C*) scapular-Y view, and (*D*) axillary view revealing a stable coracoclavicular ligament reconstruction anatomically aligned without evidence of disruption of the CC ligament, acute hardware complication, or acute osseous abnormality.

assisted CC ligament reconstruction using the technique described in this article. The patient was discharged without complication.

He presented 2 weeks later for a routine postoperative follow-up. Overall, the patient was doing well. His pain was well-controlled. He denied fever/chills, and problems with the surgical incisions. He was compliant with sling use. He was scheduled to begin physical therapy the same week. Four radiographs of the right shoulder were obtained, demonstrating CC ligament reconstruction with an anatomic reduction. There was no evidence of disruption of the CC ligament, acute hardware complication, or acute osseous abnormality (**Fig. 6**A–D).

The patient was compliant with his sling use which was discontinued after 6 weeks. He also met expectations and progressed with physical therapy per the CC reconstruction protocol. He presented for his 6-month postoperative visit and had repeat imaging revealing a stable CC ligament reconstruction still in anatomic alignment (**Fig. 7**A–D). The patient was cleared to return to all activities and will follow-up as needed.

SUMMARY

AC joint injuries are common shoulder injuries that require prompt recognition, diagnosis, and treatment. Deciding on a treatment algorithm relies on a detailed knowledge of anatomy and a thorough understanding of the specific functional demands of the patient in question. When repair or reconstruction is indicated, arthroscopic assistance can be a helpful tool to ensure a safe, anatomic reconstruction that minimizes morbidity and maximizes the potential return to high-level function.

CLINICS CARE POINTS

- Acromioclavicular (AC) joint injuries have been reported to comprise almost half of all shoulder injuries in contact sports.
- Many AC joint injuries can be treated nonoperatively, but some patients require surgery to reconstruct the coracoclavicular ligaments.
- Understanding the injury pattern, natural history, and patient expectations is crucial for proper clinical care of AC joint injuries.
- The AC ligaments and joint capsule are the primary restraint to the posterior translation of the distal clavicle.
- The coracoclavicular ligaments account for over 50% of the resistance capacity and up to 70% with large AC joint displacements.
- The trapezoid ligament primarily functions to resist compression of the AC joint, whereas the conoid is responsible mainly for resisting superior translation of the distal clavicle.
- The cross-body adduction test has the highest sensitivity for AC joint injury, whereas O'Brien's/active compression test has the highest specificity.
- The Zanca view is preferred for AC joint imaging to optimize penetration while reducing the overlap of the clavicle and scapula.
- Glenohumeral joint pathology is present in up to 57% of high-grade AC joint separation, most commonly rotator cuff injury.
- The Rockwood classification system grades injury and guides treatment.
- Type I and II injuries are treated nonoperatively through immobilization, anti-inflammatory medication, and cryotherapy.

- Type III injuries demonstrate good outcomes with nonoperative treatment, but some high-risk patients may require acute surgery.
- Surgical reduction and stabilization are almost always recommended for type IV–VI injury.
- The 70° arthroscopic camera assistance is the preferred method of the senior author for safe and thorough exposure for arthroscopic reconstruction.

DISCLOSURE

Dr R.M. Frank reports consultant fees from Allosource, Arthrex, Inc, and JRF Ortho; speaking fees from Allosource, Arthrex, Inc, JRF Ortho, and Ossur; research support from Arthrex, United States and Smith & Nephew, United Kingdom; publishing royalties from Elsevier, outside the submitted work.

ACKNOWLEDGMENTS

The authors would like to thank Kevin K Shinsako, PA-C, for his assistance with photographs for this chapter.

REFERENCES

1. Willimon SC, Gaskill TR, Millett PJ. Acromioclavicular joint injuries: anatomy, diagnosis, and treatment. Phys Sportsmed 2011;39(1):116–22.
2. Klimkiewicz JJ, Williams GR, Sher JS, et al. The acromioclavicular capsule as a restraint to posterior translation of the clavicle: a biomechanical analysis. J Shoulder Elbow Surg 1999;8(2):119–24.
3. Corteen DP, Teitge RA. Stabilization of the clavicle after distal resection: a biomechanical study. Am J Sports Med 2005;33(1):61–7.
4. Fukuda K, Craig EV, An KN, et al. Biomechanical study of the ligamentous system of the acromioclavicular joint. J Bone Joint Surg Am 1986;68(3):434–40.
5. Rios CG, Arciero RA, Mazzocca AD. Anatomy of the clavicle and coracoid process for reconstruction of the coracoclavicular ligaments. Am J Sports Med 2007;35(5):811–7 [published Online First: 20070209].
6. Chronopoulos E, Kim TK, Park HB, et al. Diagnostic value of physical tests for isolated chronic acromioclavicular lesions. Am J Sports Med 2004;32(3):655–61.
7. Krill MK, Rosas S, Kwon K, et al. A concise evidence-based physical examination for diagnosis of acromioclavicular joint pathology: a systematic review. Phys Sportsmed 2018;46(1):98–104 [published Online First: 20171213].
8. Frank RM, Cotter EJ, Leroux TS, et al. Acromioclavicular Joint Injuries: Evidence-based Treatment. J Am Acad Orthop Surg 2019;27(17):e775–88.
9. Tossy JD, Mead NC, Sigmond HM. Acromioclavicular separations: useful and practical classification for treatment. Clin Orthop Relat Res 1963;28:111–9.
10. Rockwood C. Injuries to the acromio-clavicular joint. Fracture in adalts 1984;1.
11. Petri M, Warth RJ, Greenspoon JA, et al. Clinical Results After Conservative Management for Grade III Acromioclavicular Joint Injuries: Does Eventual Surgery Affect Overall Outcomes? Arthroscopy 2016;32(5):740–6 [published Online First: 20160204].
12. Schlegel TF, Burks RT, Marcus RL, et al. A prospective evaluation of untreated acute grade III acromioclavicular separations. Am J Sports Med 2001;29(6):699–703.
13. Beitzel K, Cote MP, Apostolakos J, et al. Current concepts in the treatment of acromioclavicular joint dislocations. Arthroscopy 2013;29(2):387–97.

14. Tang G, Zhang Y, Liu Y, et al. Comparison of surgical and conservative treatment of Rockwood type-III acromioclavicular dislocation: A meta-analysis. Medicine (Baltim) 2018;97(4):e9690. https://doi.org/10.1097/md.0000000000009690.
15. Nolte PC, Lacheta L, Dekker TJ, et al. Optimal Management of Acromioclavicular Dislocation: Current Perspectives. Orthop Res Rev 2020;12:27–44 [published Online First: 20200305].
16. Krul KP, Cook JB, Ku J, et al. Successful Conservative Therapy in Rockwood Type V Acromioclavicular Dislocations. Orthopaedic Journal of Sports Medicine 2015; 3(3_suppl). 2325967115S00017.
17. Rolf O, Hann von Weyhern A, Ewers A, et al. Acromioclavicular dislocation Rockwood III-V: results of early versus delayed surgical treatment. Arch Orthop Trauma Surg 2008;128(10):1153–7.
18. Peeters I, Braeckevelt T, Palmans T, et al. Differences between Coracoclavicular, Acromioclavicular, or Combined Reconstruction Techniques on the Kinematics of the Shoulder Girdle. Am J Sports Med 2022;50(7):1971–82.
19. Voss A, Imhoff AB. Editorial Commentary: Why We Have To Respect The Anatomy In Acromioclavicular Joint Surgery And Why Clinical Shoulder Scores Might Not Give Us The Information We Need. Arthroscopy 2019;35(5):1336–8.
20. Milewski MD, Tompkins M, Giugale JM, et al. Complications related to anatomic reconstruction of the coracoclavicular ligaments. Am J Sports Med 2012;40(7): 1628–34.
21. Borbas P, Churchill J, Ek ET. Surgical management of chronic high-grade acromioclavicular joint dislocations: a systematic review. J Shoulder Elbow Surg 2019;28(10):2031–8.
22. Chang HM, Wang CH, Hsu KL, et al. Does Weaver-Dunn procedure have a role in chronic acromioclavicular dislocations? A meta-analysis. J Orthop Surg Res 2022;17(1):95.
23. Patel MS, Hill BW, Casey P, et al. Modified Weaver-Dunn Technique Using Transosseous Bone Tunnels and Coracoid Suture Augmentation. J Am Acad Orthop Surg 2022;30(3):111–8.
24. Moatshe G, Kruckeberg BM, Chahla J, et al. Acromioclavicular and Coracoclavicular Ligament Reconstruction for Acromioclavicular Joint Instability: A Systematic Review of Clinical and Radiographic Outcomes. Arthroscopy 2018;34(6): 1979–95.
25. Verstift DE, Somford MP, van Deurzen DFP, et al. Review of Weaver and Dunn on treatment of acromioclavicular injuries, especially complete acromioclavicular separation. J ISAKOS 2021;6(2):116–9.
26. Lädermann A, Gueorguiev B, Stimec B, et al. Acromioclavicular joint reconstruction: a comparative biomechanical study of three techniques. J Shoulder Elbow Surg 2013;22(2):171–8.

Risk for Fracture with Acromioclavicular Joint Reconstruction and Strategies for Mitigation

Nikolaos Platon Sachinis, PhD[a],*, Knut Beitzel, PhD[b]

KEYWORDS

- Acromioclavicular reconstruction • Fracture • AC joint • Risk factors • Review

KEY POINTS

- Depending on the type of reconstruction technique used and the location of the fracture, the rate of fractures after acromioclavicular joint reconstruction can reach 20%.
- Fracture risk factors include: osteoporosis, open approach, large bone drill holes, number of clavicle drill holes, poor drilling technique, the "cheese wire" effect from non-absorbable grafts.
- Mitigation strategies include proper patient selection, adequate view of the coracoid base (arthroscopic techniques), graft choice, small diameter tunnels on clavicle/coracoid or use of single tunnel techniques.

INTRODUCTION

Acromioclavicular (AC) joint injuries are a common cause of shoulder pain and disability, especially among athletes involved in contact sports or activities that require repetitive overhead motion. Surgical options may be considered when nonoperative management fails or in patients with high-demand shoulder function.[1,2] Reconstruction techniques are numerous, and include anatomic or nonanatomic coracoclavicular (CC) ligament reconstruction, with open or arthroscopic methods, with or without the use of autograft or allograft, and coracoacromial ligament transfer or other additional procedures that attempt to provide AC stability. However, these techniques can be associated with complications such as coracoid or clavicle fractures, which can negatively impact the patient's outcome.

a First Orthopaedic Department of Aristotle University of Thessaloniki, "Georgios Papanikolaou" Hospital, Exohi, 57010, Thessaloniki, Greece; b Orthoparc Klinik, Aachener Street, 1021B, 50858, Cologne, Germany
* Corresponding author. "Georgios Papanikolaou" Hospital, Exohi, 57010, Thessaloniki, Greece.
E-mail address: nick.sachinis@gmail.com

Clin Sports Med 42 (2023) 613–619
https://doi.org/10.1016/j.csm.2023.05.010
0278-5919/23/© 2023 Elsevier Inc. All rights reserved.

Fractures during AC ligament reconstruction have been reported as early as 1982.[3] These complications may lead to pain, loss of reduction, and shoulder range of motion and may require revision of the operation. The incidence of fractures after AC joint (ACJ) reconstruction may rise up to 20%, depending on the type of reconstruction technique and the location of the fracture.[2,4] The purpose of this review is to discuss the risk factors for coracoid fractures associated with ACJ reconstruction (**Table 1**), as well as the strategies that can be used to mitigate this risk (**Table 2**).

RISK FACTORS

In general, the coracoid process's mineral density decreases with age.[5] This reduction thus increases the risk of osteoporosis and osteoporosis-related iatrogenic fractures. Therefore, osteoporosis and factors that induce loss of bone density (increasing age, smoking, sarcopenia, other metabolic diseases) should be taken into account when considering an ACJ reconstruction technique that requires drill holes or passes a nonabsorbable suture around the coracoid base.

Coracoid Fractures

Drilling holes through the coracoid or passing a graft underneath as a loop for implantation and fixation as part of CC ligament reconstruction (synthetic sutures and button) increases the risk of coracoid fracture and cutout.[4,6] These fractures, while rare, have been reported with using open procedures for the past 3 decades.[3] Milewski and colleagues[4] found a 7.4% occurrence of coracoid fractures (2/27 patients) in a retrospective evaluation of patients having CC ligament restoration with either coracoid tunneling or loop. On a large cohort study of 279 cases by Chen and colleagues[7] in 2023, they described the complication profile of surgical management of ACJ separations utilizing a variety of reconstruction strategies. They found 2 coracoid fractures and 7 clavicle fractures; however, the specific technique that was used in these cases in not reported.

The techniques that use grafts that are passed under the coracoid process may cause a fracture due to a "cheese wire effect."[3,6,8,9] In 1982, Moneim and Balduini[3] described a coracoid fracture with postoperative infection and bone degradation between the clavicle's drill holes. Tomlinson and colleagues[9] described a fracture in a high-level baseball pitcher months after surgery from pitching a ball. In the early postoperative phase, Jeon and colleagues[8] reported a fracture caused by the patient's noncompliant heavy lifting.

With arthroscopic techniques, the prevalence of coracoid process fractures, although rarer, has also been reported. Gerhardt and colleagues,[6] in 2011, described it with arthroscopic techniques that involved small diameter bone tunnels. Clavert and colleagues[10] prospectively evaluated on 116 cases the complication rates following

Table 1
Fracture risk factors during acromioclavicular reconstruction

	Coracoid	Clavicle
Low bone mineral density	✔	✔
Surgical approach (open)	✔	
Graft choice	✔	✔
Drilling technique	✔	✔
Number of drill holes		✔

Table 2
Fracture mitigation strategies during acromioclavicular reconstruction

	Coracoid	Clavicle
Proper patient selection	✔	✔
Surgical approach/view of coracoid base (arthroscopic techniques)	✔	
Graft choice (use of autografts/allografts around bone)	✔	✔
Avoidance of multiple drilling/proper positioning of holes	✔	✔
Single tunnel techniques	✔	

arthroscopic acute AC dislocation stabilization. On a follow-up radiograph, they discovered a coracoid process fracture in 1 patient.

Clavicle Fractures

Several case reports of clavicle fractures during CC ligament reconstruction and clavicle drilling have been published throughout the postoperative period.[11–13] In the aforementioned Milewski and colleagues study, 11.1% of patients (3/27) sustained a clavicle fracture, interestingly while using a coracoid loop technique. Although the difference between open and arthroscopic methods may explain the discrepancy, these authors attribute these fractures (especially clavicle fractures) to technical faults.

Inoue and colleagues[12] reported a clavicle fracture 7 months after an ACJ reconstruction with a suture button and a hook plate that was removed at 4 months. After plate removal, widening of the clavicle hole could be seen, probably due to movement of the suture inside the hole and the subsequent erosion effect. When the patient underwent a second operation for clavicle osteosynthesis, multiple drill holes were found near the fracture site. Following a study of related literature, the authors speculated that a clavicle fracture arising from the suture hole is a complication that can arise later, even after the CC ligament has been repaired.

In a biomechanical cadaveric study, Spiegl and colleagues[14] discovered a substantial loss in clavicle strength following CC ligament repair utilizing hamstring and 6 mm tunnels compared to a cortical button device and drilling 2.4 mm tunnels in the clavicle in a cadaver model. The insertion of a tenodesis screw into the clavicular tunnel does not appear to improve the clavicle's strength or reduce its ultimate failure.[15] Clavicular tunnel diameter more than 6 mm along with inadequate tunnel spacing less than 20 to 25 mm between clavicular tunnels and less than 10 to 15 mm between the lateral tunnel and the distal edge of the clavicle may increase the incidence of clavicle fracture.[16]

Acromion Fractures

So far, acromion fractures during AC reconstructions have only been reported as erosions from retaining the hook plate. Chiang and colleagues[17] in 2010 was the first to report such a fracture in English literature. Other similar reports highlight the impact of the stress that the plate places under the acromion, causing erosion.[18,19] In Yeo and colleagues[18] case report, the authors discovered that there were already evidence of localized osteopenia and bone erosions at the third week follow-up visit, despite of relatively modest clinical manifestations of pain. This is most likely produced by the hook plate's direct pinpoint pressure and impingement at the undersurface of the acromion, which results in a stress-riser reaction with subsequent osteolysis erosion and, in worst-case scenarios, acromial fractures.

Dyrna and colleagues[20] used a finite element analysis to simulate various bone tunnels and incoming force vectors on 45 cadaveric specimens in order to determine fracture risk variables during acromion drilling for ACJ repair. They discovered that the acromion is more prone to fracture with a superior to inferior directed incoming fall force, and that horizontal tunnels with a larger diameter (4.5 mm) had the greatest influence on load to failure reduction. A 4.5 mm diameter horizontal tunnel lowered the load to failure in the medial direction of force to 25% of the natural acromion. The identical tunnel with a diameter of 2.4 mm reduced the load to failure to 61%. However, the findings suggest a "safe zone" for placing bone tunnels within the anterior half of the acromion, which has no effect on acromion loads to failure. As a result, current procedures for anatomic ACJ repair that use graft or suture fixation at the acromion are safe within current tunnel placement and size ranges.

MITIGATION STRATEGIES

Martetschläger and colleagues[21] demonstrated a 20% combined fracture rate (of the clavicle and coracoid) in 2013 and linked the complication to technical faults in drilling technique. Particularly noteworthy was the fact that good to exceptional outcomes were only recorded in patients who did not experience such a consequence; thus, avoiding this complication through careful placement of bone tunnels or the use of a loop approach should be strongly addressed. Considering the loop approaches however, it could be hypothesized that thin synthetic grafts or nonabsorbable sutures may be more prone to creating a "cheese wire" effect on the coracoid through continuous stress appliance under the coracoid base.

A biomechanical study compared the stability of the coracoid process after an anatomic double-tunnel technique using two 4 mm drill holes or a single-tunnel technique using one 4 mm or one 2.4 mm drill hole on 18 fresh-frozen cadavers.[22] Although there was no significant difference regarding load-to-failure testing between groups, the failure mechanism analysis showed that one 2.4 mm drill hole led to less destabilization of the coracoid than one or two 4 mm drill holes. Therefore, techniques with small, 2.4 mm drill holes might decrease the risk of severe iatrogenic fracture complications.

Accurate coracoid tunnel placement, particularly in the center-center or medial-center position of the coracoid, minimizes the probability of bone failure.[23] The combination of minimizing the tunnel diameter in the coracoid and proper visualization is thus recommended to help minimize coracoid fracture or cutout in transcoracoid fixation procedures.

Ma and colleagues[24] examined complications following ACJ repair or reconstruction surgery. They postulated that modern arthroscopy instrumentation has also lowered the diameter necessary to pass and fix the suture-button construct through the coracoid process. Furthermore, good vision of the entire coracoid base is essential; this is why arthroscopic procedures have so far showed a lower coracoid fracture percentage. Milewski and colleagues[4] found only a 10% fracture rate (1 of 10 arthroscopic patients) when an arthroscopic technique was utilized.

Regarding clavicle fractures, Milewski and colleagues[4] suggested that both a wider distance between tunnels and from the tunnel to the lateral edge of the clavicle may help decrease the risk of clavicle fracture. Banffy and colleagues[25,26] proposed a single-tunnel technique for CC and AC ligament reconstruction, which reduces the number of screws required in the clavicle. Inoue and colleagues[12] suggested that in order to prevent clavicle fractures at the suture hole, it is essential to avoid excessive drilling of the suture hole during ACJ reconstruction and pay attention to the widening of suture holes at radiography images. Overtensioning of the sutures, osteolysis from a soft tissue reaction, and proper management of technical/iatrogenic factors such as multiple entry-point drilling or suture holes that are not located in the center of the bone have to be minimized to reduce the risk of clavicle fractures.

REVISION OPTIONS

Dyrna and colleagues on their scoping review of revision cases for ACJ stabilization highlighted the need of aiming to restore native joint biomechanics, when possible.[27] However, they pointed that for clavicular fractures, conservative therapy may be possible if the fracture is not significantly displaced and does not result in loss of reduction of the reconstructed ACJ. Otherwise, surgical treatments may include an open reduction and internal fixation (ORIF) of the clavicle in conjunction with a CC ligament reconstruction employing a suture pulley system or an extra biologic tendon graft.[27]

Coracoid drill holes have been shown to have an impact on stability and increase the chance of fracture. Martetschläger and colleagues[22] reported that this correlates positively with both an increased number and larger size of holes. The vast majority of coracoid fractures however may be treatable without surgery. If the fracture results in subsequent instability, it must be properly evaluated. If the tunnel was placed too far anteriorly or if a blow-out occurred medially or laterally as a result of faulty tunnel placement, a new tunnel cannot be installed in the correct anatomic position near to the base of the coracoid.[27] Otherwise, a graft can be directed around the coracoid.

SUMMARY

ACJ reconstruction is a commonly performed surgical procedure with potential risks such as coracoid and clavicle fractures. The risks associated with ACJ reconstruction can be mitigated through careful technique selection and appropriate suture/anchor/graft placement. Surgeons should consider the advantages and disadvantages of each technique to minimize complications and achieve optimal clinical outcomes.

CLINICS CARE POINTS

- Low bone mineral density, open approach, large grafts with large drill holes on the coracoid/clavicle, number of drill holes in clavicle, poor drilling technique, and nonabsorbable grafts causing a "cheese wire" effect are all risk factors for inducing coracoid/clavicle fractures.

- Mitigation options include: correct patient selection, a clear view of the coracoid base (arthroscopic techniques), graft selection, small diameter tunnels on the clavicle/coracoid, or the use of single tunnel techniques.

- Conservative therapy may be an option if the fracture is not considerably displaced. ORIF of the clavicle in conjunction with a CC ligament reconstruction, or/and a new tunnel or graft around the coracoid if a new hole cannot be appropriately placed are suitable revision options.

DISCLOSURE

Both authors declare that they have no relevant or material financial interests that relate to the research described in this article.

REFERENCES

1. Phadke A, Bakti N, Bawale R, et al. Current concepts in management of ACJ injuries. J Clin Orthop Trauma 2019;10(3):480–5.

2. Martetschläger F, Kraus N, Scheibel M, et al. The diagnosis and treatment of acute dislocation of the acromioclavicular joint. Dtsch Arztebl Int 2019;116(6): 89–95.

3. Moneim MS, Balduini FC. Coracoid fracture as a complication of surgical treatment by coracoclavicular tape fixation. A case report. Clin Orthop Relat Res 1982;168:133–5.

4. Milewski MD, Tompkins M, Giugale JM, et al. Complications related to anatomic reconstruction of the coracoclavicular ligaments. Am J Sports Med 2012;40(7): 1628–34.

5. Beranger JS, Maqdes A, Pujol N, et al. Bone mineral density of the coracoid process decreases with age. Knee Surg Sports Traumatol Arthrosc 2016;24(2): 502–6.

6. Gerhardt DC, VanDerWerf JD, Rylander LS, et al. Postoperative coracoid fracture after transcoracoid acromioclavicular joint reconstruction. J Shoulder Elbow Surg 2011;20(5):e6–10.

7. Chen RE, Gates ST, Vaughan A, et al. Complications after Operative Treatment of High Grade Acromioclavicular Injuries. J Shoulder Elbow Surg. 2023:S1058-2746(23)00321-X. doi: 10.1016/j.jse.2023.03.019.

8. Jeon IH, Dewnany G, Hartley R, et al. Chronic acromioclavicular separation: the medium term results of coracoclavicular ligament reconstruction using braided polyester prosthetic ligament. Injury 2007;38(11):1247–53.

9. Tomlinson DP, Altchek DW, Davila J, et al. A modified technique of arthroscopically assisted AC joint reconstruction and preliminary results. Clin Orthop Relat Res 2008;466(3):639–45.

10. Clavert P, Meyer A, Boyer P, et al. Complication rates and types of failure after arthroscopic acute acromioclavicular dislocation fixation. Prospective multicenter study of 116 cases. Orthop Traumatol Surg Res 2015;101(8 Suppl):S313–6.

11. Ball SV, Sankey A, Cobiella C. Clavicle fracture following tight rope fixation of acromioclavicular joint dislocation. Inj Extra 2007;12(38):430–2.

12. Inoue D, Furuhata R, Kaneda K, et al. Clavicle fracture at the suture hole after acromioclavicular joint reconstruction using a suture-button: a case report. BMC Musculoskelet Disord 2019;20(1):333.

13. Turman KA, Miller CD, Miller MD. Clavicular fractures following coracoclavicular ligament reconstruction with tendon graft: a report of three cases. J Bone Joint Surg Am 2010;92(6):1526–32.

14. Spiegl UJ, Smith SD, Euler SA, et al. Biomechanical consequences of coracoclavicular reconstruction techniques on clavicle strength. Am J Sports Med 2014; 42(7):1724–30.

15. Dumont GD, Russell RD, Knight JR, et al. Impact of tunnels and tenodesis screws on clavicle fracture: a biomechanical study of varying coracoclavicular ligament reconstruction techniques. Arthroscopy 2013;29(10):1604–7.

16. Carofino BC, Mazzocca AD. The anatomic coracoclavicular ligament reconstruction: surgical technique and indications. J Shoulder Elbow Surg 2010;19(2 Suppl):37–46.

17. Chiang CL, Yang SW, Tsai MY, et al. Acromion osteolysis and fracture after hook plate fixation for acromioclavicular joint dislocation: a case report. J Shoulder Elbow Surg 2010;19(4):e13–5.

18. Yeo MHX, Lie D, Wonggokusuma E, et al. Acromion osteolysis and fracture following hook plate fixation after acute acromioclavicular joint dislocation in an elderly patient: a case report. Journal of Orthopaedic Reports 2022;1(3):100055.

19. Nadarajah R, Mahaluxmivala J, Amin A, et al. Clavicular hook–plate: complications of retaining the implant. Injury 2005;36(5):681–3.
20. Dyrna F, de Oliveira CCT, Nowak M, et al. Risk of fracture of the acromion depends on size and orientation of acromial bone tunnels when performing acromioclavicular reconstruction. Knee Surg Sports Traumatol Arthrosc 2018;26(1): 275–84.
21. Martetschläger F, Horan MP, Warth RJ, et al. Complications after anatomic fixation and reconstruction of the coracoclavicular ligaments. Am J Sports Med 2013; 41(12):2896–903.
22. Martetschläger F, Saier T, Weigert A, et al. Effect of coracoid drilling for acromioclavicular joint reconstruction techniques on coracoid fracture risk: a biomechanical study. Arthroscopy 2016;32(6):982–7.
23. Ferreira JV, Chowaniec D, Obopilwe E, et al. Biomechanical evaluation of effect of coracoid tunnel placement on load to failure of fixation during repair of acromioclavicular joint dislocations. Arthroscopy 2012;28(9):1230–6.
24. Ma R, Smith PA, Smith MJ, et al. Managing and recognizing complications after treatment of acromioclavicular joint repair or reconstruction. Curr Rev Musculoskelet Med 2015;8(1):75–82.
25. Banffy MB, van Eck CF, ElAttrache NS. Clinical outcomes of a single-tunnel technique for coracoclavicular and acromioclavicular ligament reconstruction. J Shoulder Elbow Surg 2018;27(6s). S70-s5.
26. Banffy MB, van Eck CF, Stanton M, et al. A single-tunnel technique for coracoclavicular and acromioclavicular ligament reconstruction. Arthrosc Tech 2017;6(3): e769–75.
27. Dyrna F, Berthold DP, Feucht MJ, et al. The importance of biomechanical properties in revision acromioclavicular joint stabilization: a scoping review. Knee Surg Sports Traumatol Arthrosc 2019;27(12):3844–55.

Surgical Pearls and Pitfalls for Anatomic Acromioclavicular/Coracoclavicular Ligament Reconstruction

Peter S. Chang, MD[a], Colin P. Murphy, MD[b],
Ryan J. Whalen, BS, CSCS[a], John M. Apostolakos, MD, MPH[a],
Matthew T. Provencher, MD, MBA, MC, USNR (Ret)[a,c,*]

KEYWORDS

- Acromioclavicular ligament • Coracoclavicular ligament
- Arthroscopic acromioclavicular reconstruction
- Arthroscopic coracoclavicular reconstruction

KEY POINTS

- The acromioclavicular joint should be slightly over reduced to account for creep in grafts.
- Fluoroscopy should be used to confirm appropriate tunnel position and reduction.
- Anatomic placement of bone tunnels is critical.

PRESENTATION

The most common mechanism of acromioclavicular (AC) injury is direct trauma to the superolateral aspect of the adducted shoulder, typically from a fall.[1] Indirect trauma through a fall on an outstretched hand, whereby the humeral head translocates superiorly into the acromion, is also reported.[2] Iatrogenic injuries to the AC joint, most commonly caused by excessive distal clavicle excision and disruption of the posterosuperior ligaments, can also occur.[3,4] Patients with AC injuries typically report pain about the superolateral shoulder in the area of the AC joint; the pain can sometimes be referred to the trapezius and anterior deltoid. Shoulder motion will often be painful, especially in crossbody activities.

[a] Steadman Philippon Research Institute, 181 West Meadow Drive, Suite 400, Vail, CO 81657, USA; [b] University of North Dakota Orthopaedic Surgery Residency Program, 1919 Elm Street North, Fargo, ND 58102, USA; [c] The Steadman Clinic, 181 West Meadow Drive, Suite 400, Vail, CO 81657, USA
* Corresponding author. 181 West Meadow Drive, Suite 400, Vail, CO 81657.
E-mail address: mprovencher@thesteadmanclinic.com

Clin Sports Med 42 (2023) 621–632
https://doi.org/10.1016/j.csm.2023.05.011
0278-5919/23/© 2023 Elsevier Inc. All rights reserved.

Physical examination tends to reveal ecchymosis or deformity around the AC joint, with abnormalities easier assessed by comparing with the contralateral shoulder. Patients report tenderness to palpation of the AC joint, exacerbation of pain with cross-body adduction, superficial pain with the O'Brien's active compression test, horizontal resisted extension, and passive internal rotation in adduction.[1,2,5–7] The joint should be tested for instability in both the anteroposterior and superoinferior planes; horizontal instability or irreducible deformity may indicate a need for surgical intervention.[5]

IMAGING

Plain radiographs are necessary for accurate diagnosis and classification of AC joint injuries. Radiographic evaluation should include bilateral shoulder anteroposterior (AP) view, axillary view, and Zanca view of the involved shoulder.

MANAGEMENT

The treatment of AC joint injuries depends on the grade and severity of the injury. Generally, grade I and II AC joint separations can be treated nonoperatively. There is debate on the treatment of grade III and V injuries in the literature. Surgical treatment is generally required for type IV and VI injuries. For type III and V injuries, we recommend initial nonoperative treatment with a targeted return to play in 4 to 8 weeks. If the patient/athlete cannot tolerate nonoperative treatment or if they are having trouble returning to play, then surgery is offered.

Nonoperative

Type I and II AC joint injuries can be managed initially and usually definitively with nonoperative treatment.[8] Type I AC joint injuries can be treated with sling immobilization for 2 weeks and anti-inflammatories. Type II AC joint injuries generally require a longer period of sling immobilization for around 2 to 3 weeks, as well as anti-inflammatories. Physical therapy can be started when pain resolution occurs around the 1 to 2 week mark.[9] The overall initial focus is on pain control, followed by exercises focused on core/trunk and lower body control.[9] Full mobility and flexibility should then be the focus, followed by strengthening of the shoulder and periscapular muscles with first "short-lever" exercises (exercises with the arm in an adducted position) and then with "long-lever" exercises (exercises with the arm abducted from the body).[10] Overall, there is a paucity of literature on return to play after type I and II AC joint injuries. The literature has focused on the return to play after operatively managed AC joint injuries.[11] Frank and colleagues[1] advise that for these injuries, contact sports be avoided for 1 month, and return to play can be expected around the 2 to 3 month point.[1] Symptoms may persist for up to 6 weeks for both type I and II AC joint injuries.[12] For those athletes with persistent symptoms or those wanting to return to earlier play, we have used a corticosteroid injection under ultrasound guidance in the AC joint to relieve pain at the 1 month to 6 weeks timeframe. As many as half of the patients may experience symptoms up to 10 years after a type I or II AC joint injury.[13] For patients with residual symptoms, it has been our experience that an arthroscopic or open distal clavicle excision can reduce pain.

Type III Acromioclavicular Joint Injuries

Among the management of AC joint injuries, the management of type III AC joint injuries is the most controversial and difficult to manage. With a type III injury, both the AC and coracoclavicular (CC) ligaments are torn, and thus, higher energy is imparted on the AC joint compared with type I and II AC joint injuries in which the

AC and CC ligaments are respectively sprained (Rockwood). In general, uncomplicated type III AC joint injuries can be managed successfully with nonoperative treatment. In a study by Nissen and colleagues,[14] a survey sent to American Society for Sports Medicine (AOSSM) members about managing type III AC joint injuries, 81% of AOSSM members opted for nonsurgical management of uncomplicated type III AC joint injuries. The nonsurgical management of type III AC joint injuries includes sling immobilization for up to 4 weeks, non-steroidal anti-inflammatory drugs (NSAIDs), and physical therapy (PT).[1] In patients with successful nonsurgical management of these injuries, it is important to counsel patients that they will likely still have a bump, cosmetic defect over the AC joint. A study by Dias and colleagues[15] found that 82% of patients treated nonsurgical with type III AC joint injuries had a deformity at that AC joint. Some authors advocate that for patients who are young, active, and participate in overhead activities, surgical management may be the preferred method of treatment for these injuries.[16] For patients managed with surgery, an anatomic or nonanatomic reconstruction technique may be used to reconstruct the AC joint, which will be discussed later in the paper. In a meta-analysis by Smith and colleagues,[17] there were no statistically significant differences in patients with type III AC joint injuries that were treated nonoperatively versus with surgery in clinical (strength, pain, ability to throw overhead) or radiographic outcomes (AC joint arthritis) (Smith). The nonoperatively managed group had a statically poorer rate of cosmetic results compared to the operative cohort. In the surgically treated group, there was a statistically significant higher rate of sick leave.[17] Current literature supports surgical versus nonsurgical management of these injuries on a case-by-case basis with an emphasis on a trial of initial nonoperative management.[18,19]

Operative

In general, surgical management is recommended for type IV and VI injuries; like type III injuries, the management of type V injuries is controversial.[1] Because of the severe soft tissue injury and morbidity associated with type V injuries, surgical management is the generally accepted treatment for these injuries.[20] However, similar to type III injuries, type V injuries should be taken on a case-by-case basis when the decision between surgical and nonsurgical treatment is needed taking into account the patient's functional goals, soft-tissue injury, skin, handedness, and participation in contact sports.[1] There are more than 60 surgical techniques that have been described to address AC joint injury.[1] This article will focus on the pearls and pitfalls of surgical techniques used to address AC joint dislocations/injuries. Surgical techniques range from open reduction internal fixation, repair of injured ligaments, anatomic reconstruction, to nonanatomic reconstruction. Historically, open reduction internal fixation techniques have been described with screws, pins, k-wires, plates, hook plates, and sutures.[1] These have largely fallen out of favor due to complications with this type of hardware, as well as the need for plate removal in the case of the use of hook plates.[1,10,21] We will discuss our preferred surgical techniques to address AC joint dislocations in acute, chronic, and revision settings.

ANATOMIC ACROMIOCLAVICULAR AND CORACOCLAVICULAR LIGAMENT RECONSTRUCTION

For type III and V AC joint injuries that fail nonoperative management and for type IV and VI AC joint injuries, surgical management is offered. There are many surgical techniques available to the treating surgeon. However, it is recommended that anatomic reconstruction techniques be favored and that biologic augmentation in the form of tendon grafts be used.[20] The senior author's preferred technique (MTP) will be described below, which involves an anatomic AC joint reconstruction with the use of 2 allografts and tight-rope fixation. The full surgical technique has been previously described, but this review will highlight key points and focus on pearls and pitfalls.[22]

SURGICAL TECHNIQUE

Under ultrasound guidance, the patient will initially get a catheter-infused regional anesthesia interscalene block in the perioperative holding area. The patient is then placed supine on the operating room table, and general anesthesia is induced. The patient is then placed in the beach chair position with all bony prominences padded. Placing a small towel bump behind the scapula is important to bring the operative shoulder forward. Antibiotic prophylaxis is administered, and the shoulder is prepped and draped in the typical sterile fashion. An anteroposterior saber-type incision is used from the coracoid to the posterior aspect of the AC joint, 3 cm medial to the AC joint. The deltotrapezial fascia approach is used to expose the coracoid, and full-thickness subperiosteal dissection is used on the distal clavicle and medial aspect of the acromion. The superior and inferior aspects of the coracoid are also exposed with Metzenbaum scissors. The grafts are then prepared. Two grafts are used, which can be either semitendinosus (semi-t) allo- or auto-graft or tibialis anterior (tib-ant) allograft. The grafts are prepared so that they easily fit through a 4.5 mm sizing block, and each free end is whipstitched with a FiberTape (Arthrex, Naples, FL, USA). The reconstruction consists of an AC Tight-Rope (Arthrex) and a 2-graft reconstruction to recreate the conoid and trapezoid ligaments. The AC Tight-Rope (Arthrex) is placed first, which consists of 2 Dog Bone Buttons and a loop of braided ultrahigh-molecular-weight polyethylene and polyester No. 5 FiberTape suture (Arthrex). A Hohmann retractor is placed along the inferior aspect of the coracoid, and an AC drill guide (Arthrex) is placed 25 to 30 mm posterior to the anterior tip of the coracoid at the base of the coracoid. A 3 mm cannulated guide pin is drilled through the coracoid. A suture-lasso SD Wire Loop (Arthrex) through the cannulated guide pin is used to shuttle a suture from inferior to superior for later tight-rope passage. Then a curved suture lasso is passed from medial to lateral underneath the coracoid to pass a passing suture from lateral to medial for the semi-t or tib-ant grafts, as seen in **Figs. 1** and **2**.

The AC guide (Arthrex) is then placed on the clavicle 35 mm medial to the AC joint and slightly posterior to recreate the conoid ligament. The 3 mm cannulated drill bit is used to drill through the guide. A 4.5 mm unicortical reamer is placed over the drill bit, and a few millimeters of the top of the clavicle is reamed to recess the button. A suture-lasso SD Wire Loop is passed through the cannulated guide pin to shuttle a suture from inferior to superior for tight-rope passage. A guide pin and a 4.5 mm cannulated

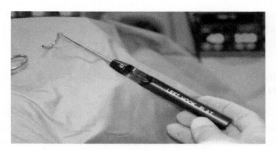

Fig. 1. Curved suture lasso for passage underneath coracoid.

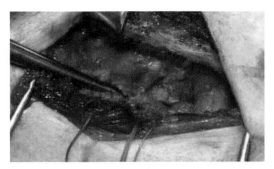

Fig. 2. Curved suture lasso underneath coracoid.

reamer are used to create an additional bone tunnel in the distal clavicle approximately 20 to 25 mm medial to the AC joint, which recreates the trapezoid ligament. Next, the acromion tunnel is drilled with a 4.5 mm drill and guide pin positioned 10 to 15 mm lateral to the AC joint. Passing sutures are placed through these 2 bone tunnels. An additional passing suture is passed from superior to inferior along the posterior aspect of the clavicle, approximately 45 mm medial to the AC joint. These sutures will be used to pass the tendon grafts. The FiberTape limbs used for the AC TightRope construct are placed into the slots of a Dog Bone Button. The FiberTape limbs are then loaded through the SutureLasso SD Wire Loop and pulled from inferior to superior through the coracoid and clavicle bone tunnels. A cobb is then used to reduce the clavicle to the acromion with a slight overreduction as there is creep in the reconstruction. The clavicle Dog Bone Button is then loaded to the suture and tensioned securely against the superior clavicle, as seen in **Fig. 3**. The reduction is confirmed with fluoroscopy.

The 2 allografts are passed around the inferior aspect of the coracoid, as seen in **Fig. 4**. One of the allografts ("graft 1") is passed through the trapezoid tunnel. The other ("graft 2") is wrapped around the clavicle just medial to the Dog Bone Button, crossing on the superior surface of the clavicle with one strand anterior and the other lateral.

A 4.75 mm Tenodesis Screw (Arthrex) is used to secure graft 1 into the superior clavicle, and the remainder of the graft is passed through the posterior acromion tunnel from inferior to superior. A 4.75 mm Tenodesis Screw (Arthrex) is used to secure graft 1 into the acromion from superior to inferior. The 2 strands of graft 2 are then tensioned across the superior clavicle and sutured together with FiberWire suture; one strand is

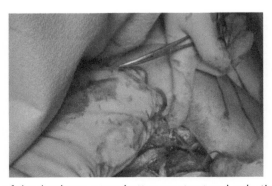

Fig. 3. Tensioning of the dog bone suture button construct and reduction of the AC joint.

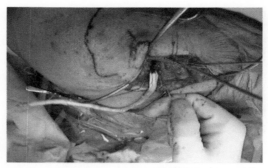

Fig. 4. Passing the tibialis anterior allografts under the coracoid.

cut at this time. The remaining limbs of graft 1 are crossed, tensioned, and sutured together with FiberWire; one strand is cut. The remnant strands of grafts 1 and 2 are then crossed, tensioned, and sutured together with FiberWire; all graft strands are then cut. The shoulder is evaluated for stability through a full arc of motion, closure is carried out in a classic layered fashion, and the operative arm is placed in a padded abduction sling with elbow support. A final postoperative X-ray is shown in **Fig. 5**.

Pearls and pitfalls

Pearls

    Slight over-reduction of the AC joint should be undertaken as these have the tendency to stretch with time postoperatively

    If the reduction cannot be achieved or the AC joint has some arthritic changes, a distal clavicle excision can be used by resecting 3 mm of the distal clavicle with the closing of the superior AC joint capsule after the reconstruction

    Anatomic placement of bone tunnels is critical for anatomic CC ligament reconstruction

    The center of the coracoid is drilled with a 3.0 mm pin in the center of the coracoid. This ensures that coracoid fracture risk is minimized, as only one drill hole is used

Pitfalls

    If the coracoid tunnel is drilled too far medially or laterally, coracoid fracture can occur or propagate postoperatively

    Injury to the brachial plexus or axillary artery can occur with drilling deep to the clavicle or medial to the coracoid

    The rotator cuff should be protected with a cobb or other instrument when drilling through the acromion

---

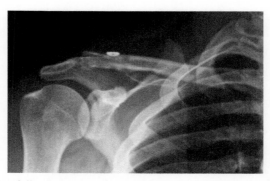

Fig. 5. Postoperative follow-up X-ray after anatomic AC/CC ligament reconstruction.

Revision Anatomic Acromioclavicular and Coracoclavicular Ligament Reconstruction

Complications necessitating revision surgery are present in roughly 22% of patients who undergo surgical repair of AC joint injuries.[23,24] The most common indications for revision surgery include loss of reduction, fracture of coracoid or clavicle, heterotopic ossification, symptomatic hardware, adhesive capsulitis, and infection.[23,24] Treatment of AC joint instability in the revision setting requires a thorough understanding of the anatomy and pathology causing the failure.

The procedure is again performed under general anesthesia supplemented with a regional interscalene block with the patient in the beach chair position. The previous incision is generally used; however, this may need to be extended for adequate exposure. Typically, the incision is centered approximately 2 to 3 cm medial to the AC joint and made in a curvilinear fashion toward the coracoid process, measuring 8 cm in total. Dissection is carried out to the level of the deltotrapezial fascia using Metzenbaum scissors and electrocautery to maintain hemostasis. A transverse incision is made through the deltotrapezial fascia beginning at the midline of the clavicle and extended across the AC joint to the acromion; dissection medial to the coracoid should be avoided to protect the musculocutaneous nerve. The periosteum is then elevated from the clavicle and acromion, preserving full-thickness flaps for eventual closure. Scar tissue and previous suture/hardware are removed as encountered during the approach. The graft is prepared on the back table during the approach. Graft options include semitendinosus allograft, semitendinosus autograft, or anterior tibialis allograft; the senior author (MTP) prefers 2 anterior tibialis grafts. Regardless of graft choice, the graft should be whipstitched on both ends with a goal diameter of 5 to 7 mm.

Once dissection is complete, and all previous hardware is removed, the previous bone tunnels should be evaluated for position, size, and lysis. Two tunnels are used in the clavicle to reconstruct the conoid ligament and the trapezoid ligament, respectively. The conoid process tunnel is positioned 45 mm medial to the distal end of the clavicle in a posterior orientation, whereas the trapezoid tunnel is placed more anteriorly, 30 mm medial to the distal end of the clavicle. If new tunnels are to be drilled, a 3.0 mm drill is drilled from superior to inferior with a retractor under the inferior clavicle to protect adjacent neurovascular structures. Passing sutures are shuttled through the tunnels. A single bone tunnel is placed in the coracoid, 25 to 30 mm posterior to the anterior tip; if drilling a new tunnel, the surgeon should ensure there is enough bone bridge from the previous tunnel to prevent any fracture. Two bone tunnels are placed in the acromion approximately 7 to 10 mm lateral to the AC joint, one about the anterior aspect of the acromion and the other 15 to 20 mm posterior to that. If drilling new tunnels, the retractor should be placed under the acromion to prevent iatrogenic rotator cuff injury.

The Dog Bone Button construct with FiberTape is passed through the coracoid tunnel from inferior to superior, whereas the 2 anterior tibialis allografts are passed around the inferior of the coracoid. The FiberTape is then passed through the conoid ligament tunnel of the clavicle from inferior to superior, and one of the allografts ("graft 1") is passed through the trapezoid tunnel. The other ("graft 2") is wrapped around the clavicle just medial to the Dog Bone Button, crossing on the superior surface of the clavicle with one strand anterior and the other lateral. The AC and CC joints are reduced manually under fluoroscopy, and the Dog Bone Button is tensioned and secured. A 4.75 mm Tenodesis Screw (Arthrex) is used to secure graft 1 into the superior clavicle, and the remainder of the graft is passed through the posterior acromion tunnel from inferior to superior. The 2 strands of graft 2 are then tensioned across the superior clavicle and sutured together with FiberWire suture, and one strand is cut at this time. The remaining limbs of graft 1 are crossed, tensioned, and sutured together with FiberWire; one strand is cut. The remnant strands of grafts 1 and 2 are then crossed, tensioned, and sutured together with FiberWire; all graft strands are then cut. The remaining free ends of FiberTape from the Dog Bone Button are then passed through the anterior acromion tunnel and secured using a Tenodesis Screw to create an internal brace construct. The shoulder is evaluated for stability through a full arc of motion, closure is carried out in a classic layered fashion, and the operative arm is placed in a padded abduction sling with elbow support.

Pearls and pitfalls

Pearls

    The AC joint should be slightly over-reduced to account for the inevitable creep in the grafts

    Fluoroscopy should be used to confirm appropriate tunnel positions and reduction of the AC joint

    Anatomic placement of bone tunnels is critical for anatomic CC ligament reconstruction

    Old bone tunnels should be critically evaluated. The old drill tunnel position, size, and lysis should be scrutinized. If a prior tunnel is malpositioned, a new tunnel should be drilled. If there is not enough space between the tunnels or a tunnel is too large, the screws can be up-sized.

Pitfalls

    If a new coracoid tunnel is drilled too far medially, laterally, or too close to the original tunnel, coracoid fracture can occur. If a coracoid fracture does occur intraoperatively, it can be fixed with a single 3.5 mm cortical screw

    Injury to the brachial plexus or axillary artery can occur with drilling deep to the clavicle or medial to the coracoid

    The rotator cuff should be protected with a cobb or other instrument when drilling through the acromion

---

REHABILITATION

Following primary surgical intervention for AC joint injury, patients are placed in a sling for 4 weeks. During this time, patients are encouraged to perform elbow, wrist, and hand range of motion exercises. Active range of motion is initiated once the sling is discontinued, and strengthening may begin once full active range of motion is achieved, typically 6 to 8 weeks postoperatively. Full return to activities and sport is typically restricted until 4 to 6 months postoperatively once full range of motion and strength are achieved. In our experience, noncontact athletes tend to return at roughly 4 to 5 months, whereas contact athletes tend to return closer to 5 to 6 months.

In the case of revision AC and CC joint reconstruction, the patient remains in their sling for a total of 6 weeks without weight bearing through the operative arm. Gentle passive range of motion of the elbow, wrist, and hand is encouraged during this time. At 4 weeks postoperatively, the patient begins physical therapy with passive shoulder range of motion and pendulum exercises. At 6 weeks postoperatively, the patient may begin active range of motion. Strengthening exercises do not begin until 3 months postoperatively. Patients typically return to full activities, including sport, at 5 to 6 months.

COMPLICATIONS

Complications can arise regardless of treatment modality; however, complications are both more common and more severe following operative management (Frank 2019).[1]

Reported complications following nonoperative management include persistent AC joint instability, cosmetic deformity, distal clavicle osteolysis, and eventual development of AC joint arthritis.[2,25] Postoperative complications include loss of reduction, hardware failure, fracture of coracoid, symptomatic hardware, infection, neurovascular damage, and persistent pain.[22] Loss of reduction and fixation, as seen in **Fig. 6**, can cause not only deformity but also pain and may warrant a revision surgery, as previously discussed.

A cadaveric biomechanical study by Mazzocca and colleagues[26] comparing anatomic CC ligament reconstruction with a modified arthroscopic Weaver–Dunn procedure and an arthroscopic method found that the anatomic coracoacromial reconstruction had significantly less anterior and posterior translation than the modified Weaver–Dunn procedure. The modified Weaver–Dunn procedure also showed greater laxity than the anatomical CC or arthroscopic reconstructions.[26] In Millett and colleagues's series of 31 patients who underwent anatomic CC ligament reconstruction, 7 patients (22.6%) had a complication that required a subsequent surgical procedure, including 2 graft ruptures/attenuation, 2 clavicle fractures, 2 distal clavicle hypertrophy, and 1 patient with adhesive capsulitis.[24] However, in this series, in patients who did not have a complication, excellent postoperative outcomes were achieved.[24] A study by Choi and colleagues[27] in a series of 30 patients with acute, unstable AC joint injuries treated with a single-tunnel CC ligament reconstruction with an autograft semitendinosus tendon graft, 47% developed a loss of reduction, and final clinical scores were significantly lower in patients with complications.

Fractures, as seen in **Fig. 7**, especially through tunnels of the clavicle or coracoid, can occur after AC joint reconstruction. In the series by Thangaraju and colleagues,[28] in a cohort of 80 patients who underwent arthroscopic-assisted AC stabilization, 4 patients presented with late fracture complications. All of the patients were male, and fracture morphology differed between the patients, including fractures of the clavicle and coracoid.[28] Three of these fractures were treated conservatively, and one was treated with open reduction internal fixation.[28] Traumatic peri-implant fractures can occur even 2 years after arthroscopically assisted AC joint reconstruction.[28] Pearls for avoiding fracture include utilization of appropriately sized drills/reamers and anatomic positioning of tunnel placement. Alternative surgical techniques could be used such as reducing the number and size of drill holes/tunnels and/or using a looped technique with the graft instead of additional tunnels.

A study by Cook and colleagues[29] looking at a clavicular bone tunnel malposition in AC joint reconstruction found that medial tunnel placement for the re-creation of the conoid and trapezoid ligaments were a significant risk factor for early failure. The authors recommended preoperative templating to optimize the placement of clavicular bone tunnels.[29] It is paramount to anatomically reconstruct the conoid and trapezoid ligaments when placing the bone tunnels in the clavicle.

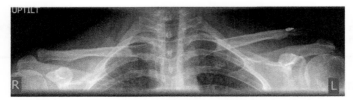

Fig. 6. Loss of reduction after AC joint reconstruction.

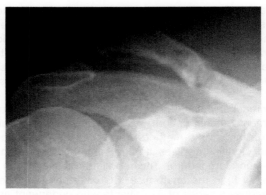

Fig. 7. Example of clavicular fracture postoperatively after CC ligament reconstruction.

Historically, hardware migration led to catastrophic complications,[1,2] leading to the abandonment of fixation with smooth pins. Although most patients report good to excellent outcomes following AC joint reconstruction, failure rates have been reported to be 21% to 28%.[23,30] Higher failure rates have been reported in patients with higher body mass index and in those where surgery was delayed. Spencer and colleagues[30] found that combined allograft loop with cortical button fixation had lower failure rates when compared to other reconstruction techniques.

Finally, postoperative instability can occur not only in the superior-inferior direction but also in the horizontal plane. Weaver–Dunn style reconstructions of the CC ligaments have not shown to adequately address horizontal instability of the AC joint (Aliberti).[31] AC joint suture cord cerclage, combined AC/CC ligament reconstruction, and Twin Tail TightRope triple button techniques have been shown to address horizontal instability (Aliberti).[31]

SUMMARY

Many AC joint injuries can be managed nonoperatively. However, for those who require surgical treatment, it is important anatomically reconstruct the CC ligaments. For those patients undergoing an AC joint reconstruction, patient outcomes are excellent postoperatively if there are no complications.

CLINICS CARE POINTS

- Injury types I and II are typically treated nonoperatively, whereas types IV, V, and VI are treated with operative intervention. Type III injuries are managed on a case-by-case basis.
- The AC ligaments provide horizontal stability to the joint.
- The CC ligaments to provide vertical stability to the joint.
- This text describes the pearls and pitfalls of an anatomic surgical technique for AC joint reconstruction using 2 grafts and tightrope fixation.

DISCLOSURE

The authors have nothing to disclose pertaining to this work.

Other disclosures: Dr M.T. Provencher receives royalties from Arthrex, Inc. and Elsevier, Inc., consulting fees from Arthrex, Inc., Joint Restoration Foundation, and SLACK, Inc., and is an honoraria for Arthrosurface. He is currently a Board or Committee member of the following: AAOS: Board or Committee member; AANA: Board or Committee member; AOSSM: Board or Committee member; ASES: Board or Committee member; Arthroscopy: Editorial or governing board; ISAKOS: Board or Committee member; Knee: Editorial or governing board; Orthopedics: Editorial or governing board; San Diego Shoulder Institute: Board or Committee member; SLACK Inc: Editorial or governing board; Society of Military Orthopaedic Surgeons: Board or Committee member.

REFERENCES

1. Frank RM, Cotter EJ, Leroux TS, et al. Acromioclavicular Joint Injuries: Evidence-based Treatment. J Am Acad Orthop Surg 2019;27(17):e775–88.
2. Mazzocca AD, Arciero RA, Bicos J. Evaluation and treatment of acromioclavicular joint injuries. Am J Sports Med 2007;35(2):316–29.
3. Renfree KJ, Wright TW. Anatomy and biomechanics of the acromioclavicular and sternoclavicular joints. Clin Sports Med 2003;22(2):219–37.
4. Klimkiewicz JJ, Williams GR, Sher JS, et al. The acromioclavicular capsule as a restraint to posterior translation of the clavicle: a biomechanical analysis. J Shoulder Elbow Surg 1999;8(2):119–24.
5. Beitzel K, Mazzocca AD, Bak K, et al. ISAKOS upper extremity committee consensus statement on the need for diversification of the Rockwood classification for acromioclavicular joint injuries. Arthroscopy 2014;30(2):271–8.
6. O'Brien SJ, Pagnani MJ, Fealy S, et al. The active compression test: a new and effective test for diagnosing labral tears and acromioclavicular joint abnormality. Am J Sports Med 1998;26(5):610–3.
7. Chronopoulos E, Kim TK, Park HB, et al. Diagnostic value of physical tests for isolated chronic acromioclavicular lesions. Am J Sports Med 2004;32(3):655–61.
8. Stucken C, Cohen SB. Management of acromioclavicular joint injuries. Orthop Clin North Am 2015;46(1):57–66.
9. Sciascia A, Bois AJ, Kibler WB. Nonoperative Management of Traumatic Acromioclavicular Joint Injury: A Clinical Commentary with Clinical Practice Considerations. Int J Sports Phys Ther 2022;17(3):519–40.
10. Sethi GK, Scott SM. Subclavian artery laceration due to migration of a Hagie pin. Surgery 1976;80(5):644–6.
11. Kay J, Memon M, Alolabi B. Return to Sport and Clinical Outcomes After Surgical Management of Acromioclavicular Joint Dislocation: A Systematic Review. Arthroscopy 2018;34(10):2910–2924 e1.
12. Park JP, Arnold JA, Coker TP, et al. Treatment of acromioclavicular separations. A retrospective study. Am J Sports Med 1980;8(4):251–6.
13. Mikek M. Long-term shoulder function after type I and II acromioclavicular joint disruption. Am J Sports Med 2008;36(11):2147–50.
14. Nissen CW, Chatterjee A. Type III acromioclavicular separation: results of a recent survey on its management. Am J Orthop (Belle Mead NJ) 2007;36(2):89–93.
15. Dias JJ, Steingold RF, Richardson RA, et al. The conservative treatment of acromioclavicular dislocation. Review after five years. J Bone Joint Surg Br 1987;69(5):719–22.

16. Gstettner C, Tauber M, Hitzl W, et al. Rockwood type III acromioclavicular dislocation: surgical versus conservative treatment. J Shoulder Elbow Surg 2008; 17(2):220–5.
17. Smith TO, Chester R, Pearse EO, et al. Operative versus non-operative management following Rockwood grade III acromioclavicular separation: a meta-analysis of the current evidence base. J Orthop Traumatol 2011;12(1):19–27.
18. Trainer G, Arciero RA, Mazzocca AD. Practical management of grade III acromioclavicular separations. Clin J Sport Med 2008;18(2):162–6.
19. Murena L, Canton G, Vulcano E, et al. Scapular dyskinesis and SICK scapula syndrome following surgical treatment of type III acute acromioclavicular dislocations. Knee Surg Sports Traumatol Arthrosc 2013;21(5):1146–50.
20. Beitzel K, Cote MP, Apostolakos J, et al. Current concepts in the treatment of acromioclavicular joint dislocations. Arthroscopy 2013;29(2):387–97.
21. Lyons FA, Rockwood CA Jr. Migration of pins used in operations on the shoulder. J Bone Joint Surg Am 1990;72(8):1262–7.
22. Haber DB, Spang RC, Sanchez G, et al. Revision Acromioclavicular-Coracoclavicular Reconstruction: Use of Precontoured Button and 2 Allografts. Arthrosc Tech 2017;6(6):e2283–8.
23. Clavert P, Meyer A, Boyer P, et al. Complication rates and types of failure after arthroscopic acute acromioclavicular dislocation fixation. Prospective multicenter study of 116 cases. Orthop Traumatol Surg Res 2015;101(8 Suppl):S313–6.
24. Millett PJ, Horan MP, Warth RJ. Two-Year Outcomes After Primary Anatomic Coracoclavicular Ligament Reconstruction. Arthroscopy 2015;31(10):1962–73.
25. Simovitch R, Sanders B, Ozbaydar M, et al. Acromioclavicular joint injuries: diagnosis and management. J Am Acad Orthop Surg 2009;17(4):207–19.
26. Mazzocca AD, Santangelo SA, Johnson ST, et al. A biomechanical evaluation of an anatomical coracoclavicular ligament reconstruction. Am J Sports Med 2006; 34(2):236–46.
27. Choi NH, Lim SM, Lee SY, et al. Loss of reduction and complications of coracoclavicular ligament reconstruction with autogenous tendon graft in acute acromioclavicular dislocations. J Shoulder Elbow Surg 2017;26(4):692–8.
28. Thangaraju S, Tauber M, Habermeyer P, et al. Clavicle and coracoid process periprosthetic fractures as late post-operative complications in arthroscopically assisted acromioclavicular joint stabilization. Knee Surg Sports Traumatol Arthrosc 2019;27(12):3797–802.
29. Cook JB, Shaha JS, Rowles DJ, et al. Clavicular bone tunnel malposition leads to early failures in coracoclavicular ligament reconstructions. Am J Sports Med 2013;41(1):142–8.
30. Spencer HT, Hsu L, Sodl J, et al. Radiographic failure and rates of re-operation after acromioclavicular joint reconstruction: a comparison of surgical techniques. Bone Joint Lett J 2016;98-B(4):512–8.
31. Aliberti GM, Kraeutler MJ, Trojan JD, et al. Horizontal Instability of the Acromioclavicular Joint: A Systematic Review. Am J Sports Med 2020;48(2):504–10.

Midshaft Clavicle Fractures

When Is Surgical Management Indicated and Which Fixation Method Should Be Used?

Myra Trivellas, MD, Jocelyn Wittstein, MD*

KEYWORDS

- Midshaft clavicle fracture • Operative versus nonoperative treatment management
- Intramedullary fixation • Malunion

KEY POINTS

- Operative treatment is recommended for displaced midshaft clavicle fractures, as this provides earlier return to work and sport, greater patient-reported satisfaction with appearance, and significantly decreased incidence of nonunion and malunion when compared with conservative treatment.
- Nonoperative treatment is recommended for nondisplaced fractures or minimally displaced fractures without significant shortening.
- Overall cost data analysis has shown increased cost-effectiveness with operative treatment for displaced clavicle fractures.
- Athletes can benefit significantly from operative treatment.

INTRODUCTION

Clavicle fractures are common traumatic injuries in adults and are caused by a direct impact to the shoulder; 75% to 80% of all clavicle fractures occur in the middle third segment of the clavicle, commonly referred to as midshaft.[1] The Allman classification of clavicle fractures published in 1967 in Journal of Bone and Joint Surgery (JBJS) describes types by location of the fracture along the shaft broken up by thirds: type I middle (most common), type II lateral, and type III medial (least common).[2] The most commonly fractured middle third of the bone lacks strong muscular or ligamentous attachments compared with the medial and lateral aspects of the bone and adjacent joints. Therefore, this section is prone to injury and displacement following trauma. When fractured, the medial fragment is pulled posterosuperiorly by the sternocleidomastoid muscle and the lateral fragment is pulled inferomedially by the pectoralis major tendon and the weight of arm[3] (**Fig. 1**).

Department of Orthopaedic Surgery, Duke University School of Medicine, 3475 Erwin Road, Durham, NC 27705, USA
* Corresponding author.
E-mail address: jocelyn.wittstein@duke.edu

Clin Sports Med 42 (2023) 633–647
https://doi.org/10.1016/j.csm.2023.05.005

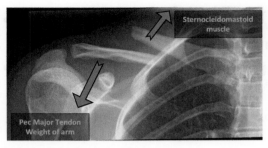

Fig. 1. Midshaft clavicle fracture displacing forces.

Clavicle fractures are associated with significant pain and dysfunction during the acute injury phase and in cases of significant malunion can contribute to chronic shoulder dysfunction. Decision-making regarding care of midshaft clavicle fractures has long been controversial, with the pendulum swinging from nonoperative treatment to more operative treatment for significantly displaced fractures in light of many well-done comparative studies.

DIAGNOSIS

Diagnosis is made with history, physical examination, and radiographs. As with most acute fractures, a history of some trauma, physical examination showing point tenderness, possible deformity and ecchymosis, and abnormal motion at the fracture site are all clear indicators of an underlying fracture. Radiographs will show the evidence of fracture and any comminution, displacement, and shortening. In addition to standard upright anteroposterior (AP) radiographs of bilateral shoulders, clavicle-specific radiographs can be helpful to obtain views along the anatomic axis of the clavicle, perpendicular to the maximal deforming forces, and to eliminate overlapping scapula in the view. An AP with a 30° cephalic tilt of the radiography beam is recommended to best depict true displacement of midshaft fractures (**Fig. 2**). Other clavicle views such as a Zanca view, which is done with the radiography beam angled with a 15° cephalic tilt, are helpful for distal third clavicle fractures, and a Serendipity view, using a 45° cephalic tilt, is recommended to show the medial clavicle and sternoclavicular

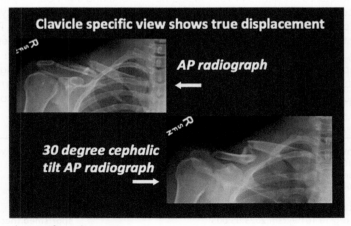

Fig. 2. Clavicle-specific radiographs.

(SC) joint best. These can help demonstrate true displacement and allow for specific comparison in follow-up images. Radiographic interval follow-up depends on fracture type and treatment. For example, minimally displaced fractures are generally not expected to displace further, and therefore, nonoperative management with radiographic follow-up at 6 and again at 10 to 12 weeks is reasonable. Significantly displaced, shortened fractures would require operative treatment. After operative treatment, radiographs are checked at 2, 6, and again at 10 to 12 weeks after fixation.

TREATMENT OPTIONS

Nonoperative treatment of clavicle fractures has long been an accepted treatment option; however, treatment algorithms have shifted from nonoperative to more operative management of displaced midshaft fractures in the era of randomized prospective trials. Nonoperative treatment is still considered the standard of care for nondisplaced or minimally displaced fractures (displaced <100%) in the absence of neurovascular injury or skin threatening.[4,5] In addition, time to presentation to a medical professional with interval healing, combined with potentially limited resources for surgical intervention among some patient populations, can be reasons for nonoperative management. Conservative treatment consists of a sling for 4 to 6 weeks with progression to light strengthening starting at 6 to 10 weeks. Consistent radiographic follow-up throughout the initial 2 to 6 weeks is necessary to ensure no further displacement and appropriate healing.

Nonoperative treatment with completely displaced midshaft fractures has shown to harbor certain healing risks. In addition, significant shortening has historically resulted in worse patient satisfaction and higher risk of nonunion when treated conservatively.[6,7] Nonunion can occur in 10% to 18% of fractures treated conservatively.[8,9] Clavicle fractures treated nonoperatively, even in the adolescent population, have been shown to have a malunion rate of 10% to 20%.[10] When planning treatment options, the patient and provider must consider patient activity level, occupation, and demands, in addition to overall physiologic propensity for healing. Furthermore, the biomechanical risk factors for malunion or nonunion must be considered, including degree of displacement, shortening, and comminution of the fracture.[11] Nonunion presents as continued or unresolving pain in some patients or can present as increased fatigue after activities. Malunion affects patients on a spectrum of reported severity, and although might not be painful, residual deformity of the fracture sight can be bothersome to patients cosmetically or with certain clothing or pack/bag wear.

If nonoperative treatment is not indicated, options and reasons for operative treatment should be thoroughly discussed with the patient and their family. All stabilization methods require an implant that may or may not be permanent. These include open reduction and internal fixation (ORIF) with plates and intramedullary (IM) fixation. The advantages of operative fixation are immediate postoperative stability and decreased fracture-associated pain from movement of fragments and restoration of anatomy and length of the clavicle. Absolute indications for operative intervention are associated vascular injury, open fracture, or impending skin compromise due to displaced bone tenting the overlying skin. Other indications for patients older than 12 year old with less remodeling potential include shortening of greater than 2 cm.[12] Females achieve 80% of their clavicle length by 9 years of age and boys by 12 years of age[13]; therefore, angulation would result in some permanent amount of shortening.

Furthermore, in polytrauma patients, with multiply fractured extremities, it can be helpful in rehabilitation and recovery efforts to stabilize all upper-extremity fractures to allow for assisted weight-bearing and mobilization.

ORIF can be performed with either single or dual-plating technique. Historically, a single plate (commonly a 3.5-mm compression plate), placed superiorly along the clavicle (**Fig. 3**), has led to durable and predictable results for stabilization and healing. With advances in implants, pre-contoured and anatomic clavicle-specific plate designs with locking screw options have been introduced with success. Varying the type and thickness of the plate can assist in decreasing plate prominence and symptomatic hardware. Positioning of the plate has also been shown to affect symptomatic hardware and subsequent removal rates. Anterior plating has been shown to have lower incidence of hardware removal when compared with superior plate positioning, but in biomechanical testing has been shown to be less stiff in axial and torsion forces when compared with superior plating.[14,15] Dual-plating techniques are also an option and allow for stabilization of the bone with lower profile and thinner plates while still providing enough strength to stabilize the bone.[16] This can be done using minifragment plates that can be easily contoured to fit the clavicle.

INTRAMEDULLARY FIXATION

IM fixation for clavicles was first reported in the 1940s using wires.[17] Historically, the technique was developed using various pin-type implants.[18,19] More recently due to desire for increased strength and stability, surgeons have transitioned to using titanium elastic nails (TENs)[20] similar to those used in pediatric fractures or threaded IM devices (**Fig. 4**). There are various implants including IM screw options with compression. Hardware prominence can depend on the implant and technique. The TEN and Rockwood pin can require subsequent surgery for implant removal due to prominence or potential for migration.[21] IM implants are frequently removed for these reasons, but this is done only after complete fracture healing. IM techniques provide appropriate stability as the longitudinal design can counteract the deforming forces of the posterosuperior pull of the sternocleidomastoid on the medial fragment and the inferomedial pull of the lateral fragment by the pectoralis major. IM options adequately maintain length and allow for early use of the arm. Simple fracture patterns that are displaced with minimal comminution and minimal obliquity to the fracture are more amenable biomechanically to IM devices.[22]

The advantages of IM fixation are smaller, more cosmetic incisions and less disruption to surrounding tissues and periosteum, which provide the majority of the blood supply to the midshaft clavicle. Infection rate and refracture rate after implant removal have also been shown to be lower when using IM devices compared with plate fixation.[21,23,24]

Therefore, patients can theoretically safely return to sports faster after removal of an IM device compared with a plate. IM fixation is more technically demanding than standard plate fixation. Furthermore, it is not a practical treatment option for patients that

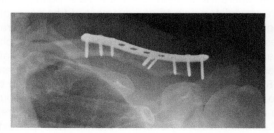

Fig. 3. Superior plate.

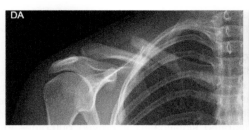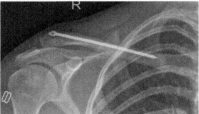

Fig. 4. Intramedullary fixation of clavicle fracture.

are delayed in presentation for fracture care if the fracture fragments are relatively nonmobile.

FRACTURE-ASSOCIATED PATIENT FACTORS

Sleep positioning can be difficult with upper extremity fractures, and pain and disrupted sleep can lead to difficulties with mood changes, productivity decreases, and sequela associated with psychologic stress and fatigue. Owing to the faster stability achieved with internal fixation, pain relief and function can usually be restored faster with operative treatment.[25] Likewise, a gentle range of motion and even return to functional weight-bearing can be allowed after operative fixation, allowing patients to restore some basic activities of daily living.[26]

Of note, clavicle fractures are not as severe or disruptive as lower extremity fractures, and postponed presentation to a provider can influence injury management. Delay in seeking medical attention could make open reduction and internal fixation more difficult due to callus formation and deformity or drive the patient to elect a trial of nonoperative treatment. With late presentation, the patient could have already undergone a significant portion of the healing process, which is usually expected by 3 to 4 weeks after injury depending on patient age. The initial phases of injury are the most debilitating and painful part of recovery. Therefore, if the patient has already suffered through the hardest weeks, continued nonsurgical treatment can frequently be a practical management option, as this would avoid an operation that would restart the healing process, cause additional pain, and impart the risk of surgical complications.

RECENT TRENDS

Studies of trends from the early 2000s showed that the incidence of clavicle fractures has been increasing both in and outside of the United States. Moreover, the rate of operative fixation has disproportionally been increasing with a reported 300% to 700% increase in operative fixation of clavicle fractures.[27,28] Further investigation of trends in clavicle fracture surgeries in the United States found that patients who were white, privately insured, and of high-income status had higher rates of surgical fixation of their fractures. Whereas delay in surgery was associated with patients of lower income status, suggesting varied access to care.[28]

DISCUSSION
Current Evidence for Operative Versus Nonoperative Intervention

A review of published evidence in the last 15 years supports surgical intervention for midshaft clavicle fractures in adults that are either completely displaced, shortened greater than 2 cm, or are significantly comminuted.[29] Most of this literature reports on open reduction and plate fixation and shows improved functional outcomes, patient-reported satisfaction with appearance, and significantly decreased incidence of nonunion and malunion when compared with conservative treatment without surgery.

The Canadian Orthopaedic Trauma Society (COTS) published their multicenter, prospective randomized clinical trial of 132 patients with a displaced midshaft clavicle fracture. They randomized patients to either operative treatment with plate fixation or nonoperative treatment with a sling and evaluated radiographic and functional outcomes using the Constant and disabilities of the arm, shoulder, and hand (DASH) scores. Both functional scores demonstrated significantly improved outcomes in operatively treated fractures compared with their nonoperative counterparts. Timing until radiographic union was also significantly decreased in the operatively treated fractures by an average of 12 weeks faster in the surgical group. In this RCT, the COTS reported a mean time to radiographic union of 28.4 weeks in the nonoperative group compared with 16.4 weeks in the operative group. They found this to be statistically significant with a P-value = .001. In addition, nonunions and symptomatic malunions occurred significantly more frequently in the nonoperatively treated fractures compared with the operatively treated group. Although there were more complications reported in the operatively treated fractures, these were generally due to prominent hardware and could be treated with hardware removal. Ultimately, patients who underwent surgery were more likely to be satisfied with the appearance of their shoulder at 1 year post-op.[11]

Similarly, Fuglesang and colleagues published a report reviewing 59 patients with 2.7 year outcome data who underwent conservative treatment of their completely displaced midshaft clavicle fractures. They showed fair to poor clinical results and patient-reported DASH scores. Patients with 100% or greater displacement of the fracture fragments reported significantly lower upper extremity function in those treated conservatively versus operatively. Moreover, the investigators found a significantly increased rate of nonunions in conservatively treated patients. This risk for nonunion increased with age.[30]

In a JBJS 2017 randomized controlled trial (RCT) of 160 adults, Woltz and colleagues published their findings on plate fixation compared with nonoperative treatment for displaced midshaft clavicular fractures. Their primary outcome was to evaluate union at 1 year, and the group found that open reduction and plate fixation provided more reliable healing compared with nonsurgical treatment. They also evaluated DASH and Constant scores for all patients at different time points, but in contrast to prior research discussed, they did not find any statistically significant differences in these functional scores between the two groups at all time points.[31]

A randomized clinical trial out of Denmark, published in 2018, in The Bone and Joint Journal, again evaluated operative versus nonoperative treatment of displaced midshaft clavicle fractures. They randomized 146 adult patients to operative versus nonoperative treatment of displaced clavicle fractures and evaluated union and function scores (DASH and Constant scores) at different time points during the first year. Early function scores, both DASH and Constant scores, were improved in the operative group, which was statistically significant at 3 months. After 6 months and at 1 year, the investigators found no statistically significant differences between the surgically and conservatively treated patients. Nonunion rates were significantly lower in the operatively treated patients. Twenty-five percent of the surgically treated patients underwent hardware removal in their study.[25]

Qin and colleagues performed a meta-analysis of nine randomized clinical trials comparing open reduction and plate fixation versus nonsurgical treatment for displaced midshaft clavicle fractures. They found that the surgical treatment of fractures showed significant advantages over conservative treatment when analyzing for nonunion rate, malunion rate, and appearance dissatisfaction rate. The analysis of the nonoperative treatment group showed the lower rate of reported complications. The analysis did not find a significant difference in functional outcome when comparing reported DASH scores among the RCTs. Overall, they found that in regard to complete healing and appearance, patients reported better outcomes with ORIF over nonsurgical treatment.[32]

Level 1 evidence from Axelrod and colleagues also showed surgical intervention had improvements in all outcomes evaluated, most notably union rates, when compared with conservative treatments. They do acknowledge that although operative treatment showed statistically superior upper extremity function results versus conservative treatment, these results were not always above the minimal clinically important differences. In their 2020 report: What Is the Best Evidence for Management of Displaced Midshaft Clavicle Fractures? A Systematic Review and Network Meta-analysis of 22 RCTs, they analyzed studies that totaled over 1000 patients with midshaft clavicle fractures to identify which treatment had the highest union rate, lowest revision rate, and highest functional outcomes at 1 year. Union rates were significantly higher in the surgically treated group, with the number needed to treat being 10 patients to avoid one nonunion. When counseling patients, they recommend discussing the evidence that union rates are more predictable after an operation, but that patients should understand a second operation might be needed to remove symptomatic hardware once the fracture has healed.[8]

In 2022, investigators from The University of Hong Kong published a systematic review and meta-analysis of RCTs comparing operative and nonoperative management of midshaft clavicle fractures. Their study analyzed a total of 3094 adult patients across all 31 RCTs that included among the operatively treated fractures both plate fixation and IM fixation. DASH and Constant scores, time to union, and risk of treatment related complications were compared between the surgically treated and conservatively treated patients. Overall, they found that surgical intervention led to better functional outcome scores and decreased time to union. They further analyzed available data for comparison of short-term results (3 months), intermediate-term (6–12 months), and long-term (>24 months) clinical outcomes. From their subgroup analysis, they reported that not only did they see improvements in DASH and Constant scores in the early term results, but these higher functional scores were still noted in the operatively treated groups after 24 months.[33]

DIFFERENCES IN FIXATION TECHNIQUES

Described fixation techniques for midshaft clavicle fractures include IM fixation and various plating options including superior, anterior inferior, and dual min-fragment plating. Each of these techniques has specific advantages and disadvantages specific to biomechanical strength, wound problems, hardware prominence, and need for removal of hardware.

Superior plating has been shown to be a biomechanically stronger construct that is stiffer in axial compression than anteroinferior positioning.[15] However, it is associated with more hardware prominence and irritation. Clinically, when comparing superior and anteroinferior fixation positioning, there are no significant differences in regard to stabilization and complete healing. A meta-analysis study published in 2017, in the Journal of Orthopedic Trauma, analyzed surgical fixation methods comparing anteroinferior plating versus superior plating. In their analysis of 34 articles, there were no statistically significant differences detected in union, malunion, or nonunion rates. Their study showed that anteroinferior plating was associated with significantly lower rates of symptomatic hardware and therefore lower subsequent implant removal when compared with superior plating. They found no differences in postoperative shoulder function scores when examining DASH and Constant scores among the two interventions.[14]

Dual mini-fragment orthogonal plating has been shown to have similar biomechanical strength as superior plating using a single larger plate.[16,34] Dual-plating techniques as previously described allow for lower profile hardware and less prominence and therefore lower rates of symptomatic hardware removal.[16] You and colleagues published a systematic review and meta-analysis of single plate versus dual plating and reported a 4% rate of removal of symptomatic hardware in the dual plating. In contrast, the single-plate group had a 3.9 times higher implant removal rate due to symptomatic hardware. Healing was the same between both groups.[35]

A systematic review and meta-analysis of RCTs of plate fixation or IM fixation for midshaft clavicle fractures published in Journal of Shoulder Elbow Surgery (JSES) in 2016 showed no differences in union, infection, or wound problems between the two treatment options. They found that hardware removal was common in both fixation techniques, but that IM nailing had significantly higher rates of secondary surgery for implant removal (mean of 73% for TEN vs 38% for plate). Their study also showed that refracture after removal of hardware was more common with plate fixation.[36] Ju and colleagues published another systematic review and meta-analysis of RCTs comparing plate fixation and IM fixation of midshaft clavicle fractures analyzing 10 RCTs. They evaluated DASH and Constant function scores and found no statistically significant difference between the two groups. They found an associated slight increase in the risk of infection and less satisfaction with cosmetic appearance with plate fixation when compared with IM fixation. Overall, their analysis results did not suggest any difference between the two groups in long-term functional outcomes.[37]

In a 2020 study of 94 adolescents evaluating clinical and radiographic outcomes of midshaft clavicle fractures, Kim and colleagues evaluated four different treatment options: conservative figure-of-8 brace, open reduction and internal fixation with a plate (OPL), minimally invasive plate osteosynthesis (MIPO), and IM nail fixation with a threaded Steinmann pin (TSP). They found that all groups had satisfactory outcomes and obtained full fracture union, but Constant scores were higher in the surgically treated groups compared with nonoperative treatment. Angulation and bone length was closest to normal in OPL and TSP groups. TSP and MIPO groups had faster bone healing. Scar appearance satisfaction was highest in the TSP group as expected.[38]

COST-EFFECTIVENESS

The cost of injury is associated not only with the cost of treatment interventions but also in the time required for recovery and return to full activity in addition to the value placed on quality of life. Although less quantifiable, time lived without pain and dysfunction can be considered more valuable in terms of quality of life. A 2013 JSES study of 204 patients showed that patients with displaced clavicle fractures obtain significant improvements both clinically and financially from operative fixation. Althausen and colleagues found significantly less chronic pain, deformity, weakness, and better range of motion reported in patients who underwent operative stabilization. This led the surgically treated patients to return to work faster (missing 8.4 vs 35.2 days of work), require less assistance at home, and incurred less physical therapy costs ($971.76 vs $1820). Overall, although the initial hospital bill was higher due to surgical costs, the total cost savings for patients was reported as $5091.33 of less cost in favor of operative treatment.[39] This cost analysis highly depends on the resources available to a patient. A study published in JBJS in 2019 by Liu and colleagues also reported on cost-effectiveness of operative versus nonoperative treatment of displaced midshaft clavicle fractures. They did this by analyzing calculated quality-adjusted life years (QALYs) and Medicare costs for operative and nonoperative treatment of substantially displaced midshaft clavicle fractures. The investigators used a Markov model to evaluate clinical results at 5 years and predicted lifetime results. They used this model in their cost-effectiveness analysis to determine how long clinical benefits in operatively treated patients must persist for operative intervention to be more cost-effective than nonoperative treatment for displaced midshaft clavicle fractures. They found that the cost per QALY with operative management was less than $38,000 in the first 5-year and less than $8000 in the lifetime analyses. These costs were below the willingness-to-pay threshold of $50,000 per QALY. They therefore concluded that for operative treatment to be cost-effective, patients must see clinical benefits for at least 3 years postoperative fixation.[40]

RETURN TO SPORT

In athletes, return to sport can be a significant driver of treatment, as a critical aspect of their quality-of-life centers around ability to participate in their sport. Their conditioning and strength are dependent on consistent training, and days missed are important considerations in a patient-specific treatment algorithm. A systematic review of 10 studies on midshaft clavicle fractures showed that return to sports was significantly decreased with operative treatment (mean of 10 weeks missed vs mean of 21 weeks missed with conservative management) of displaced midshaft fractures.[41] For patients who participate in contact sports, the investigators recommend at least 6 weeks of no contact after fixation. If the removal of hardware is desired by the athlete, this should be done after the season has ended to limit the risk of refracture after initial implant removal. Return to sport for nonoperatively treated clavicles is recommended only after union is clearly seen on radiographs, and the athlete has no pain along the clavicle. Depending on the fracture type and patient's desired activities, that is, high-level contact sports, this could be longer than 12 weeks if radiographic union is not proven. Athletes may return to lower extremity training and cardio conditioning during the early postoperative period to allow for fitness maintenance. In addition to the physical benefits of continued training, encouragement of lower extremity work outs, cross-training, and continued team involvement provides the athlete connection and psychological benefits, allowing them to return to play with more mental preparedness and less effects on quality of life that are associated with an injured mentality.

CASE STUDY: RECURRENT CLAVICLE FRACTURE AFTER NONOPERATIVE TREATMENT
Presentation

We present a case of an 18-year-old high school football player, running back, who presented to the author's clinic 5 weeks after sustaining a mildly displaced midshaft clavicle fracture. He had been treated with nonoperative management at outside facility and presented to clinic for a second opinion. There were no concerning neurovascular or skin findings on examination, and his pain was improving. Radiographs showed early bridging callus formation, mild deformity, and a clearly visible fracture line (Fig. 5). The patient reported that he had no pain and was eager to return to play.

As he showed signs of healing with mild deformity and no concerning findings on examination, the decision was made to continue with nonoperative management. At

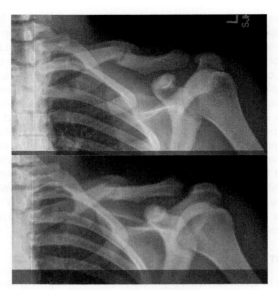

Fig. 5. Case: Presenting radiographs 5 weeks after initial injury.

12 weeks following his initial injury, he returned to clinic for routine follow-up. He reported no pain and on questioning, he admitted to pain-free to return to full-weight bench press, contrary to the recommendations of conservative management from the provider. On examination, the fracture site was non-tender and without crepitus or motion. Radiographs showed bridging bone across the deformity (**Fig. 6**). The patient was cleared to return to contact play after 12 weeks of nonoperative care. On return to play, a contact injury was sustained, and the patient suffered a refracture at the prior site. Subsequent radiographs showed refracture with additional displacement at the fracture site (**Fig. 7**).

Treatment Options

At this point, a discussion was had with the athlete and his family in regard to treatment options, and surgical treatment was recommended to expedite healing and reduce nonunion and malunion risk. Open reduction and internal fixation with orthogonal dual mini-fragment plating yielded anatomic results (**Fig. 8**). The athlete subsequently healed the fracture, was able to return to sport, and had no further issues.

Discussion

The duration of nonoperative treatment before return to play must be individualized based on the type of sport, clinical examination, and serial imaging demonstrating healing. Patients returning to high-risk sports may benefit from CT imaging as an additional modality before return to contact play to reduce the risk of refracture. The argument can be made that for athletes whose main goal is to return to sport expeditiously and reliably, operative treatment is the best choice to give them a strong construct and predictable results. Shared decision-making should include discussion of risk of refracture with nonoperative treatment, risks of surgical treatment, and reduced time to return to play with surgical treatment.

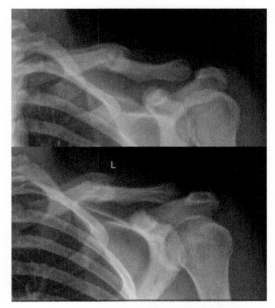

Fig. 6. Case: Radiographic follow-up 12 weeks after initial injury.

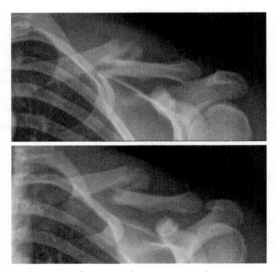

Fig. 7. Case: Radiographs with refracture after return to play.

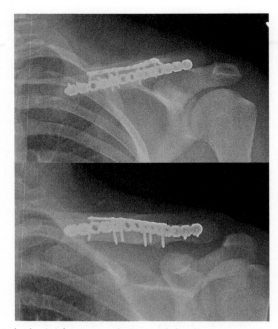

Fig. 8. Status post dual mini-fragment plating with healing.

SUMMARY

The recent literature has continued to evaluate management options for midshaft clavicle fractures and various outcome data. For fractures that are significantly displaced, operative treatment either with open reduction and plate fixation or with IM fixation has been shown to provide improved functional outcomes, earlier return to work, greater patient-reported satisfaction with appearance, and significantly decreased incidence of nonunion and malunion when compared with conservative treatment without surgery. Return to sport has also been shown to be faster in operatively treated fractures. When considering return to contact sports, even minimally or mildly displaced fractures should be considered for surgical stabilization, as this can have significant benefits for athletes and their training and can protect the original injury site from reinjury. However, as with all surgical management, operative intervention is not without risk that otherwise is avoided with conservative treatment. Although initially more expensive, the opportunity for more time with improved quality-of-life and return to productivity makes operative fixation an attractive option when evaluating cost-effectiveness data. Ultimately, shared decision-making with the patient and their support system combined with understanding patient goals allows the provider to recommend a management option to achieve a satisfactory outcome.

CLINICS CARE POINTS

Pros and cons of operative versus nonoperative treatment of midshaft clavicle fractures	
Operative	**Nonoperative**
Advantages	
Improved short-term function	Avoids complications associated with surgical risk

Earlier return to work and sport	Acceptable and practical option if delayed presentation
Lower rate of malunion and nonunion	Avoids symptomatic hardware
Cost-effective when considering less time lost, of productivity and quality of life (QOL)	
Equivocal improvements in long-term function	Equivocal improvements in long-term function
Disadvantages	
Symptomatic hardware commonly can require secondary surgery for implant removal	Varying cosmetic deformity and shortening
Additional risks of surgery (numbness in supraclavicular nerve distribution, wound healing problems, infection)	Higher rate of malunion and nonunion

DISCLOSURE

The authors have no conflicts of interest to disclose that pertain to this topic.

REFERENCES

1. Kihlström C, Möller M, Lönn K, et al. Clavicle fractures: epidemiology, classification and treatment of 2,422 fractures in the Swedish Fracture Register; an observational study. BMC Musculoskelet Disord 2017;18(1):82.
2. Allman FL Jr. Fractures and ligamentous injuries of the clavicle and its articulation. J Bone Joint Surg Am 1967;49(4):774–84.
3. Hyland S, Charlick M, Varacallo M. Anatomy, Shoulder and Upper Limb, Clavicle. Updated 2022 Jul 25. In: StatPearls. Treasure Island (FL): StatPearls Publishing; 2022. Available from: https://www.ncbi.nlm.nih.gov/books/NBK525990/.
4. Khan LA, Bradnock TJ, Scott C, et al. Fractures of the clavicle. J Bone Joint Surg Am 2009;91(2):447–60.
5. Jones SD, Bravman JT. Midshaft clavicle fractures—when to operate. Ann Joint 2021;6:21.
6. Lazarides S, Zafiropoulos G. Conservative treatment of fractures at the middle third of the clavicle: the relevance of shortening and clinical outcome. J Shoulder Elbow Surg 2006;15(2):191–4.
7. McKee MD, Pedersen EM, Jones C, et al. Deficits following nonoperative treatment of displaced midshaft clavicular fractures. J Bone Joint Surg Am 2006; 88(1):35–40.
8. Axelrod DE, Ekhtiari S, Bozzo A, et al. What Is the Best Evidence for Management of Displaced Midshaft Clavicle Fractures? A Systematic Review and Network Meta-analysis of 22 Randomized Controlled Trials. Clin Orthop Relat Res 2020; 478(2):392–402.
9. Murray Ir, Foster Cj, Robinson Cm. Risk factors for non-union in displaced midshaft clavicle fractures treated non operatively. Orthop Proc 2012;94-B-(SUPP_XXXIII):16.
10. McIntosh AL. Surgical Treatment of Adolescent Clavicle Fractures: Results and Complications. J Pediatr Orthop 2016;36:S41–3.
11. Canadian Orthopaedic Trauma Society. Nonoperative treatment compared with plate fixation of displaced midshaft clavicular fractures. A multicenter, randomized clinical trial. JBJS 2007;89(1):1–10. What Is the Best Evidence for Management of Displaced Midshaft Clavicle Fractures? A Systematic Review and Network Meta-analysis of 22 Randomized Controlled Trials.

12. Nowak J, Holgersson M, Larsson S. Can we predict long-term sequelae after fractures of the clavicle based on initial findings? A prospective study with nine to ten years of follow-up. J Shoulder Elbow Surg 2004;13(5):479–86.
13. McGraw MA, Mehlman CT, Lindsell CJ, et al. Postnatal growth of the clavicle: birth to 18 years of age. J Pediatr Orthop 2009;29(8):937–43.
14. Nourian A, Dhaliwal S, Vangala S, et al. Midshaft Fractures of the Clavicle: A Meta-analysis Comparing Surgical Fixation Using Anteroinferior Plating Versus Superior Plating. J Orthop Trauma 2017;31(9):461–7.
15. Toogood P, Coughlin D, Rodriguez D, et al. A biomechanical comparison of superior and anterior positioning of precontoured plates for midshaft clavicle fractures. Am J Orthop (Belle Mead NJ) 2014;43(10):E226–31.
16. Prasarn ML, Meyers KN, Wilkin G, et al. Dual mini-fragment plating for midshaft clavicle fractures: a clinical and biomechanical investigation. Arch Orthop Trauma Surg 2015;135:1655–62.
17. Eichinger JK, Balog TP, Grassbaugh JA. Intramedullary Fixation of Clavicle Fractures: Anatomy, Indications, Advantages, and Disadvantages. J Am Acad Orthop Surg 2016;24(7):455–64.
18. Enneking TJ, Hartlief MT, Fontijne WP. Rushpin fixation for midshaft clavicular nonunions: good results in 13/14 cases. Acta Orthop Scand 1999;70(5):514–6.
19. Hoogervorst P, van Schie P, van den Bekerom MP. Midshaft clavicle fractures: Current concepts. EFORT Open Rev 2018;3(6):374–80.
20. Assobhi JE. Reconstruction plate versus minimal invasive retrograde titanium elastic nail fixation for displaced midclavicular fractures. J Orthop Traumatol 2011;12(4):185–92.
21. van der Meijden OA, Houwert RM, Hulsmans M, et al. Operative treatment of dislocated midshaft clavicular fractures: plate or intramedullary nail fixation? A randomized controlled trial. J Bone Joint Surg Am 2015;97(8):613–9.
22. Park JS, Ko SH, Hong TH, et al. Plate fixation versus titanium elastic nailing in midshaft clavicle fractures based on fracture classifications. J Orthop Surg 2020;28(3). https://doi.org/10.1177/2309499020972204.
23. Li Ying MD, Helvie Peter BS, Farley Frances AMD, et al. Complications After Plate Fixation of Displaced Pediatric Midshaft Clavicle Fractures. J Pediatr Orthop 2018;38(7):350–3.
24. Smith SD, Wijdicks CA, Jansson KS, et al. Stability of mid-shaft clavicle fractures after plate fixation versus intramedullary repair and after hardware removal. Knee Surg Sports Traumatol Arthrosc 2014;22(2):448–55.
25. Qvist AH, Væsel MT, Jensen CM, et al. Plate fixation compared with nonoperative treatment of displaced midshaft clavicular fractures: a randomized clinical trial. Bone Joint Lett J 2018;100-B(10):1385–91.
26. Brian C, Jennifer T, Hrayr B, et al. Immediate Weight-bearing as Tolerated has Improved Outcomes Compared to Non–weight-bearing after Surgical Stabilisation of Midshaft Clavicle Fractures in Polytrauma Patients. J Orthop Trauma Rehabil 2018;25(1):16–20.
27. Schairer WW, Nwachukwu BU, Warren RF, et al. Operative Fixation for Clavicle Fractures socioeconomic Differences Persist Despite Overall Population Increases in Utilization. J Orthop Trauma 2017;31(6):e167–72.
28. Huttunen TT, Launonen AP, Berg HE, et al. Trends in the Incidence of Clavicle Fractures and Surgical Repair in Sweden: 2001-2012. J Bone Joint Surg Am 2016;98(21):1837–42.
29. Song HS, Kim H. Current concepts in the treatment of midshaft clavicle fractures in adults. Clin Shoulder Elb 2021;24(3):189–98.

30. Fuglesang HF, Flugsrud GB, Randsborg PH, et al. Radiological and functional outcomes 2.7 years following conservatively treated completely displaced midshaft clavicle fractures. Arch Orthop Trauma Surg 2016;136(1):17–25.
31. Woltz S, Stegeman SA, Krijnen P, et al. Plate Fixation Compared with Nonoperative Treatment for Displaced Midshaft Clavicular Fractures: A Multicenter Randomized Controlled Trial. J Bone Joint Surg Am 2017;99(2):106–12.
32. Qin M, Zhao S, Guo W, et al. Open reduction and plate fixation compared with non-surgical treatment for displaced midshaft clavicle fracture: A meta-analysis of randomized clinical trials. Medicine (Baltim) 2019;98(20):e15638.
33. Yan MZ, Yuen WS, Yeung SC, et al. Operative management of midshaft clavicle fractures demonstrates better long-term outcomes: A systematic review and meta-analysis of randomised controlled trials. PLoS One 2022;17(4):e0267861.
34. Ziegler CG, Aman ZS, Storaci HW, et al. Low-Profile Dual Small Plate Fixation Is Biomechanically Similar to Larger Superior or Anteroinferior Single Plate Fixation of Midshaft Clavicle Fractures. Am J Sports Med 2019;47(11):2678–85.
35. You DZ, Krzyzaniak H, Kendal JK, et al. Outcomes and complications after dual plate vs. single plate fixation of displaced mid-shaft clavicle fractures: A systematic review and meta-analysis. J Clin Orthop Trauma 2021;17:261–6 [Erratum in: J Clin Orthop Trauma. 2021 Jul 30;20:101538].
36. Houwert RM, Smeeing DP, Ahmed Ali U, et al. Plate fixation or intramedullary fixation for midshaft clavicle fractures: a systematic review and meta-analysis of randomized controlled trials and observational studies. J Shoulder Elbow Surg 2016;25(7):1195–203.
37. Ju W, Mohamed SO, Qi B. Comparison of plate fixation vs. intramedullary fixation for the management of mid-shaft clavicle fractures: A systematic review and meta-analysis of randomised controlled trials. Exp Ther Med 2020;20(3):2783–93.
38. Kim HY, Yang DS, Bae JH, et al. Clinical and Radiological Outcomes after Various Treatments of Midshaft Clavicle Fractures in Adolescents. Clin Orthop Surg 2020; 12(3):396–403.
39. Althausen PL, Shannon S, Lu M, et al. Clinical and financial comparison of operative and nonoperative treatment of displaced clavicle fractures. J Shoulder Elbow Surg 2013;22(5):608–11.
40. Liu J, Srivastava K, Washington T, et al. Cost-Effectiveness of Operative Versus Nonoperative Treatment of Displaced Midshaft Clavicle Fractures: A Decision Analysis. J Bone Joint Surg Am 2019;101(1):35–47.
41. Robertson GA, Wood AM. Return to sport following clavicle fractures: a systematic review. Br Med Bull 2016;119(1):111–28.

Getting Athletes Back on the Field

Management of Clavicle Fractures and Return to Play

Wade Gobbell, MD, Christopher M. Edwards, BS,
Samuel R. Engel, MA, Katherine J. Coyner, MD, MBA*

KEYWORDS

- Clavicle • Fracture • Athlete • Return to sport

KEY POINTS

- Defining return to sport timelines for athletes with clavicle fractures depends on time to radiographic union, level of competition, type of sport, and injury timing within the season.
- Fixation of clavicle fractures in contact athletes may necessitate the use of fixation constructs with higher biomechanical strengths, including larger superior plates or dual plating.
- Postinjury or postoperative rehabilitation timelines should be guided by restoration of functional range of motion, strength, and sport-specific exercises.

INTRODUCTION

Clavicle fractures are common injuries at all levels of sports participation, with the mechanism usually involving a medially directed blow to the lateral shoulder. Treatment may be conservative or surgical, with either option necessitating significant time away from sports participation. Given the prevalence of clavicle fractures among athletes and the significant impact they can have on collegiate and professional careers, it is imperative that orthopedic sports medicine physicians can competently diagnose and manage these injuries to enable athletes to safely and efficiently return to a high level of play. One must be equipped with a data-driven approach to counsel athletes and their families, coaches, and/or agents on the timeline for return to sport, their expectations for performance after return, and the risk of returning to play prior to fracture union. This review will cover broadly clavicle injuries in sports, the diagnosis

UConn Health Department of Orthopedic Surgery, 263 Farmington Avenue, Farmington, CT 06030, USA
* Corresponding author.
E-mail address: coyner@uchc.edu

Clin Sports Med 42 (2023) 649–661
https://doi.org/10.1016/j.csm.2023.05.006
0278-5919/23/© 2023 Elsevier Inc. All rights reserved.

and management of clavicle fractures in athletes, and guidelines for return to play. We will review findings of both recent and historical studies and share our approach to rehabilitating athletes after operative treatment of clavicle fractures. The technical aspects of open reduction and internal fixation (ORIF) of clavicle fractures will be described in detail in other chapters within this text.

Epidemiology of Sports-Related Clavicle Fractures

Clavicle fractures represent 4% of fractures for all age groups based on a study of more than 2000 cases at a large urban hospital.[1] Other studies have reported clavicle fracture prevalence between 2.6% and 10%.[2,3] Isolated clavicle fractures comprise more than 40% of all fractures involving the shoulder girdle.[3]

Approximately 30% to 50% of clavicle fractures are attributable to sports participation.[4–6] Clavicle fractures are the most prevalent of all fractures among athletes, contributing close to 10% of all sport-related fractures.[4,7] At the 2004 National Football League Combine, clavicle injuries were the fourth most common injury reported by elite college football players.[8] Clavicle fractures are common among both adults and adolescents, but patients between 10 and 19 years of age have the highest risk of injury.[5,6,9] Multiple studies have found that male athletes are disproportionately affected by clavicle fractures and are up to 3 times more likely to sustain a clavicle fracture than women.[6,9] Overall, clavicle fractures have the highest prevalence in football followed by soccer, snowboarding, bicycling, wrestling, and snow skiing as demonstrated by a study of over 2000 fractures.[9] Another study found that male athletes in high school were most likely to sustain clavicle fractures in ice hockey followed by lacrosse, football, and wrestling.[10] For female athletes, the high school sports with the highest rate of clavicle fracture were soccer followed by lacrosse and basketball.[10]

Clavicle fractures are prevalent in winter sports and are the third most common injury to recreational snowboarders, representing 6.5% of over 5500 reported injuries.[11,12] Interestingly, clavicle fracture rates for snowboarding are much higher than those for skiing despite both sports having similar participation risks.[13]

For both professional and recreational cyclists participating in road, mountain, or trail biking, clavicle fractures are the most prevalent among acute injuries.[14–18] Clavicle fractures were the most common traumatic injury among Tour de France participants over 7 years.[19] An analysis of all clavicle fractures assessed at an emergency department over a 10-year period identified cycling as the most common source of injury with an increase in incidence during the study period.[20] One study has even demonstrated that the increase in bicycle use among commuters in New York City is correlated with increased clavicle fracture incidence.[21]

ANATOMY AND BIOMECHANICS

The clavicle is a sigmoid-shaped bone that lies horizontally between the sternum and acromion. It serves as an important connection between the axial skeleton and upper limbs. The clavicle articulates medially with the sternum at the sternoclavicular (SC) joint and laterally with the acromion at the acromioclavicular (AC) joint. The AC joint enables gliding movement of the shoulder. The AC ligament connects the clavicle and acromion process of the scapula and restricts motion (see Perry and colleagues' article, "Acromioclavicular Joint Anatomy and Biomechanics: the Significance of Posterior Rotational and Translational Stability," in this issue for a detailed review). The SC joint facilitates several movements including protraction-retraction, depression-elevation, and rotation. The SC joint is stabilized by the anterior and posterior SC joint ligaments in addition to the anterior interclavicular ligament and posterior costoclavicular ligament (see Gobbell and colleagues' article, "Atraumatic Sternoclavicular Joint Instability: Prevalence, Etiology, and Management," in this issue for a detailed review). The trapezius and deltoid muscles attach along the lateral surface of the clavicle. The sternocleidomastoid, pectoralis major, subclavius, and sternohyoid muscles attach along the medial surface of the clavicle. Below the middle third of the clavicle are the subclavian and axillary vessels, as well as the nerves of the brachial plexus.

Epidemiological studies have found the most common mechanism of fracture to be direct fall onto the shoulder.[1,22,23] Biomechanical studies of the forces involved in clavicle fractures demonstrated that a direct injury may exceed the critical buckling load of the bone at a compressive force equal to the individual's body weight.[23] Athletes are prone to clavicle fractures from contact with playing surfaces during competition and contact with other players resulting in a direct blow to the shoulder.[23]

Most clavicle fractures involve the middle third of the bone.[3,24] When grouping sports-related and other traumatic mechanisms, approximately 70% to 80% of fractures are mid-diaphyseal, 48% have any displacement, and 19% are comminuted.[3,25]

Classification of Clavicle Fractures

There are numerous methods for classification of clavicle fractures, and the most frequently used systems are outlined in this section. Currently, most practitioners follow the methodology published by Allman, but it is not uncommon to hear references to other systems such as Neer and Robinson. For this reason, we thought it was relevant to include the following information for reference.

The Allman Classification system classifies fractures of the clavicle into three groups. Group 1 represents fractures of the middle third and are the most common form. Group 2 fractures are distal to coracoclavicular ligament, and nonunion is common in these cases. Group 3 fractures are located at the proximal end of the clavicle.[26]

The Neer Classification is similarly grouped into three types. Type 1 involves the middle third and represents approximately 80% of fractures. Type 2 involves the distal end and accounts for 15% of fractures. Type 3 or medial third clavicle fractures account for only 5% of fractures.[27]

The Robinson Classification consists of three broad categories with further subdivision. Type 1 are fractures of the medial fifth and can be undisplaced (a) or displaced (b). Type 1a1 and 1a2 are nondisplaced extra-articular and intra-articular, respectively. Similarly, Type 1b1 and 1b2 are displaced extra-articular and intra-articular, respectively. Type 2 are fractures of the middle three-fifths of the clavicle. Type 2a1 are nondisplaced cortical alignment fractures, whereas Type 2a2 are angulated cortical alignment fractures. Type 2b are displaced fractures and can be simple, wedge comminution (b1) or multifragmented and segmental (b2). Type 3 fractures involve the lateral fifth of the clavicle and can be nondisplaced extra-articular (a1), nondisplaced intra-articular (a2), displaced extra-articular (b1), or displaced intra-articular (b2).[2]

DIAGNOSIS AND MANAGEMENT
History and Physical Examination

Clavicle fractures occur during acute injuries or trauma. Patients will present with localized pain, swelling, crepitus, deformity, and occasionally, tenting of the skin. When evaluating a patient for clavicle fracture, clinicians should acknowledge the possibility of vascular or neurological damage due to the proximity of vascular structures and the brachial plexus as it may impact the decision to elect surgical or nonsurgical treatment. Assessing the structural integrity of the AC and SC joints is also important. In most cases, there will be a deformity directly over the location of the fracture although this is less common with lateral and nondisplaced medial fractures. The fracture may be mobile and may be associated with crepitus.

In addition to musculoskeletal testing, thorough neurologic examination should be performed for both motor and sensory nerves. In particular, the medial branch of the supraclavicular nerve is at the highest risk of injury.[24] A purely sensory nerve injury to this branch results in numbness of the skin overlying the clavicle. While uncommon, brachial plexus injuries can occur due to acute elongation of nerve fibers or compression from bone fragments or soft-tissue edema.[28]

The lungs and subclavian artery can also be involved in cases of traumatic fracture. It is estimated that pneumothorax may occur in 3% of midclavicular fractures and hemothorax in 1% of midclavicular fractures.[24] These pathologies are often detected during the primary trauma survey with diagnosis confirmed by radiographs. Injury to the subclavian artery is another rare complication of the clavicle fracture that can be life-threatening. Penetrating or blunt trauma can cause rupture, pseudoaneurysm, dissection, or thrombosis.[29] Evaluation of the subclavian artery can be performed using the brachial-brachial index as well as vascular ultrasound or computed tomography (CT) scan.

Diagnostic Imaging

Radiographic evaluation for all clavicle fractures should include an anteroposterior radiograph as well as an apical oblique radiograph with 15° to 40° of cephalic angulation.[30] For evaluation of the AC joint and clavicle, the Zanca view requires 10° to 15° of cephalic angulation to remove the overlap between the AC joint and acromion.[30] Upright positioning as compared to supine positioning better demonstrates clavicle fracture displacement and shortening.[31] Weighted views can help identify inconspicuous fractures but are rarely performed because they provide limited information for management and increase patient discomfort.[32] CT angiogram should be performed when neurological or vascular damage is suspected, especially for proximal fractures. CT can also be useful for preoperative planning to assess the degree of displacement, comminution, and shortening of the clavicle.

Management

Detailed discussion of treatment of clavicle fractures is found in other chapters within this text and will be only briefly included here. Above all, absolute and relative indications for surgery should inform treatment decisions. While a trial of conservative treatment in nonathletes may help most patients avoid surgery and its associated risks, the stakes are higher for an athlete. Time sidelined by injury equates to at least loss of a hobby for the recreational athlete and, at worst, loss of salary/career opportunities for the professional. The higher union rate (95% vs 64% at 1 year for distal one-third fractures) and faster time to radiographic union (mean 28.4 vs 16.4 weeks for midshaft fractures) for surgical treatment quantify its improved reliability compared with conservative management.[33,34]

When opting for surgical management, fracture location and orientation will guide implant choice. The increased load placed on the fixation construct by the contact athlete compared to the general population would indicate the use of more robust hardware such as larger plates or dual plate constructs.

Minimizing time from injury to surgery not only facilitates fracture reduction intraoperatively but also accelerates the recovery timeline. Regardless of surgical or nonsurgical treatment, a period of rest and immobilization is prescribed before physical therapy begins. Although there is no clear consensus on duration or type of immobilization with nonoperative treatment, a period of immobilization of at least 3 to 4 weeks is typically recommended to allow fracture union.[35] With surgical treatment, active-assisted range-of-motion exercises may begin after 1 week in our postoperative protocol. To maintain the chronological advantage of surgical stabilization in the early healing stages, we recommend surgery within the first 1 to 2 weeks after injury.

RETURN TO PLAY

The detrimental effects of a clavicle fracture can be underappreciated. Although approximately 80% of patients return to their preinjury level of sports participation, return to sport times vary widely depending on the election of surgical management and rehabilitation protocols.[36] For athletes with a clavicle fracture, minimizing the time away from sports participation must be balanced with the safety of return to play. Important factors to consider include the age and skeletal maturity of the patient, the severity and complexity of the fracture, and the type and level of sport the patient participates in, as well as his or her position(s). Before clearing an athlete for sports participation, it is important to ensure there is evidence of complete healing of the clavicle based on radiographs and clinical assessment. Evidence of healing based on radiographs is demonstrated by consolidation or callus at the fracture site. The adequacy of clinical healing is marked by minimal tenderness to palpation, complete range of motion, and normal strength when compared to the contralateral side.

For patients who undergo surgical management, a period of immobilization following surgery is recommended followed by a gradually progressive course of physical therapy. Many protocols call for 2 to 3 weeks of immobilization with physical therapy and strengthening starting around 6 weeks postoperatively.[33,37] Other recommendations are more aggressive, mandating only 10 days of immobilization in a sling, followed by range-of-motion exercises, and strengthening and gradual return to sport starting at 6 weeks postoperatively.[38] In general, earlier rehabilitation is associated with earlier return to play, but individualized protocols should be designed based on fracture characteristics and patient factors.

The type of sport in which the patient participates factors significantly in the return-to-sport time, with contact sports generally taking the longest. Return to sport may be recommended as early as 3 to 6 weeks for noncontact sports and 8 to 12 weeks for contact sports.[14,39] For professional cyclists treated with plate fixations of clavicle fractures, the return time to activity and competition can be as early as 10 days and 3 weeks, respectively.[14] Vora and colleagues found that 17 National Football League (NFL) players who sustained clavicle fractures experienced a 3.5-month return to competition, albeit without impact on subsequent performance.[40]

Return to sport with conservatively managed clavicle fractures is dependent on time to union prior to commencing range-of-motion exercises, and refracture risk is incurred with early return. In a study of clavicle fractures among NFL athletes over 5 seasons, 4 out of 7 displaced midshaft clavicle fractures treated without surgery went on to refracture within 1 year of the initial injury.[41] As a result, athletes may experience delayed return times and lose opportunities to participate in competition. The 4 athletes who sustained a refracture in this cohort lost a mean of 1.5 seasons as a result of their original and subsequent injuries.[41]

Early operative stabilization of the fracture site facilitates earlier initiation of range of motion and return to competition.[24] In a retrospective review of 54 athletes, Ranalletta and colleagues found that operative treatment of clavicle fractures enabled early and safe return to sport at a mean of 68 days, with over 90% of patients returning to the same level of sport.[42] Similarly, Meisterling and colleagues reviewed 29 athletes who underwent surgical treatment for midshaft clavicle fractures and found the average time for return to sport was 83 days.[43] Over 20% of patients were participating in sports before 6 weeks, without increased risk of complication for the accelerated return.[43]

In a systematic review of clavicle fractures treated conservatively and operatively, Robertson and Wood found that approximately 80% of athletes will have the capacity to play at their preinjury level of activity.[36] However, return rates to preinjury level of play for conservatively managed displaced midshaft fractures were significantly lower than those for operatively managed fractures. For patients who received operative treatment, there was no significant difference between the return rates to preinjury level of play for plate fixation versus intramedullary nailing. The study also found a statistically significant 12-week difference in return times for conservatively managed displaced midshaft fractures as compared to operatively managed fractures (21.5 vs 9.4 weeks, respectively), but no difference between conservatively managed nondisplaced midshaft fractures and operatively managed fractures.[36]

Assessing clavicle fractures treated by ORIF in NFL players, two separate studies found that 50% and 44% of players were able to return to play in the same 18-week season.[41,44] In the athletes with displaced midshaft clavicle fractures, 4 of 13 athletes were able to return to football during the same season. In the surgical group, 3 athletes returned at a mean of 8 weeks postoperatively, while 1 conservatively treated athlete returned at 10 weeks after injury and sustained a refracture 1 week after return.[41]

Jack and colleagues found that clavicle fractures managed operatively returned at 211 ± 145 days on average.[44] In another study by the same authors, conservatively managed clavicle fractures returned after a mean 245 ± 120 days.[45] Because the authors defined return to sport as return to game participation, the large standard deviation was likely due to the time within the season that the injury occurred. This difference of almost 5 weeks can significantly impact an individual's ability to return within an 18-week regular season.

Other studies have found similar relationships between surgical treatment and quicker return to play. One study of 188 clavicle fractures in professional road cyclists found an average return time of 54 days for surgically treated fractures versus 59 days for conservatively managed fractures.[17] Looking at the safety of return to play in National Hockey League ice hockey players, researchers found that the average time from injury to return to sport was 65 days in the operative group and 98 days in the nonoperative group.[46]

Implant choice for fixation of the clavicle is discussed in depth in other chapters, but here, we highlight considerations for return to play. Time to return to play and return rates were shown to be similar between midshaft fractures treated with plate and those treated with intramedullary fixation.[36] A systematic review and meta-analysis of biomechanical studies showed that superior plating had higher stiffness and greater load to failure in bending and torsion than intramedullary fixation, with no differences in rotational strength.[47] The bending failure torque was greater for the clavicle after removal of the intramedullary device than after removal of the plate and screws.[47] Another biomechanical study showed no significant differences in bending, torsional, or axial compression strength of dual mini-fragment plate fixation compared with larger anterior or superior plating.[48]

After healing is demonstrated by radiographic and clinical indices, hardware management varies by fixation method. If pinning is elected, routine removal of intramedullary pins is recommended after radiographic union.[49] Otherwise plate and screw constructs are usually left in place unless there is irritation. In that case, the hardware can be removed after complete fracture healing. Return to play after intramedullary pin removal may occur after 4 weeks assuming stable radiographic appearance of the fracture site.[49] A systematic review and meta-analysis found that refracture after hardware removal was more common with plate and screw fixation than with intramedullary fixation.[50] There is no published consensus regarding return to play after plate and screw removal, but the risk of refracture is rate-limiting. The authors recommend return to play once the surgical incision has appropriately healed assuming radiographs show adequate union after hardware removal; this may be as early as 2 weeks for noncontact sports and 4 weeks for contact athletes. Risk factors for refracture after removal of clavicle plate and screws have been found to include female sex and lower body mass index[51] and simple or segmental fracture patterns.[52] Other than fracture pattern, neither study determined any radiographic parameters conferring increased risk for refracture after hardware removal.

OUR APPROACH TO REHAB AFTER ORIF

Goals for the immediate postoperative period include maintaining stability of the fracture and pain control. The use of a sling for immobilization and the judicious use of narcotic medication is recommended for the first week. A progressive rehab course is initiated by week 2, with the ultimate objective of regaining normal shoulder range of motion, restoring normal upper-extremity strength and endurance, and allowing the patient to return to at least the preinjury level of sports participation. The following protocol (**Fig. 1**) is composed of general guidelines that may be adjusted by the

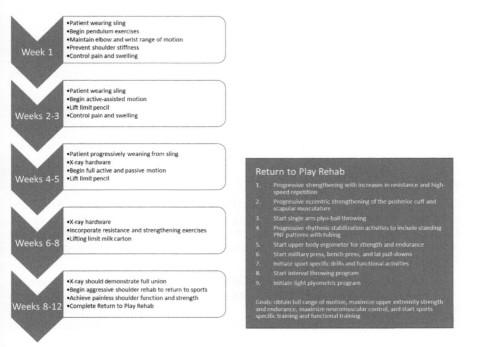

Week 1
• Patient wearing sling
• Begin pendulum exercises
• Maintain elbow and wrist range of motion
• Prevent shoulder stiffness
• Control pain and swelling

Weeks 2-3
• Patient wearing sling
• Begin active-assisted motion
• Lift limit pencil
• Control pain and swelling

Weeks 4-5
• Patient progressively weaning from sling
• X-ray hardware
• Begin full active and passive motion
• Lift limit pencil

Weeks 6-8
• X-ray hardware
• Incorporate resistance and strengthening exercises
• Lifting limit milk carton

Weeks 8-12
• X-ray should demonstrate full union
• Begin aggressive shoulder rehab to return to sports
• Achieve painless shoulder function and strength
• Complete Return to Play Rehab

Return to Play Rehab
1. Progressive strengthening with increases in resistance and high-speed repetition
2. Progressive eccentric strengthening of the posterior cuff and scapular musculature
3. Start single arm plyo-ball throwing
4. Progressive rhythmic stabilization activities to include standing PNF patterns with tubing
5. Start upper body ergometer for strength and endurance
6. Start military press, bench press, and lat pull-downs
7. Initiate sport specific drills and functional activities
8. Start interval throwing program
9. Initiate light plyometric program

Goals: obtain full range of motion, maximize upper extremity strength and endurance, maximize neuromuscular control, and start sports specific training and functional training

Fig. 1. An overview of the rehabilitation program for operative management of clavicle fractures.

athletic trainer or physical therapist based on individual patient progression and capabilities. Radiographic healing should also be monitored throughout the rehabilitation process.

Ultimately, safe return to sport for the patient requires adequate strength, flexibility, and endurance. Return following ORIF of the clavicle requires complete fracture union to minimize risk of reinjury and return of strength and shoulder motion on functional testing. Symptoms such as pain, swelling, or instability should be closely monitored by the patient throughout rehabilitation and as he or she reinitiates sport activities.

After ORIF, we recommend an intensive 12-week protocol for complete recovery of strength and range of motion. Physical therapy should be initiated within the first week postoperatively. Many of the early stages can be performed at home after being taught proper form.

Week 1

The patient is in a sling that may be removed for pendulum exercises. The patient should have no active shoulder motion but can perform elbow and wrist range-of-motion exercises without resistance. The goals for this phase of rehabilitation include maintaining elbow and wrist range of motion, preventing shoulder stiffness, and controlling pain and swelling. It is imperative that the repair is protected.

Weeks 2 to 3

The patient should continue to wear the sling, but it may be removed for exercises. The patient can begin active-assisted motion and should continue pendulum exercises. The rope and pulley can be used for flexion and scaption. The patient should not lift anything heavier than a pencil in the operative hand. Goals for this phase include initiating shoulder range of motion and preventing pain. The repair should continue to be protected.

Weeks 4 to 5

The patient should progressively wean from sling. If radiographs demonstrate no change to the hardware, the patient may begin full active and passive motion. However, there is no lifting of anything heavier than a pencil.

Weeks 6 to 8

If radiographs are showing signs of union, the patient may begin to slowly incorporate resistance and strengthening exercises. Lifting limitations are a carton of milk.

Weeks 8 to 12

Once radiographs demonstrate union and 2 weeks of resistance exercises have been performed, the patient should work on aggressive shoulder rehab to return to sports. Once painless shoulder function has been achieved and strength has returned, an athlete may return to play when he or she has completed the return-to-play rehab. This consists of the following steps.

1. Progressive strengthening with increases in resistance and high-speed repetition
2. Progressive eccentric strengthening of the posterior cuff and scapular musculature
3. Start single arm plyo-ball throwing
4. Progressive rhythmic stabilization activities to include standing PNF patterns with tubing
5. Start upper-body ergometer for strength and endurance
6. Start military press, bench press, and lat pull-downs

7. Initiate sport-specific drills and functional activities
8. Start an interval throwing program
9. Initiate a light plyometric program

The goals of this final phase are obtaining full range of motion, maximizing upper-extremity strength and endurance, maximizing neuromuscular control, and starting sports-specific training and functional training.

More aggressive rehabilitation protocols have been described in the literature. A case report of a football player demonstrated safe return to the field in 6 weeks following surgical treatment and accelerated rehabilitation.[53] The authors initiated early and progressive rehabilitation focused on strength and range of motion, as well as maintaining cardiovascular fitness. Weekly radiographs were obtained to monitor healing. By week 4, the athlete was working on advanced strengthening exercises and participating in noncontact practices. By week 5, he demonstrated full strength and range of motion and was cleared for full contact.[53] Further studies should be conducted to demonstrate the effectiveness and reliability of an accelerated approach. The safety of expedited rehabilitation protocols has not been directly compared to more conservative approaches, and rehabilitation should always be individualized to the patient and sport.

CASE PRESENTATION

A 22-year-old collegiate football player sustained a displaced, middle one-third left clavicle fracture when landing on his shoulder after diving for a successful touchdown reception. This injury occurred during the season opener. He had no skin compromise or clinical evidence of neurologic injury. Radiographs were obtained, showing a displaced, angulated Type 1 clavicle fracture (**Fig. 2**), and he was scheduled for ORIF on postinjury day #2. The timing of the injury during the college football "Week 0" allowed potential return to football during the same season, and the cited evidence regarding higher rates of return to play and lower refracture rate influenced our decision to recommend surgery. We also considered that his position as a wide receiver and that the injury affected his nondominant upper extremity would impart more stability than the same injury in the dominant arm of a throwing athlete. In this case, the inferior cortex was found to be intact intraoperatively. A 3.5-mm plate was contoured to the superior surface of the clavicle. He was placed in a sling and placed in the standard postoperative protocol. He attended daily therapy sessions with the team athletic trainers.

Radiographs at 8 weeks postoperatively showed fracture union (**Fig. 3**), and he demonstrated full strength and range of motion in therapy. He participated in receiving

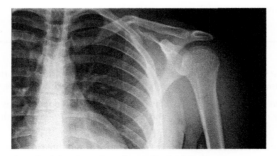

Fig. 2. Anteroposterior clavicle view showing left clavicle fracture.

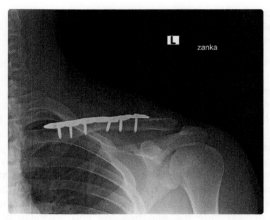

Fig. 3. Anteroposterior clavicle radiograph at 8 weeks postoperatively, showing reduction and fixation with a 3.5-mm superior plate and screws and consolidation at the fracture site.

drills prior to return to game situations. He was cleared for return to football for the team's final 4 games of the regular season. He ultimately returned to his previous level of performance, catching two passes for 67 yards receiving in the team's end-of-season bowl game at just under 4 months postoperatively.

SUMMARY

Clavicle fractures are some of the most common fractures among athletes. The type of sport is directly related to fracture risk, with athletes participating in football, soccer, snowboarding, bicycling, wrestling, and snow skiing having the highest risk of clavicle injury. Surgical versus nonoperative treatment of clavicle fractures in the athlete is determined primarily from physical examination and imaging studies, with special consideration of the importance of attempting return to sport within the same season, if feasible. Surgical strategies for successful early return to sport and prevention of reinjury include early timing of surgery, maximizing the biomechanical strength of the fixation construct, and a graduated progression through rehabilitation protocols. Guidelines for return to athletic competition are influenced by radiographic and clinical evidence of fracture healing, restoration of functional range of motion and strength, and sport-specific drills.

CLINICS CARE POINTS

Pearls

- For displaced fractures, surgical intervention results in higher rates of return to play, shorter return-to-play times, and lower incidence of refracture than nonoperative treatment.

- Use of a 3.5-mm superior contoured plate or a dual-plate construct has been shown to provide superior resistance to bending and torsional forces compared with intramedullary fixation.

- When plate removal is indicated, refracture risk is higher than that of intramedullary implant removal but remains low overall.

Pitfalls

- While pressure to accelerate return to play may be applied by the athlete and his or her parents, coaches, and/or agents, resumption of contact before radiographic and clinical healing carries an increased risk of reinjury that diminishes with increased time from stabilization.
- Conservative treatment avoids risks of surgery on the front end but results in increased risks of symptomatic nonunion and refracture, which double loss of playing time and may ultimately require surgery.

DISCLOSURE

K.J.C. reports speaking fees from Arthrex, Inc. and Smith & Nephew and research support from Arthrex, Inc. and Food and Drug Administration (FDA) outside the submitted work. The other authors have no disclosures.

REFERENCES

1. Nordqvist A, Petersson C. The incidence of fractures of the clavicle. Clin Orthop Relat Res 1994;300:127–32.
2. Robinson CM. Fractures of the clavicle in the adult. Epidemiology and classification. J Bone Joint Surg Br 1998;80(3):476–84.
3. Postacchini F, Gumina S, De Santis P, et al. Epidemiology of clavicle fractures. J Shoulder Elbow Surg 2002;11(5):452–6.
4. Court-Brown CM, Wood AM, Aitken S. The epidemiology of acute sports-related fractures in adults. Injury 2008;39(12):1365–72.
5. DeFroda SF, Lemme N, Kleiner J, et al. Incidence and mechanism of injury of clavicle fractures in the NEISS database: Athletic and non athletic injuries. J Clin Orthop Trauma 2019;10(5):954–8.
6. Van Tassel D, Owens BD, Pointer L, et al. Incidence of clavicle fractures in sports: analysis of the NEISS Database. Int J Sports Med 2014;35(1):83–6.
7. Aitken SA, Watson BS, Wood AM, et al. Sports-related fractures in South East Scotland: an analysis of 990 fractures. J Orthop Surg 2014;22(3):313–7.
8. Kaplan LD, Flanigan DC, Norwig J, et al. Prevalence and variance of shoulder injuries in elite collegiate football players. Am J Sports Med 2005;33(8):1142–6.
9. Twomey-Kozak J, Whitlock KG, O'Donnell JA, et al. Epidemiology of Sports-Related Clavicle Fractures in the United States: Injuries From 2015 to 2019. Orthop J Sports Med 2022;10(10). https://doi.org/10.1177/23259671221126553. 23259671221126553.
10. McCarthy MM, Bihl JH, Frank RM, et al. Epidemiology of Clavicle Fractures Among US High School Athletes, 2008-2009 Through 2016-2017. Orthop J Sports Med 2019;7(7). https://doi.org/10.1177/2325967119861812. 2325967119861812.
11. Ishimaru D, Ogawa H, Wakahara K, et al. Hip pads reduce the overall risk of injuries in recreational snowboarders. Br J Sports Med 2012;46(15):1055–8.
12. Oberle L, Pierpoint L, Spittler J, et al. Epidemiology of Clavicle Fractures Sustained at a Colorado Ski Resort. Orthop J Sports Med 2021;9(5). 23259671211006722.
13. Kim S, Endres NK, Johnson RJ, et al. Snowboarding injuries: trends over time and comparisons with alpine skiing injuries. Am J Sports Med 2012;40(4):770–6.
14. van der Ven DJC, Timmers TK, Broeders IAMJ, et al. Displaced Clavicle Fractures in Cyclists: Return to Athletic Activity After Anteroinferior Plate Fixation. Clin J Sport Med 2019;29(6):465–9.

15. Fancourt HS, Vrancic S, Neeman T, et al. Serious cycling-related fractures in on and off-road accidents: A retrospective analysis in the Australian Capital Territory region. Injury 2022;53(10):3233–9.

16. Bigdon SF, Hecht V, Fairhurst PG, et al. Injuries in alpine summer sports - types, frequency and prevention: a systematic review. BMC Sports Sci Med Rehabil 2022;14(1):79.

17. Konarski A, Walmsley M, Jain N. Return to competition following clavicle fractures in professional road cyclists. J Orthop 2022;34:100–3.

18. Edler C, Droste JN, Anemüller R, et al. Injuries in elite road cyclists during competition in one UCI WorldTour season: a prospective epidemiological study of incidence and injury burden. Phys Sportsmed 2023;51(2):129–38.

19. Haeberle HS, Navarro SM, Power EJ, et al. Prevalence and Epidemiology of Injuries Among Elite Cyclists in the Tour de France. Orthop J Sports Med 2018; 6(9). 2325967118793392.

20. Herteleer M, Winckelmans T, Hoekstra H, et al. Epidemiology of clavicle fractures in a level 1 trauma center in Belgium. Eur J Trauma Emerg Surg 2018;44(5): 717–26.

21. Kugelman D, Paoli A, Mai D, et al. Urban Cycling Expansion is Associated with an Increased Number of Clavicle Fractures. Bull Hosp Jt Dis 2020;78(2):101–7.

22. Nowak J, Mallmin H, Larsson S. The aetiology and epidemiology of clavicular fractures. A prospective study during a two-year period in Uppsala, Sweden. Injury 2000;31(5):353–8.

23. Stanley D, Trowbridge EA, Norris SH. The mechanism of clavicular fracture. A clinical and biomechanical analysis. J Bone Joint Surg Br 1988;70(3):461–4.

24. Rowe CR. An atlas of anatomy and treatment of midclavicular fractures. Clin Orthop Relat Res 1968;58:29–42.

25. Aitken SA. The epidemiology of fractures of the upper limb, lower limb and pelvis in adults. University of Edinburgh; 2013.

26. Allman FL Jr. Fractures and ligamentous injuries of the clavicle and its articulation. J Bone Joint Surg Am 1967;49(4):774–84.

27. Neer CS 2nd. Fractures of the distal third of the clavicle. Clin Orthop Relat Res 1968;58:43–50.

28. Fozzato S, Petrucci QA, Passeri A, et al. Brachial plexus paralysis in a patient with clavicular fracture, medico-legal implications. Acta Biomed 2022;93(4):e2022285.

29. Buchanan DAS, Owen D, Angliss R, et al. Acute subclavian artery occlusion with associated clavicle fracture managed with bypass graft alone. BMJ Case Rep 2018;2018. bcr2018224719.

30. Sandstrom CK, Gross JA, Kennedy SA. Distal clavicle fracture radiography and treatment: a pictorial essay. Emerg Radiol 2018;25(3):311–9.

31. Backus JD, Merriman DJ, McAndrew CM, et al. Upright versus supine radiographs of clavicle fractures: does positioning matter? J Orthop Trauma 2014; 28(11):636–41.

32. Yap JJ, Curl LA, Kvitne RS, et al. The value of weighted views of the acromioclavicular joint. Results of a survey. Am J Sports Med 1999;27(6):806–9.

33. Canadian Orthopaedic Trauma Society. Nonoperative treatment compared with plate fixation of displaced midshaft clavicular fractures. A multicenter, randomized clinical trial. J Bone Joint Surg Am 2007;89(1):1–10.

34. Hall JA, Schemitsch CE, Vicente MR, et al. Operative Versus Nonoperative Treatment of Acute Displaced Distal Clavicle Fractures: A Multicenter Randomized Controlled Trial. J Orthop Trauma 2021;35(12):660–6.

35. Postacchini R, Gumina S, Farsetti P, et al. Long-term results of conservative management of midshaft clavicle fracture. Int Orthop 2010;34(5):731–6.
36. Robertson GA, Wood AM. Return to sport following clavicle fractures: a systematic review. Br Med Bull 2016;119(1):111–28.
37. Robinson CM, Goudie EB, Murray IR, et al. Open reduction and plate fixation versus nonoperative treatment for displaced midshaft clavicular fractures: a multicenter, randomized, controlled trial. J Bone Joint Surg Am 2013;95(17):1576–84.
38. McKee RC, Whelan DB, Schemitsch EH, et al. Operative versus nonoperative care of displaced midshaft clavicular fractures: a meta-analysis of randomized clinical trials. J Bone Joint Surg Am 2012;94(8):675–84.
39. Pujalte GG, Housner JA. Management of clavicle fractures. Curr Sports Med Rep 2008;7(5):275–80.
40. Vora D, Baker M, Pandarinath R. Impact of Clavicle Fractures on Return to Play and Performance Ratings in NFL Athletes. Clin J Sport Med 2019;29(6):459–64.
41. Morgan RJ, Bankston LS Jr, Hoenig MP, et al. Evolving management of middle-third clavicle fractures in the National Football League. Am J Sports Med 2010; 38(10):2092–6.
42. Ranalletta M, Rossi LA, Piuzzi NS, et al. Return to sports after plate fixation of displaced midshaft clavicular fractures in athletes. Am J Sports Med 2015;43(3): 565–9.
43. Meisterling SW, Cain EL, Fleisig GS, et al. Return to athletic activity after plate fixation of displaced midshaft clavicle fractures. Am J Sports Med 2013;41(11): 2632–6.
44. Jack RA 2nd, Sochacki KR, Navarro SM, et al. Performance and Return to Sport After Clavicle Open Reduction and Internal Fixation in National Football League Players. Orthop J Sports Med 2017;5(8). 2325967117720677.
45. Jack RA 2nd, Sochacki KR, Navarro SM, et al. Performance and Return to Sport After Nonoperative Treatment of Clavicle Fractures in National Football League Players. Orthopedics 2017;40(5):e836–43.
46. Hebert-Davies J, Agel J. Return to elite-level sport after clavicle fractures. BMJ Open Sport Exerc Med 2018;4(1):e000371.
47. Hulsmans MH, van Heijl M, Houwert RM, et al. Surgical fixation of midshaft clavicle fractures: A systematic review of biomechanical studies. Injury 2018;49(4): 753–65.
48. Ferguson DP, Baker HP, Dillman D, et al. Dual mini-fragment plate fixation of midshaft clavicle fractures is biomechanically equivalent to anatomic pre-contoured plating [published online ahead of print, 2022 Apr 12]. Eur J Orthop Surg Traumatol 2022. https://doi.org/10.1007/s00590-022-03268-1.
49. Fritz EM, van der Meijden OA, Hussain ZB, et al. Intramedullary Fixation of Midshaft Clavicle Fractures. J Orthop Trauma 2017;31(Suppl 3):S42–4.
50. Houwert RM, Smeeing DP, Ahmed Ali U, et al. Plate fixation or intramedullary fixation for midshaft clavicle fractures: a systematic review and meta-analysis of randomized controlled trials and observational studies. J Shoulder Elbow Surg 2016;25(7):1195–203.
51. Tsai SW, Ma HH, Hsu FW, et al. Risk factors for refracture after plate removal for midshaft clavicle fracture after bone union. J Orthop Surg Res 2019;14(1):457.
52. Park HY, Kim SJ, Sur YJ, et al. Refracture after locking compression plate removal in displaced midshaft clavicle fractures after bony union: a retrospective study. Clin Shoulder Elb 2021;24(2):72–9.
53. Rabe SB, Oliver GD. Clavicular fracture in a collegiate football player: a case report of rapid return to play. J Athl Train 2011;46(1):107–11.

Clavicle Nonunion and Malunion

Surgical Interventions for Functional Improvement

Alirio J. deMeireles, MD, MBA, Natalia Czerwonka, MD,
William N. Levine, MD*

KEYWORDS

- Clavicle • Clavicle nonunion • Clavicle malunion • Bone grafting
- Clavicle shortening • Revision surgery

KEY POINTS

- Clavicle nonunion or malunion occurs in 5% to 15% of clavicle fractures treated nonoperatively and can cause significant shoulder pain and dysfunction.
- At our institution, nonunions and malunions are typically addressed with superiorly positioned, precontoured compression plating.
- The need for biological augmentation, whether autograft or allograft, is debated. The authors prefer to use allograft augmentation particularly in the setting of atrophic nonunion.
- With careful preoperative planning and meticulous surgical technique, radiographic union and good to excellent clinical outcomes are reliably achieved after operative management of these complex injuries.

INTRODUCTION

Clavicle fractures are common injuries, comprising 2% to 10% of all fractures in adults, with roughly 75% occurring at the middle third of the bone, 20% at the distal third, and the remaining occurring medially.[1,2] Owing to excellent early outcomes studies, most of these fractures were treated nonoperatively.[3,4] Nonunions of the clavicle have been historically considered as rare, with Neer referring to the clavicle as the "invincible bone."[3] However, more recent evidence demonstrates variability in healing by subtype and suggests there are specific subsets of patient and fracture characteristics associated with higher risk of poor outcome, including nonunion or malunion. Modern studies have shown that nonunion after nonoperative treatment occurs in

Department of Orthopedic Surgery, Columbia University Irving Medical Center-NewYork Presbyterian Hospital, New York, NY, USA
* Corresponding author. 622 West 168th Street, PH-1130, New York, NY 10032
E-mail address: wnl1@cumc.columbia.edu

Clin Sports Med 42 (2023) 663–675
https://doi.org/10.1016/j.csm.2023.05.012
0278-5919/23/© 2023 Elsevier Inc. All rights reserved.

5.9% to 15% of patients depending on fracture subtype.[1,5] As more detailed patient-reported outcome measures become the standard, there seems to be a greater recognition of functional deficits in this patient population than previously considered.[6] Thus, it is important for surgeons to understand the treatment principles of these challenging pathologic conditions. To that end, the purpose of this article is to provide a brief overview of the diagnosis and workup of clavicle nonunion and malunion, followed by a comprehensive review of the surgical techniques used to address this condition.

BACKGROUND

Malunion and nonunion of the clavicle can severely affect its function.[7] Although most clavicle fractures treated nonoperatively go on to some degree of malunion, most of these are mild and asymptomatic.[6] However, particularly with large initial displacement, significant malunion and subsequent deformity can occur. In this setting, the native kinematics of the clavicle are altered, and patients may experience pain, decreased strength and endurance, and dissatisfaction with cosmesis.[8] Further, computational studies have demonstrated that with progressive shortening of the clavicle, there is a resultant decrease in the moment-generating capacity of the shoulder, leading to impaired shoulder abduction, flexion, and internal rotation.[9]

Similar to symptomatic malunion, nonunion can cause a significant deleterious effect on patient outcomes. Subsequently, many studies have attempted to highlight patient-specific and fracture-specific risk factors that predispose to nonunion. Patient-specific risk factors are potentially modifiable variables and are imperative to optimize. Advanced age, female gender, obesity, poor functional status, malnutrition, vitamin deficiencies, smoking, infection, and certain medications or treatment modalities such as radiation and chemotherapy increase the odds of a poor outcome.[10,11] Fracture-specific factors include shortening greater than 2 cm, high degree of fracture comminution, and Neer type II fractures.[6,12,13] Although neither the aforementioned patient nor fracture characteristics represent an absolute indication for surgery, they should be discussed with the patient during the shared decision-making process and can help guide initial operative versus nonoperative management decisions.

CLINICAL SYMPTOMS, DIAGNOSIS, AND WORKUP

Patients with clavicle malunion will often present with weakness, easy fatiguability, and cosmetic complaints. More rarely, they may present with scapular winging or symptoms of thoracic outlet syndrome. Similarly, symptomatic nonunion patients commonly complain of pain, impaired shoulder function, easy fatigability with overhead activity, and suboptimal mobility.[14,15]

A comprehensive history and physical examination are essential when evaluating patients with clavicle malunions and nonunions. A thorough interview should clarify the details surrounding the injury itself, medical comorbidities, surgical history, current and recent medications, and the patient's social situation. Understanding patient-specific risk factors allows the surgeon to both identify the root cause(s) of nonunion and to optimize the chance of successful treatment. The physical examination includes the evaluation of the injured and contralateral clavicle, ipsilateral upper extremity, and cervical spine.

Routine laboratory work is not considered mandatory for cases of malunion. In cases of nonunion, surgeons should consider obtaining a complete blood count, erythrocyte sedimentation rate, c-reactive protein, vitamin D level, and calcium levels because these may provide important information regarding infection and bone health. Malnutrition laboratories, including serum albumin, total lymphocyte count, and ferritin can be considered, although we do not send these routinely for all patients. Cotinine testing has been shown in the arthroplasty literature to both aid in smoking cessation programs as well as to verify patient compliance with smoking cessation.[16]

Plain radiographs are often sufficient to diagnose nonunion or malunion. A standard radiographic series involves anteroposterior view of the bilateral clavicles and a 45° cephalic tilt radiograph of the injured clavicle. If available, serial plain radiographs from the time of initial injury should be evaluated to understand the evolution of the fracture.

Computed tomography (CT) scans are not routinely used to evaluate clavicle non-unions and malunions, although they can provide details in multiple planes that may be beneficial in surgical decision-making and planning in the setting of complex deformities. CT scans also allow for a more precise understanding of the degree of fracture healing, if any. In our practice, we obtain a CT scan for patients who have undergone previous open reduction and internal fixation of a clavicle where nonunion is suspected on plain radiographs. In addition, for any patient who wishes to proceed with hardware removal (minimum 2 years postoperatively), we obtain a CT to ensure that their "pain" is truly from the hardware, and not an unrecognized nonunion.

TREATMENT
Overview

The goal of treatment is to ensure a stable clavicle that is painless through full active range of motion. To achieve this, it is helpful to determine why the fracture did not heal and subsequently, how it can be treated based on the possible causes of nonunion.

Clavicle malunions or nonunions that are asymptomatic often do not require surgical intervention.[13,17] Patients with painful malunion, painful nonunion, those with decreased function, associated thoracic outlet syndrome, brachial plexus neuropathy, or associated vascular injury should be considered for surgery.[18]

Resection Procedure

Partial or entire clavicle resection has largely fallen out of favor because it negatively affects shoulder stability and function. Historically, it was used in the treatment of concomitant thoracic outlet syndrome or subclavian vascular compression, with the intent of removing the clavicle to increase costoclavicular space.[19] However, with the improvement of implants and a large body of literature supporting excellent outcomes for modern plating systems, resection is now uncommon.[20–24]

However, in the setting of distal clavicle nonunion or malunion, excision of the distal fragment can be considered if the fragment is too small for fixation, if there is poor bone stock, and if acromioclavicular arthrosis is present.[25,26] There is no general consensus regarding the size of the lateral fragment that dictates whether excision or reconstruction is the appropriate route.

Reconstruction Procedures

Reconstruction techniques for clavicle nonunions include reconstruction plates, locking compression plates, hook plates, coracoclavicular screws, intramedullary fixation, bone grafting, and several combinations of the above.[27–29]

Plating—midshaft clavicle
Biomechanical studies have demonstrated that superior plating provides significantly greater stiffness and fracture rigidity as compared with anterior plating; this has been

attributed to its tension-bearing face and greater moment of resistance because it sits farther away from the inferior cortex compared with the anterior plate.[5,30,31] However, the superior plate has been associated with hardware prominence due to the subcutaneous position of the plate, and consequently has been linked to higher rates of reoperation and hardware removal.[32] Although there are potential downstream disadvantages, superior plating has been shown to result in high levels of bony union following clavicle nonunion. A recent prospective randomized control trial demonstrated that there was no difference in union rates between locking and nonlocking superior plate fixation for displaced midshaft clavicle nonunions; however, there was a statistically significant decreased time to union observed in the locking plate cohort (13 weeks vs 17 weeks, respectively, $P = .009$).[33]

Anterior plates have classically been associated with decreased hardware prominence and improved soft tissue coverage compared with superior plates.[34,35] Recent studies have demonstrated anterior plating to have similar functional outcomes and union rates to superior plating.[32,32,35] Further, both plate locations have similar risks of iatrogenic neurovascular injury, and one has not been proven to be greater than the other at decreasing risks to the brachial plexus and its branches or the subclavian vein and artery.[36,37]

Dual plating is less commonly used to treat clavicle nonunion. The literature is mixed regarding the biomechanical properties of dual plating compared with traditional single plating. Ziegler and colleagues demonstrated that no significant difference in bending stiffness or load to failure was observed among dual mini-plating, superior plating, and anteroinferior plating of midshaft clavicle fractures in 18 cadavers.[38] Prasarn and colleagues also found dual mini-plating to be relatively similar to anterior and superior plating in terms of axial and torsional stiffness, although significantly superior to both in terms of bending stiffness.[20] Recently, Boyce and colleagues investigated the stiffness and survivorship of a combination plate construct (traditional superior plate with additional mini anterior plate) compared with single superior plating and dual mini-plating. This biomechanical study demonstrated that in a comminuted clavicle fracture sawbones model, dual mini-plating demonstrated the lowest stiffness and survivorship of the 3 cohorts, whereas the combination of an anterior mini plate and the conventional superior plate was significantly stiffer and had higher load to failure than the other 2 cohorts.[39] Clinically, dual plating has shown excellent outcomes in terms of achieving bony union after clavicle fracture.[20] However, the literature is lacking on long-term outcomes of dual plating in clavicle nonunions specifically.[40]

Plating—distal clavicle

It has been well established that nonoperative treatment of distal clavicle fractures has a higher relative risk of nonunion, particularly the unstable Neer type II.[41] Fixation is often challenging due to the small size of the lateral fracture fragment, the often-poor bone stock, concurrent coracoclavicular ligament disruption, and potential for iatrogenic trauma to the acromioclavicular joint. Common techniques include hook plating, plate and screw osteosynthesis alone, plating with coracoclavicular reconstruction, and suture fixation.

Hook plates are commonly used for distal clavicle fractures and have been shown to have excellent union rates although with a high rate of postoperative hardware pain and subsequent plate removal.[42,43] More specifically, several studies have shown that after fracture, hook plates result in high union rates ranging from 94% to 100%, similar to that of anterior/superior plates, suture, or pin fixation.[42–46] However, some studies have shown that higher complication and revision rates are associated with hook plates compared with locking plates and coracoclavicular fixation.[42,44] Common complications include rotator cuff impingement, subacromial inflammation, and acromial fractures. Hook plates are removed after a minimum of 3 months from date of implantation to prevent the development of subacromial impingement or iatrogenic rotator cuff pathologic condition. This should be considered and counseled on during the preoperative visit.

As with midshaft clavicle fractures, superior, anterior, and dual plating can be used to treat distal clavicle nonunions as well. Ideally, 3 bicortical screws are needed to achieve adequate plate fixation, which can be challenging if the fracture fragment is small.[47] When there is sufficient bone stock, the fragment is large, and the coracoclavicular ligaments are disrupted, plate fixation is appropriate. In a cadaveric study, Worhacz and colleagues demonstrated that superior precontoured locking plates have significantly greater stiffness and load to failure compared with superior nonlocking and anterior locking constructs in distal Neer type IIA fractures.[48] Conversely, Wilkerson and colleagues showed in 6 cadavers with type IIB fractures that anterior dynamic compression plates had a statistically significant higher load to failure than superior dynamic compression plates. In a clinical case series on unstable distal clavicle fractures, Shin and colleagues found that precontoured anatomic plate fixation has high union rates and satisfactory clinical outcomes, thus demonstrating the utility of precontoured plates in maintaining fixation of unstable distal fractures.[45]

In fracture patterns that involve disruption of the coracoclavicular ligaments, reconstruction of the ligament reconstruction can yield positive outcomes. Yagnik and colleagues demonstrated that all 21 patients with unstable distal clavicle fractures who were treated with a combination of cortical button fixation and coracoclavicular (CC) ligament reconstruction achieved union within 4 months.[49] Further, all patients were reported to have achieved good functional outcomes and satisfaction with their surgery, based on mean improvements in American Shoulder and Elbow Surgeons (ASES) scores and University of California Los Angeles (UCLA) scores.[49] Still, further investigation is warranted before this technique can be recommended over plate fixation. Similarly, though CC ligament reconstruction in combination with plating is an option, it has not been well studied in the setting of distal clavicle nonunion. Rieser and colleagues demonstrated in 21 cadavers that biomechanically, a distal-third locking plate combined with CC ligament reconstruction had increased stiffness, decreased displacement, and maximal resistance to compression compared with either construct alone.[50] A construct that provides greater stiffness and stability may be better suited to prevent hypertrophic nonunion. Clinically, Schliemann and colleagues demonstrated that a combination of locking plate fixation and CC ligament reconstruction led to bony union within 6 to 10 weeks in 14 patients with unstable distal clavicle fractures.[51] Finally, in a case series of 38 patients with distal clavicle nonunion, Robinson and colleagues found that locking plate fixation combined with a tunnel suspensory device led to the achievement of bony union for all patients and low complication rates across the cohort.[52]

It should be noted that there are few studies in the literature directly comparing these fixation techniques and their outcomes in the setting of distal clavicle nonunion. Most of the literature focuses on outcomes following distal clavicle fracture.

Bone Grafting

The need for supplemental bone grafting is the subject of debate in the literature.[53] This is typically recommended with atrophic clavicle nonunions or to achieve appropriate length when segmental defects are present. Autogenous bone grafting (commonly from the iliac crest bone graft [ICBG]) is the gold standard, given its trifecta of osteoinductive, osteoconductive, and osteogenic healing.[22,54–57] In a retrospective review of 34 clavicle nonunions treated with plate fixation and ICBG, all 34 patients achieved bony union.[56] Known disadvantages to this technique include increased operative time, neurogenic injury, donor site pain, hematoma formation, and iliac fracture.[24,58] In a retrospective study, Beirer and colleagues demonstrated that radiographic bony union was achieved in all 14 patients with clavicle nonunion or malunion who were treated with precontoured locking plates and ICBG, with one patient refracturing 3 years after surgery.[59] However, 14% of patients sustained secondary fracture of their anterior superior iliac spine following grafting. Although rare, iliac crest fractures following harvest can be avoided through minimally invasive, percutaneous methods.[60] Bone grafting can be used to treat distal clavicle nonunions as well. In a case series of 10 patients with distal clavicle nonunion, Villa and colleagues found all nonunions healed within 4 months of surgery, after either dual mini-plating with bone graft and single plating with bone graft.[61]

Demineralized bone matrix (DBM) and bone morphogenic protein (BMP) can be used as alternatives to ICBG. Although these methods eliminate donor-site and harvest complications, neither is osteogenic and BMP is solely osteoinductive. Yet, studies thus far have largely demonstrated excellent outcomes whether autograft or allograft is used. Wiss and colleagues reported a series of 78 clavicle nonunions treated with superior plating or dual plating, with or without bone graft via either autogenous ICBG, BMP-2, or BMP-7. The study found that there were no statistically significant differences in healing rates between the type of plate or bone graft used to treat the nonunion. Further, 87.5% of patients healed after their primary nonunion surgery.[24]

Vascularized Bone Grafting

Rarely, vascularized bone graft may be used in settings of chronic or persistent nonunion that have failed to respond to operative reconstruction or atrophic nonunions with significant bone loss. Vascularized bone graft bypasses the process of creeping substitution observed in nonvascularized bone grafting, thus allowing for potentially improved healing processes and revascularization of necrotic bone.[62] Commonly, the vascularized periosteal graft is taken from the medial femoral condyle, iliac crest, fibula, or radius and then anastomosed with the thoracoacromial trunk.[63] There is limited information in the literature regarding the use of vascularized bone reconstruction in clavicle nonunion. In a retrospective series of 7 patients with symptomatic recalcitrant clavicular nonunion who were treated with medial femoral condyle graft, all patients achieved clinical and radiographic union by an average of 15 months; shoulder motion and pain scores improved, and minimal donor site morbidity was observed.[64] Fuchs and colleagues described vascularized medial femoral condyle transfer in 3 patients with atrophic nonunion of the clavicle.[65] In each case, patients achieved bony union by a minimum of 5 months and sustained improvements in their shoulder function, range of motion, and pain levels. Similarly, Momberger and colleagues also demonstrated that vascularized fibular grafting for segmental clavicular nonunion in 3 patients was a successful salvage procedure, which led to radiographic healing and improvements in pain and shoulder function.[63] Ultimately, the results of these studies indicate that vascularized bone grafting is a useful tool for addressing recalcitrant bony nonunion in the clavicle, although we recommend its use as a salvage method.

Intramedullary Procedures

Intramedullary fixation of clavicle nonunion and malunion can be achieved through a variety of methods, such as Kirschner wires, elastic titanium nails, Steinmann pins, or external fixation. Current available literature indicates that intramedullary fixation can achieve similar union rates and clinical outcomes to plating. However, many of these studies have a small sample size or are retrospective in nature. In patients with clavicle malunion, Smekal and colleagues demonstrated that elastic stable intramedullary nailing with corrective osteotomy resulted in 100% bony union and improved disabilities of the arm, shoulder, and hand (DASH) outcomes compared with preoperative levels; however, this case series only consisted of 5 patients.[66] Kleweno and colleagues demonstrated in a retrospective study comparing patients with midshaft clavicle fracture treated with intramedullary pinning versus plating, that patients in the pin group all achieved bony union, with 28% of patients experiencing associated complications. However, the study only included simple and wedge clavicle fractures, raising the point that pinning may not be amenable to fixation of every type of clavicle fracture or nonunion.[67] Ultimately, from a biomechanical perspective, intramedullary fixation results in decreased rigidity compared with plating, and in the setting of nonunion, stable and rigid fixation is the goal. With the paucity of evidence in the current available literature regarding intramedullary fixation in the setting of clavicle nonunion or malunion and the decreased rigidity that intramedullary fixation affords, we recommend plating and its adjuvants for the treatment of clavicle nonunion or malunion.

MALUNION

Similar to nonunions, surgical indications for malunion include pain, functional limitations, and neurologic problems such as brachial plexus compression and thoracic outlet syndrome. Patient dissatisfaction with cosmesis and appearance is also an important consideration not to be overlooked. The standard approach to clavicle malunions is osteotomy through the original fracture plane followed by subsequent plate osteosynthesis. Osteotomy is critical to restore anatomic length, alignment, and rotation. This can be technically challenging because it requires realignment of the bony segments in 3 orthogonal planes and, if not correctly performed, may lead to persistent malunion. The contralateral, uninjured side can be used to gauge the proper length, alignment, and rotation.[68] Both anterior and superior plating can be used. Compression plating, with or without bone grafting, is commonly used. In a case series on 15 patients with midshaft clavicle malunion, McKee and colleagues performed corrective osteotomy and subsequent compression plating; 14 of the patients achieved bony union, clavicle length, and alignment.[7] Further, patient-reported outcomes as measured by DASH were found to improve for all patients ($P = .0001$).[7] Similarly, Hillen and colleagues found that corrective osteotomy followed by posterior-superior plate and screw fixation resulted in 9 out of 10 patients achieving union and significant improvements in patient-reported outcomes as measured by DASH.[69] However, in that study, 7 of the 10 patients did require plate and screw removal due to pain and irritation from the hardware.

COMPLICATIONS

Many of the complications seen with operative management of clavicle nonunion or malunion are the same or similar to the complications of clavicle fractures. Persistent hardware irritation or pain, hardware breakage, or infection can occur.[70] Much of the available literature has shown that union can be reasonably expected after operative management of clavicle nonunion or malunion.[7,20,33,35,51,58,61,69,70] Although infrequent, vascular compromise, thoracic outlet syndrome, or brachial plexopathy following nonunion or malunion have been reported in the literature, largely through case reports.[71] Although there are no standard guidelines for the optimal management of these complications, resection of the callus, neurolysis of brachial plexus, if involved, and the removal of any hardware that may be contributing to symptoms are advised.[72,73]

Overall, complication rates are generally reported to be low after clavicle nonunion intervention. In a systematic review and meta-analysis, Sidler-Maier and colleagues found that the complication rate across 103 patients treated surgically for clavicle

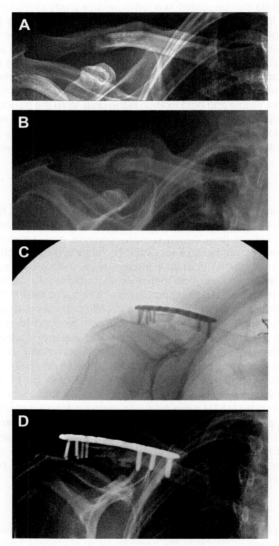

Fig. 1. Caption: Case of a 64-year-old right-hand-dominant woman, (*A*) initially sustained a minimally displaced right lateral clavicle fracture after falling onto the pavement; (*B*) 1 year after her injury, radiographs revealed hypertrophic nonunion of her lateral clavicle; (*C*) She was then treated with a precontoured locking plate (Acumed, Hillsboro, OR, USA) to obtain fixation and (*D*) went on to achieve healing of the distal clavicle nonunion at 5 months follow-up.

malunion was less than 6%.[70] Although infrequent, refracture following callus removal, loss of fixation, and infection were the reported complications.

SUMMARY

Clavicle nonunion and malunion are relatively uncommon but when symptomatic can result in pain and dysfunction that requires surgical intervention. Various reconstructive and grafting techniques are available to achieve stable fixation and union. In the setting of persistent nonunion, vascularized bone grafting may be necessary. A thorough understanding of the patient's type of nonunion and potential for healing is crucial for achieving satisfactory results, as is thoughtful preoperative planning and surgical fixation.

REPRESENTATIVE CASE—HYPERTROPHIC NONUNION

A 64-year-old right-hand-dominant woman initially sustained a minimally displaced right lateral clavicle fracture after falling onto the pavement (**Fig. 1**A). She was treated nonoperatively at an outside hospital. Five months later, she was seen by the senior author; at that time, she reported ongoing pain, and examination showed decreased strength of her right supraspinatus compared with her contralateral side. She was treated nonoperatively with trial of physical therapy for 8 months, during which she reported continued anterior pain. Twelve months after her injury, she presented to the office with pain and decreased shoulder range of motion; radiographs revealed hypertrophic nonunion of her lateral clavicle (**Fig. 1**B). Given her painful nonunion, she was indicated for surgery. She was taken to the operating room, placed in the beach chair position, and the nonunion was debrided to healthy viable bone. A precontoured locking plate (Acumed, Hillsboro, OR, USA) was used to obtain fixation (**Fig. 1**C). Autograft from the resected nonunion and DBM allograft putty (Arthrex, Naples, FL, USA) were placed around the nonunion to promote bony healing. At 5-month follow-up, the patient reported minimal pain as well as full active range of motion. Radiographs show healing of the distal clavicle nonunion (**Fig. 1**D).

CLINICS CARE POINTS

Pearls
- Use an evidence-based approach based on fracture subtype to guide recommendations and treatment with respect to nonoperative versus operative management
- In the case of nonunion, ensure preoperative optimization by counseling patients on modifiable risk factors and making appropriate referrals (ie, nutrition or smoking cessation)
- Minimize risk of hardware irritation by meticulously elevating the periosteal layer for later closure
- Counsel all operative patients on the potential need for future surgical removal of hardware

Pitfalls
- Do not treat all clavicle fractures as equal; prognosis varies widely based on subtype
- If using a hook plate for operative fixation, take care to not overreduce the clavicle with respect to the acromion. The patient should be counseled on the need for future removal of hardware with the use of this implant
- Poor drilling technique and/or excessively long screws can lead to neurovascular compromise; one can mitigate this risk by placing a retractor beneath the inferior aspect of the clavicle

---

DISCLOSURE

A.J. deMeireles has no disclosures. N. Czerwonka has no disclosures. W.N. Levine receives IP royalties and is an unpaid consultant for Zimmer Biomet.

REFERENCES

1. van der Meijden OA, Gaskill TR, Millett PJ. Treatment of clavicle fractures: current concepts review. J Shoulder Elbow Surg 2012;21(3):423–9.
2. Wiesel B, Nagda S, Mehta S, et al. Management of Midshaft Clavicle Fractures in Adults. JAAOS - J Am Acad Orthop Surg. 2018;26(22):e468.
3. Neer C 2nd. Nonunion of the clavicle. J Am Med Assoc 1960;5(172):1006–11.
4. Rowe CR. An atlas of anatomy and treatment of midclavicular fractures. Clin Orthop 1968;58:29–42.
5. Zlowodzki M, Zelle BA, Cole PA, et al. Treatment of acute midshaft clavicle fractures: Systematic review of 2144 fractures. On behalf of the Evidence-Based Orthopaedic Trauma Working Group. J Orthop Trauma 2005;19(7):504–7.
6. Martetschläger F, Gaskill TR, Millett PJ. Management of clavicle nonunion and malunion. J Shoulder Elbow Surg 2013;22(6):862–8.
7. McKee MD, Wild LM, Schemitsch EH. Midshaft malunions of the clavicle. J Bone Jt Surg 2003;85(5):790–7.
8. McKee MD, Pedersen EM, Jones C, et al. Deficits following nonoperative treatment of displaced midshaft clavicular fractures. J Bone Joint Surg Am 2006; 88(1):35–40.
9. Patel B, Gustafson PA, Jastifer J. The effect of clavicle malunion on shoulder biomechanics; A computational study. Clin Biomech 2012;27(5):436–42.
10. Gausden EB, Villa J, Warner SJ, et al. Nonunion After Clavicle Osteosynthesis: High Incidence of Propionibacterium acnes. J Orthop Trauma 2017;31(4): 229–35.
11. Clement ND, Goudie EB, Brooksbank AJ, et al. Smoking status and the Disabilities of the Arm Shoulder and Hand score are early predictors of symptomatic nonunion of displaced midshaft fractures of the clavicle. Bone Jt J 2016; 98-B(1):125–30.
12. Murray IR, Foster CJ, Eros A, et al. Risk Factors for Nonunion After Nonoperative Treatment of Displaced Midshaft Fractures of the Clavicle. J Bone Jt Surg 2013; 95(13):1153–8.
13. Robinson CM, Court-Brown CM, Mcqueen MM, et al. Estimating the risk of nonunion following nonoperative treatment of a clavicular fracture. J Bone Jt Surg-Am 2004;86(7):1359–65.
14. Chan K. Clavicle malunion. J Shoulder Elbow Surg 1999;8(4):287–90.
15. Hill JM, McGuire MH, Crosby LA. Closed treatment of displaced middle-third fractures of the clavicle gives poor results. J Bone Joint Surg Br 1997;79-B(4): 537–8.
16. Hart A, Rainer WG, Taunton MJ, et al. Cotinine Testing Improves Smoking Cessation Before Total Joint Arthroplasty. J Arthroplasty 2019;34(7S):S148–51.
17. Nordqvist A, Petersson C, Redlund-Johnell I. The natural course of lateral clavicle fracture: 15 (11–21) year follow-up of 110 cases. Acta Orthop Scand 1993;64(1): 87–91.
18. Amorosa LF, Buirs LD, Bexkens R, et al. Single-Stage Treatment Protocol for Presumed Aseptic Diaphyseal Nonunion. JBJS Essent Surg Tech 2015;5(2):e8.
19. Simpson SN, Jupiter JB. Clavicular Nonunion and Malunion: Evaluation and Surgical Management. J Am Acad Orthop Surg 1996;4(1):1–8.

20. Prasarn ML, Meyers KN, Wilkin G, et al. Dual mini-fragment plating for midshaft clavicle fractures: a clinical and biomechanical investigation. Arch Orthop Trauma Surg 2015;135(12):1655–62.

21. Chen W, Tang K, Tao X, et al. Clavicular non-union treated with fixation using locking compression plate without bone graft. J Orthop Surg 2018;13(1):317.

22. Zhang J, Yin P, Han B, et al. The treatment of the atrophic clavicular nonunion by double-plate fixation with autogenous cancellous bone graft: a prospective study. J Orthop Surg 2021;16(1):22.

23. Ballmer FT, Lambert SM, Hertel R. Decortication and plate osteosynthesis for nonunion of the clavicle. J Shoulder Elbow Surg 1998;7(6):581–5.

24. Wiss DA, Garlich JM. Clavicle nonunion: plate and graft type do not affect healing rates—a single surgeon experience with 71 cases. J Shoulder Elbow Surg 2021; 30(3):679–84.

25. Petersson CJ. Resection of the Lateral End of the Clavicle: *A 3 to 30-Year Follow-Up*. Acta Orthop Scand 1983;54(6):904–7.

26. Gokkus K, Saylik M, Atmaca H, et al. Limited distal clavicle excision of acromio-clavicular joint osteoarthritis. Orthop Traumatol Surg Res 2016;102(3):311–8.

27. Banerjee R, Waterman B, Padalecki J, et al. Management of Distal Clavicle Fractures. J Am Acad Orthop Surg 2011;19(7):392–401.

28. Khan LAK, Bradnock TJ, Scott C, et al. Fractures of the Clavicle. J Bone Jt Surg-Am 2009;91(2):447–60.

29. McKee MD, Kreder HJ, Mandel S, et al. Nonoperative treatment compared with plate fixation of displaced midshaft clavicular fractures: A multicenter, randomized clinical trial. J Bone Jt Surg 2007;89(1):1–10.

30. Iannotti MR, Crosby LA, Stafford P, et al. Effects of plate location and selection on the stability of midshaft clavicle osteotomies: A biomechanical study. J Shoulder Elbow Surg 2002;11(5):457–62.

31. Celestre P, Roberston C, Mahar A, et al. Biomechanical Evaluation of Clavicle Fracture Plating Techniques: Does a Locking Plate Provide Improved Stability? J Orthop Trauma 2008;22(4):241–7.

32. Formaini N, Taylor BC, Backes J, et al. Superior Versus Anteroinferior Plating of Clavicle Fractures. Orthopedics 2013;36(7). https://doi.org/10.3928/01477447-20130624-20.

33. Uchiyama Y, Handa A, Omi H, et al. Locking versus nonlocking superior plate fixations for displaced midshaft clavicle fractures: A prospective randomized trial comparing clinical and radiografic results. J Orthop Sci 2021;26(6):1094–9.

34. Collinge C, Devinney S, Herscovici D, et al. Anterior-inferior Plate Fixation of Middle-third Fractures and Nonunions of the Clavicle. J Orthop Trauma 2006; 20(10):680–6.

35. Nolte PC, Tross AK, Studniorz J, et al. No difference in mid-term outcome after superior vs. anteroinferior plate position for displaced midshaft clavicle fractures. Sci Rep 2021;11(1):22101.

36. Werner SD, Reed J, Hanson T, et al. Anatomic Relationships After Instrumentation of the Midshaft Clavicle With 3.5-mm Reconstruction Plating: An Anatomic Study. J Orthop Trauma 2011;25(11):657–60.

37. Hussey MM, Chen Y, Fajardo RA, et al. Analysis of Neurovascular Safety Between Superior and Anterior Plating Techniques of Clavicle Fractures. J Orthop Trauma 2013;27(11):627–32.

38. Ziegler CG, Aman ZS, Storaci HW, et al. Low-Profile Dual Small Plate Fixation Is Biomechanically Similar to Larger Superior or Anteroinferior Single Plate Fixation of Midshaft Clavicle Fractures. Am J Sports Med 2019;47(11):2678–85.

39. Boyce GN, Philpott AJ, Ackland DC, et al. Single versus dual orthogonal plating for comminuted midshaft clavicle fractures: a biomechanics study. J Orthop Surg 2020;15(1):248.

40. DeBaun MR, Chen MJ, Campbell ST, et al. Dual Mini-Fragment Plating Is Comparable With Precontoured Small Fragment Plating for Operative Diaphyseal Clavicle Fractures: A Retrospective Cohort Study. J Orthop Trauma 2020;34(7): e229–32.

41. Hall JA, Schemitsch CE, Vicente MR, et al. Operative Versus Nonoperative Treatment of Acute Displaced Distal Clavicle Fractures: A Multicenter Randomized Controlled Trial. J Orthop Trauma 2021;35(12):660–6.

42. Asadollahi S, Bucknill A. Hook Plate Fixation for Acute Unstable Distal Clavicle Fracture: A Systematic Review and Meta-analysis. J Orthop Trauma 2019;33(8): 417–22.

43. Good DW, Lui DF, Leonard M, et al. Clavicle hook plate fixation for displaced lateral-third clavicle fractures (Neer type II): a functional outcome study. J Shoulder Elbow Surg 2012;21(8):1045–8.

44. Stegeman SA, Nacak H, Huvenaars KH, et al. Surgical treatment of Neer type-II fractures of the distal clavicle: A meta-analysis. Acta Orthop 2013;84(2):184–90.

45. Shin SJ, Ko YW, Lee J, et al. Use of plate fixation without coracoclavicular ligament augmentation for unstable distal clavicle fractures. J Shoulder Elbow Surg 2016;25(6):942–8.

46. Flinkkilä T, Ristiniemi J, Lakovaara M, et al. Hook-plate fixation of unstable lateral clavicle fractures: A report on 63 patients. Acta Orthop 2006;77(4):644–9.

47. Hessmann M, Kirchner R, Baumgaertel F, et al. Treatment of unstable distal clavicular fractures with and without lesions of the acromioclavicular joint. Injury 1996;27(1):47–52.

48. Worhacz K, Nayak AN, Boudreaux RL, et al. Biomechanical Analysis of Superior and Anterior Precontoured Plate Fixation Techniques for Neer Type II-A Clavicle Fractures. J Orthop Trauma 2018;32(12):e462–8.

49. Yagnik GP, Jordan CJ, Narvel RR, et al. Distal Clavicle Fracture Repair: Clinical Outcomes of a Surgical Technique Utilizing a Combination of Cortical Button Fixation and Coracoclavicular Ligament Reconstruction. Orthop J Sports Med 2019; 7(9). 2325967119867925.

50. Rieser GR, Edwards K, Gould GC, et al. Distal-third clavicle fracture fixation: a biomechanical evaluation of fixation. J Shoulder Elbow Surg 2013;22(6):848–55.

51. Schliemann B, Roßlenbroich SB, Schneider KN, et al. Surgical treatment of vertically unstable lateral clavicle fractures (Neer 2b) with locked plate fixation and coracoclavicular ligament reconstruction. Arch Orthop Trauma Surg 2013; 133(7):935–9.

52. Robinson PG, Williamson TR, Yapp LZ, et al. Functional outcomes and complications following combined locking plate and tunneled suspensory device fixation of lateral-end clavicle nonunions. J Shoulder Elbow Surg 2021;30(11):2570–6.

53. Myeroff C, Archdeacon M. Autogenous Bone Graft: Donor Sites and Techniques. J Bone Jt Surg 2011;93(23):2227–36.

54. Baldwin P, Li DJ, Auston DA, et al. Autograft, Allograft, and Bone Graft Substitutes: Clinical Evidence and Indications for Use in the Setting of Orthopaedic Trauma Surgery. J Orthop Trauma 2019;33(4):203–13.

55. Endrizzi DP, White RR, Babikian GM, et al. Nonunion of the clavicle treated with plate fixation: A review of forty-seven consecutive cases. J Shoulder Elbow Surg 2008;17(6):951–3.

56. Schnetzke M, Morbitzer C, Aytac S, et al. Additional bone graft accelerates healing of clavicle non-unions and improves long-term results after 8.9 years: a retrospective study. J Orthop Surg 2015;10(1):2.
57. Tenpenny W, Caldwell PE, Rivera-Rosado E, et al. Arthroscopic-Assisted Bone Graft Harvest From the Proximal Humerus for Distal Third Clavicle Fracture Nonunion. Arthrosc Tech 2020;9(12):e1937–42.
58. Missiuna P. Anatomically safe and minimally invasive transcrestal technique for procurement of autogenous cancellous bone graft from the mid-iliac crest. Can J Surg 2011;54(5):327–32.
59. Beirer M, Banke IJ, Harrasser N, et al. Mid-term outcome following revision surgery of clavicular non- and malunion using anatomic locking compression plate and iliac crest bone graft. BMC Musculoskelet Disord 2017;18(1):129.
60. Morison Z, Vicente M, Schemitsch EH, et al. The treatment of atrophic, recalcitrant long-bone nonunion in the upper extremity with human recombinant bone morphogenetic protein-7 (rhBMP-7) and plate fixation: A retrospective review. Injury 2016;47(2):356–63.
61. Villa JC, van der List JP, Gausden EB, et al. Plate fixation and bone grafting of distal clavicle nonunions: radiologic and functional outcomes. Arch Orthop Trauma Surg 2016;136(11):1521–9.
62. Shin EH, Shin AY. Vascularized Bone Grafts in Orthopaedic Surgery. JBJS Rev 2017;5(10):e1.
63. Momberger NG, Smith J, Coleman DA. Vascularized fibular grafts for salvage reconstruction of clavicle nonunion. J Shoulder Elbow Surg 2000;9(5):389–94.
64. Chieh-Ting Huang T, Sabbagh MD, Lu CK, et al. The vascularized medial femoral condyle free flap for reconstruction of segmental recalcitrant nonunion of the clavicle. J Shoulder Elbow Surg 2019;28(12):2364–70.
65. Fuchs B, Steinmann SP, Bishop AT. Free vascularized corticoperiosteal bone graft for the treatment of persistent nonunion of the clavicle. J Shoulder Elbow Surg 2005;14(3):264–8.
66. Smekal V, Deml C, Kamelger F, et al. Corrective osteotomy in symptomatic midshaft clavicular malunion using elastic stable intramedullary nails. Arch Orthop Trauma Surg 2010;130(5):681–5.
67. Kleweno CP, Jawa A, Wells JH, et al. Midshaft clavicular fractures: comparison of intramedullary pin and plate fixation. J Shoulder Elbow Surg 2011;20(7):1114–7.
68. Hingsammer AM, Vlachopoulos L, Meyer DC, et al. Three-dimensional corrective osteotomies of mal-united clavicles-is the contralateral anatomy a reliable template for reconstruction?: Three-Dimensional Corrective Osteotomies of Clavicles. Clin Anat 2015;28(7):865–71.
69. Hillen RJ, Eygendaal D. Corrective osteotomy after malunion of mid shaft fractures of the clavicle. Strateg Trauma Limb Reconstr 2007;2(2–3):59–61.
70. Sidler-Maier CC, Dedy NJ, Schemitsch EH, et al. Clavicle Malunions: Surgical Treatment and Outcome—a Literature Review. HSS J ®. 2018;14(1):88–98.
71. Nicholson JA, Stirling PHC, Strelzow J, et al. Dynamic Compression of the Subclavian Artery Secondary to Clavicle Nonunion: A Report of 2 Cases. JBJS Case Connect 2019;9(1):e4.
72. Gadinsky NE, Smolev ET, Ricci MJ, et al. Two cases of brachial plexus compression secondary to displaced clavicle fractures. Trauma Case Rep 2019;23:100219.
73. McGillivray MK, Doherty C, Bristol SG, et al. Surgical management of delayed brachial plexopathy following clavicle nonunion. J Orthop Trauma 2022. https://doi.org/10.1097/BOT.0000000000002343.

Dual- Versus Single-Plate Fixation of Clavicle Fractures

Understanding the Rationale Behind both Approaches

Lisa M. Tamburini, MD, Benjamin C. Mayo, MD,
Cory Edgar, MD, PhD*

KEYWORDS

- Clavicle • Single place • Dual plate • Orthogonal plating • Precontoured plates

KEY POINTS

- Midshaft clavicle fracture is treated nonoperatively and operatively, with higher union rates and faster return to activity after operative treatment.
- Operative treatment options for clavicle fractures include a single plate placed either superiorly or anteroinferiorly or two plates placed orthogonally.
- Single- and dual-plate fixation result in acceptable union rates.
- Dual-plate constructs allow for smaller, less prominent plates to be used, which are less likely to require symptomatic implant removal.

INTRODUCTION

Clavicle fractures are a common injury accounting for 2.6% to 4% of fractures.[1,2] These fractures are typically the result of a high-energy force following a fall onto the shoulder (30%); motor vehicle accidents (12.3%); and during sporting activities (30%), such as, football (16.2%) and cycling (4.1%).[1–3] Fractures to the shaft of the clavicle make up 69% of all clavicle fractures.[1] There are two common classification systems for describing midshaft clavicle fractures: the AO Foundation/Orthopaedic Trauma Association classification and the Edinburgh classification. Using the AO Foundation/Orthopaedic Trauma Association classification system the clavicle is identified by the number 15, followed by a location qualifier, 1 for medial fractures,

Department of Orthopaedic Surgery, University of Connecticut, UConn Musculoskeletal Institute, 120 Dowling Way, Farmington, CT 06032, USA
* Corresponding author.
E-mail address: coedgar@uchc.edu

Clin Sports Med 42 (2023) 677–684
https://doi.org/10.1016/j.csm.2023.06.016
0278-5919/23/© 2023 Elsevier Inc. All rights reserved.

2 for shaft fractures, and 3 for lateral fractures. Additionally, a letter is added to describe fracture pattern: A for simple fractures, B for wedge fractures, and C for comminuted fractures.[1] The Edinburgh classification can also be used to describe clavicle fractures, type I fractures occur in the medial fifth of the clavicle, type II in the middle three-fifths, and type III in the lateral fifth. Again, two qualifiers are added: A for nondisplaced or less than 100% displaced and B for greater than 100% displacement and 1 or 2 for intra-articular fractures or fracture comminution.[1] These classification systems can help guide treatment based on known risk factors for worse outcomes.

Although many of these fractures are treated without surgical intervention with good outcomes, there are risks of nonunion, malunion, and persistent symptoms. There is also a greater ability to return to activity and perform overhead activities more quickly after surgical treatment, which may be a consideration when treating younger and more active individuals.[4,5] For those that are treated with surgery, there are risks including infection, symptoms from the implant, and the need for additional surgery. There has been an increased emphasis on reducing implant-associated complications with surgical management without sacrificing outcomes or failure rate. When choosing operative management, fixation with a single plate placed either superiorly or anteroinferiorly or dual plates placed orthogonally have been described. We discuss these treatment options, their outcomes, and the rationale behind them.

SURGICAL TREATMENT TECHNIQUES

There has been some debate with regards to management of clavicular fractures. Historically it has been thought that the degree of nonunion or malunion following nonoperative treatment was very low and therefore these fractures were often treated nonoperatively. More recently, however, data have shown a higher rate of nonunion and malunion than previously described. A meta-analysis by McKee and coworkers[6] reported a nonunion rate of 14.5% and a symptomatic malunion rate of 8.5% following nonoperative treatment of displaced midshaft clavicular fractures. This is in comparison with a 1.4% nonunion and 0% symptomatic malunion rate following operative treatment.[6] Operative treatment is generally considered for fractures with greater than 2 cm of shortening, greater than 2 cm of displacement, skin tenting, in combination with ipsilateral serial rib fractures, or a floating shoulder.[7] Additionally, a patient's desire to return to previous level of activity plays a role in this decision making. Higher rates of return to sport after operative treatment of clavicle fractures have been reported and operative treatment also allows a faster return to sport.[4,5]

SINGLE-PLATE FIXATION
Biomechanics

Traditionally, clavicle fixation has been completed through a single superiorly placed plate. A variety of plates have been used in the fixation of clavicular fractures including 3.5-mm reconstruction plates, 3.5-mm locking compression plates, 3.5-mm precontoured plates, 2.7-mm reconstruction plates, and 2.7-mm calcaneal plates. Overall, union rates and need for reoperation are not affected by the type of plate used.[8] There are, however, biomechanical differences among plate options. The 3.5-mm plates have higher bending stiffness when compared with 2.7-mm plates and are more likely to failure by plastic deformation.[8,9] The 2.7-mm plates, however, require more displacement before plastic deformation and fail by plate breakage.[8,9] Limited contact dynamic compression plates placed superiorly have better biomechanical stability when compared with reconstruction plates and dynamic compression plates. Iannotti and colleagues[10] compared limited contact dynamic compression plates, dynamic compression plates, and reconstruction plates and found limited contact dynamic compression plates to have greater biomechanical stability. Because of the S-shape of the clavicle, precontoured plates have been designed to better fit this shape. Precontoured plates with locking screws created a stiffer construct, which had a higher number of cycles to failure than noncontoured locking compression plates.[11] With many different plate choices, a plate with the appropriate characteristics can be chosen based on fracture pattern and need for absolute versus relative stability.

With the advent of precontoured plates and easier bending, anterior plating has become a popular option because of many purported benefits. When compared with superiorly placed plates, anterior plates experienced less stress when exposed to axial compression and torsion forces.[12,13] Although this is true, anteroinferiorly placed plates were found to fail at a lower load by plate bending.[13] Gilde and colleagues[14] compared reconstruction and dynamic compression 2.7-mm plates placed anteroinferiorly and found that reconstruction plates failed more often. Many single-plate options with acceptable biomechanical properties exist taking into consideration location and type of plate used.

Clinical Outcomes

Overall, single-plate fixation, either superiorly or anteroinferiorly, results in good patient-reported outcomes.[15–18] Clavicle fracture fixation with a single plate demonstrates high union rates, with anterior plating having a slightly higher union rate than superior plating.[17,19,20] Single plating is, however, associated with complications that can require reoperation including symptomatic hardware because of the thick plates frequently used and the thin soft tissue coverage, nonunion, deep infection, wound dehiscence, and broken hardware.[18,21–23] There are many studies looking at implant removal after single-plate fixation of clavicular fractures. Reports of implant removal rates vary from 37% to 61% and 7.7% to 67% in anteroinferior plating and superior plating, respectively.[17,18,20,24] Although the data show that there is a high number of patients who require implant removal, there are some data to suggest patients who undergo anteroinferior plating have less symptoms as a result of their plate.[24,25] With a similar surgical approach, operative time for anterior and superior plating is similar, around 60 ± 20 minutes.[26,27] A meta-analysis did show anteroinferior plating may reduce blood loss, operation time, and union time.[28]

Single plating, superiorly and anteroinferiorly, allow individuals to return to high levels of activity. In a study of cyclists with clavicular fractures treated with anteroinferior plates, all cyclists returned to sport, with competitive cyclists returning at an average of 10 days and recreational cyclists at an average of 2 to 3 weeks.[29] Similarly, 94% of athletes with clavicular fractures treated with a superiorly placed precontoured locking plate returned to sport at their preinjury level.[30] This study did find a wider range of time to return to activity of 5 to 180 days.[30]

DUAL-PLATE FIXATION
Orthogonal Plating

Biomechanics
Although clavicle fractures can be treated with one plate, placed superiorly or anteriorly, this plate is often larger and therefore is prominent, which can lead to implant complications and even implant removal as discussed previously. This is most appropriate when the fracture "keys" in and stability is imparted by fracture anatomy (**Fig. 1**). Additionally, this plate predominantly resists force in only one direction. The use of two

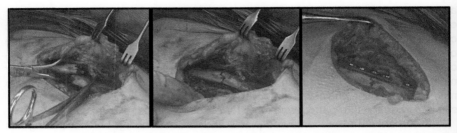

Fig. 1. Left simple clavicle fracture with stable fracture pattern, treated with 2.7-mm superior plate.

small plates, placed orthogonally, addresses rotational and pullout forces as an inferior displacement force from gravity and shoulder gridle activation is initiated (**Fig. 2**). Smaller plates are less prominent and therefore less commonly cause irritation and with two orthogonally placed plates, there is better resistance to deforming forces.

Although a 2.7-mm or 3.5-mm plate is used for single plating, dual-plate constructs can be made up of smaller plates, such as a 2.4-mm plate superiorly and a 2.7-mm plate anteriorly. In cases with larger patients or more significant comminution an anterior 3.5-mm plate is placed after length is established with a smaller superior plate (**Fig. 3**). Acceptable results have even been seen with plates of 2.4 mm and 2.0 mm.[31] As with single plating, reconstruction, locking compression, and nonlocking plates have all been used in dual-plate constructs.

Overall, no significant difference in construct stiffness has been reported when comparing dual plating to single plating for clavicular fracture fixation.[32–35] Additionally, no difference in load to failure has been noted.[33,35] Dual-plate fixation may even create a construct that is superior to single plating. Dual-plate constructs have been shown to be stiffer when exposed to bending forces in the superior and anterior direction and axial forces.[36–38] This stronger construct leads to lesser degree of fracture displacement after repeated cycling.[37]

Clinical Outcomes

Dual plating has favorable outcomes that are comparable with single plating. Similarly to clavicle fracture fixation with a single plate, dual plating has very high union rates despite the need for increased soft tissue exposure for two plates.[22,31,39–41] Although dual plating uses smaller plates, studies have shown no difference in maintenance of reduction.[31,42] In contrast to single plating, dual plating does have more favorable outcomes with regard to complications, reoperations, and implant removal. Studies have shown rates of implant removal between 0% and 15%.[21,22,31,41–43] A low number of complications, such as peri-incisional numbness, superior plate prominence, and

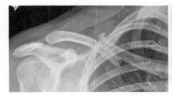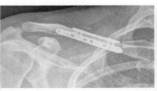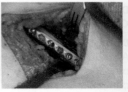

Fig. 2. Left clavicle fracture with dual-plate fixation; 2.4-mm superior plate, 2.7-mm anterior plate.

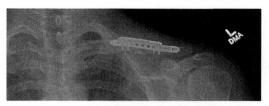

Fig. 3. Left clavicle fracture with dual-plate fixation; 2.4-mm superior plate, 3.5-mm anterior plate with comminution.

infection, have been noted with dual plating with few of these requiring reoperation.[22,40] With smaller, less prominent plates, the rate of implant removal is lower with dual plating when compared with single plating.[41,42] As may be expected, operative time is longer with dual plating than with single plating. A study by Lee and colleagues[44] reported an average operative time of 174 minutes for dual plating and 119 minutes for single plating.

SUMMARY

For clavicle fractures that indicate surgical management because of fracture or patient characteristics, plating is the method of choice for fixation. A single plate may be placed superiorly or anteriorly or two plates may be used. When a single plate is used it is often a larger, 3.5-mm plate. These plates demonstrate the ability to create strong constructs that resist deforming forces. With low levels of nonunion and good patient-reported outcomes this may seem like a great option for fixation. However, these plates are often prominent because of their size and superficial location. Single plates are often associated with symptoms that require implant removal, with reported rates of up to 67%. Dual plating is an alternative option that maintains similar or even improved construct stability, which allows for high levels of fracture union while allowing smaller plates to be used. The use of smaller plates in turn decreases the frequency and severity of symptoms experienced because of prominent implant position.

CLINICS CARE POINTS

- Clavicle fractures should be treated operatively when there is greater than 2 cm of shortening, greater than 2 cm of displacement, skin tenting, ipsilateral rib fractures, or in the presence of a floating shoulder. Operative management should also be highly considered in active, athletic individuals wishing to return to a high level of activity.

- When choosing between single and dual plating, fracture pattern, patient activity level, patient size, and patient expectations should all be taken into consideration.

- Because prominent hardware is a common problem, patients must be counseled regarding this before surgery.

- Single and dual plating for clavicle fracture provide biomechanically stable constructs with overall good clinical outcomes.

DISCLOSURES

L.M. Tamburini has no disclosures. B.C. Mayo has no disclosures. C. Edgar is a paid consultant for Mitek; is a Board member for MTF; and a full list of disclosures is found on the AAOS Web site.

REFERENCES

1. Frima H, van Heijl M, Michelitsch C, et al. Clavicle fractures in adults; current concepts. Eur J Trauma Emerg Surg 2020;46(3):519–29.
2. Khan LK, Bradnock TJ, Scott C, et al. Fractures of the clavicle. JBJS 2009;91(2): 447–60.
3. O'Neill BJ, Hirpara KM, O'Briain D, et al. Clavicle fractures: a comparison of five classification systems and their relationship to treatment outcomes. Int Orthop 2011;35(6):909–14.
4. Robertson GA, Oliver CW, Scott H. Infographic: return rates and return times to sport after middle-third clavicle fracture: important knowledge for management of these injuries in athletes. BMJ Publishing Group Ltd and British Association of Sport and Exercise Medicine 2017;52(6):412.
5. Hebert-Davies J, Agel J. Return to elite-level sport after clavicle fractures. BMJ Open Sport & Exercise Medicine 2018;4(1):e000371.
6. McKee RC, Whelan DB, Schemitsch EH, et al. Operative versus nonoperative care of displaced midshaft clavicular fractures: a meta-analysis of randomized clinical trials. JBJS 2012;94(8):675–84.
7. Waldmann S, Benninger E, Meier C. Nonoperative treatment of midshaft clavicle fractures in adults. Open Orthop J 2018;12:1.
8. Alzahrani MM, Cota A, Alkhelaifi K, et al. Are clinical outcomes affected by type of plate used for management of mid-shaft clavicle fractures? J Orthop Traumatol 2018;19(1):1–6.
9. Alzahrani MM, Cota A, Alkhelaifi K, et al. Mechanical evaluation of 2.7-versus 3.5-mm plating constructs for midshaft clavicle fractures. JAAOS-Journal of the American Academy of Orthopaedic Surgeons 2021;29(9):e440–6.
10. Iannotti M, Crosby LA, Stafford P, et al. Effects of plate location and selection on the stability of midshaft clavicle osteotomies: a biomechanical study. J Shoulder Elbow Surg 2002;11(5):457–62.
11. Worhacz K, Nayak AN, Boudreaux RL, et al. Biomechanical analysis of superior and anterior precontoured plate fixation techniques for Neer type II-A clavicle fractures. J Orthop Trauma 2018;32(12):e462–8.
12. Huang T-L, Chen W-C, Lin K-J, et al. Conceptual finite element study for comparison among superior, anterior, and spiral clavicle plate fixations for midshaft clavicle fracture. Med Eng Phys 2016;38(10):1070–5.
13. Robertson C, Celestre P, Mahar A, et al. Reconstruction plates for stabilization of mid-shaft clavicle fractures: differences between nonlocked and locked plates in two different positions. J Shoulder Elbow Surg 2009;18(2):204–9.
14. Gilde AK, Jones CB, Sietsema DL, et al. Does plate type influence the clinical outcomes and implant removal in midclavicular fractures fixed with 2.7-mm anteroinferior plates? A retrospective cohort study. J Orthop Surg Res 2014;9(1):1–7.
15. Naimark M, Dufka FL, Han R, et al. Plate fixation of midshaft clavicular fractures: patient-reported outcomes and hardware-related complications. J Shoulder Elbow Surg 2016;25(5):739–46.
16. Nourian A, Dhaliwal S, Vangala S, et al. Midshaft fractures of the clavicle: a meta-analysis comparing surgical fixation using anteroinferior plating versus superior plating. J Orthop Trauma 2017;31(9):461–7.
17. Arojuraye S, Salihu M, Mustapha I, et al. Anteroinferior versus superior plating techniques for displaced midshaft clavicle fractures: a retrospective single centre cohort study from Northern Nigeria. Surgeon 2022;20(5):e248–53.

18. Nolte P-C, Tross A-K, Studniorz J, et al. No difference in mid-term outcome after superior vs. anteroinferior plate position for displaced midshaft clavicle fractures. Sci Rep 2021;11(1):1–8.
19. Axelrod DE, Ekhtiari S, Bozzo A, et al. What is the best evidence for management of displaced midshaft clavicle fractures? A systematic review and network meta-analysis of 22 randomized controlled trials. Clin Orthop Relat Res 2020; 478(2):392.
20. Salazar LM, Koso RE, Momtaz DA, et al. Results of pre-contoured titanium anterior plating of midshaft clavicle fractures. J Shoulder Elbow Surg 2022;31(1): 107–12.
21. Charles SJ, Chen SR, Mittwede P, et al. Risk factors for complications and reoperation following operative management of displaced midshaft clavicle fractures. J Shoulder Elbow Surg 2022;31(10):e498–506.
22. Chen X, Shannon SF, Torchia M, et al. Radiographic outcomes of single versus dual plate fixation of acute mid-shaft clavicle fractures. Arch Orthop Trauma Surg 2017;137(6):749–54.
23. Jones CB, Sietsema DL, Ringler JR, et al. Results of anterior-inferior 2.7-mm dynamic compression plate fixation of midshaft clavicular fractures. J Orthop Trauma 2013;27(3):126–9.
24. Hulsmans MH, Van Heijl M, Houwert RM, et al. Anteroinferior versus superior plating of clavicular fractures. J Shoulder Elbow Surg 2016;25(3):448–54.
25. Serrano R, Borade A, Mir H, et al. Anterior-inferior plating results in fewer secondary interventions compared to superior plating for acute displaced midshaft clavicle fractures. J Orthop Trauma 2017;31(9):468–71.
26. Sohn H-S, Shon MS, Lee K-H, et al. Clinical comparison of two different plating methods in minimally invasive plate osteosynthesis for clavicular midshaft fractures: a randomized controlled trial. Injury 2015;46(11):2230–8.
27. Zhang Y, Xu J, Zhang C, et al. Minimally invasive plate osteosynthesis for midshaft clavicular fractures using superior anatomic plating. J Shoulder Elbow Surg 2016;25(1):e7–12.
28. Ai J, Kan S-L, Li H-L, et al. Anterior inferior plating versus superior plating for clavicle fracture: a meta-analysis. BMC Muscoskel Disord 2017;18(1):1–9.
29. van der Ven DJ, Timmers TK, Broeders IA, et al. Displaced clavicle fractures in cyclists: return to athletic activity after anteroinferior plate fixation. Clin J Sport Med 2019;29(6):465–9.
30. Ranalletta M, Rossi LA, Piuzzi NS, et al. Return to sports after plate fixation of displaced midshaft clavicular fractures in athletes. Am J Sports Med 2015;43(3): 565–9.
31. Chen MJ, DeBaun MR, Salazar BP, et al. Safety and efficacy of using 2.4/2.4 mm and 2.0/2.4 mm dual mini-fragment plate combinations for fixation of displaced diaphyseal clavicle fractures. Injury 2020;51(3):647–50.
32. Ferguson DP, Baker HP, Dillman D, et al. Dual mini-fragment plate fixation of midshaft clavicle fractures is biomechanically equivalent to anatomic pre-contoured plating. Eur J Orthop Surg Traumatol 2022;1–8.
33. Ruzbarsky JJ, Nolte P-C, Miles JW, et al. Does dual plating clavicle fractures increase the risk of refracture after hardware removal? A biomechanical investigation. J Shoulder Elbow Surg 2021;30(9):e594–601.
34. Zhang F, Chen F, Qi Y, et al. Finite element analysis of dual small plate fixation and single plate fixation for treatment of midshaft clavicle fractures. J Orthop Surg Res 2020;15(1):1–7.

35. Ziegler CG, Aman ZS, Storaci HW, et al. Low-profile dual small plate fixation is biomechanically similar to larger superior or anteroinferior single plate fixation of midshaft clavicle fractures. Am J Sports Med 2019;47(11):2678–85.
36. Kitzen J, Paulson K, Korley R, et al. Biomechanical evaluation of different plate configurations for midshaft clavicle fracture fixation: single plating compared with dual mini-fragment plating. JBJS Open Access 2022;7(1).
37. Pastor T, Knobe M, van de Wall BJ, et al. Low-profile dual mini-fragment plating of diaphyseal clavicle fractures. A biomechanical comparative testing. Clin Bio-Mech 2022;94:105634.
38. Boyce GN, Philpott AJ, Ackland DC, et al. Single versus dual orthogonal plating for comminuted midshaft clavicle fractures: a biomechanics study. J Orthop Surg Res 2020;15(1):1–7.
39. Zhuang Y, Zhang Y, Zhou L, et al. Management of comminuted mid-shaft clavicular fractures: comparison between dual-plate fixation treatment and single-plate fixation. J Orthop Surg 2020;28(2).
40. Rompen IF, van de Wall BJM, van Heijl M, et al. Low profile dual plating for midshaft clavicle fractures: a meta-analysis and systematic review of observational studies. Eur J Trauma Emerg Surg 2022;1–9.
41. You DZ, Krzyzaniak H, Kendal JK, et al. Outcomes and complications after dual plate vs. single plate fixation of displaced mid-shaft clavicle fractures: a systematic review and meta-analysis. Journal of clinical orthopaedics and trauma 2021;17:261–6.
42. DeBaun MR, Chen MJ, Campbell ST, et al. Dual mini-fragment plating is comparable with precontoured small fragment plating for operative diaphyseal clavicle fractures: a retrospective cohort study. J Orthop Trauma 2020;34(7):e229–32.
43. Czajka CM, Kay A, Gary JL, et al. Symptomatic implant removal following dual mini-fragment plating for clavicular shaft fractures. J Orthop Trauma 2017;31(4):236–40.
44. Lee C, Feaker DA, Ostrofe AA, et al. No difference in risk of implant removal between orthogonal mini-fragment and single small-fragment plating of midshaft clavicle fractures in a military population: a preliminary study. Clin Orthop Relat Res 2020;478(4):741.

Classification of Distal Clavicle Fractures and Indications for Conservative Treatment

Jayson Lian, MD, Ferdinand J. Chan, MD, Benjamin J. Levy, MD*

KEYWORDS

• Distal clavicle fracture • Neer classification • Clavicle • Conservative treatment

KEY POINTS

- Distal clavicle fractures are typically caused by direct force to the lateral shoulder.
- Fracture stability is governed by integrity of the acromioclavicular and coracoclavicular ligaments.
- Treatment depends on displacement and stability of the fracture.
- Although management of Neer type II fractures is controversial, types I and III can often be managed nonoperatively.
- Possible complications of nonoperative management include nonunion and acromioclavicular joint arthritis.

INTRODUCTION

Distal or lateral third clavicle fractures are a common injury treated by orthopedic surgeons, yet their nuanced and variable presentation can lead to a lack of consensus in their management. Fractures of the distal clavicle are typically caused by a fall directly onto the lateral shoulder or direct force to the shoulder.[1,2] Clavicular fractures represent 2.6% to 10% of all fractures in the body.[2–6] These fractures have a bimodal distribution, most commonly occurring in younger men and then next most commonly in both men and women aged older than 70 years.[7] Distal third clavicle fractures account for 10% to 30% of all clavicle fractures.[1,4–6,8–11]

Distal clavicle fractures are a unique subset of clavicle fractures (distinct from midshaft of medial-third clavicle fractures) because of their ligamentous attachments and articulation with the coracoid process and acromion. As such, the distal clavicle acts

Montefiore Einstein, Department of Orthopaedic Surgery, 1250 Waters Place, Tower 1, 11th Floor, Bronx, NY 10461, USA
* Corresponding author.
E-mail address: belevy@montefiore.org

Clin Sports Med 42 (2023) 685–693
https://doi.org/10.1016/j.csm.2023.05.007
0278-5919/23/© 2023 Elsevier Inc. All rights reserved.
sportsmed.theclinics.com

as an important strut between the axial skeleton and shoulder girdle and aids with shoulder strength, mobility, and function.

Historically, the vast majority of distal clavicle fractures were managed nonoperatively.[12] It was not until the 1960s, when Dr Charles Neer described the effect of distal clavicle nonunion as a disruption to the coracoclavicular (CC) ligaments[13] that operative fixation was more regularly considered. Although relatively uncommon, clavicle malunions and nonunions have long-term consequences such as persistent pain, loss of strength, and decreased range of motion.[14–17] Since then, significant research on the treatment and classification of distal clavicle fractures have been described, with ongoing work to elucidate which fracture patterns require surgical intervention and which surgical techniques may be most effective for achieving anatomic union.

When indicated, conservative management of distal clavicle fractures involves sling immobilization for 2 weeks, gradual range of motion exercises, and is a reliable method of providing excellent return of function to the extremity, with expected return to sport in 3 to 4 months.

Anatomy

Critical to understanding management of distal clavicle fractures is an understanding of its articulation with the scapula through its soft tissue attachments. Movement of the shoulder and scapulothoracic motion is governed by the articulation of the distal clavicle and scapula.[18] Specifically, glenohumeral motion is influenced by integrity of the ligamentous attachments between the distal clavicle and coracoid.[18] The distal clavicle's integrity is intimately involved with the acromioclavicular (AC) joint. The critical structures that portend stability to the AC joint include the AC capsule, AC ligament, CC ligaments, and coracoacromial (CA) ligaments.[19] The capsuloligamentous AC complex attaches to the distal clavicle approximately 6 mm medial to the AC joint.[20] The AC ligaments attach from the medial acromion to the distal clavicle and act as a primary constraint for posterior displacement of the clavicle.[21] Specifically, the posterior and superior AC ligaments are most important for providing anterior-posterior stability to the AC joint.[21] When the AC joint capsule is disrupted, the CC ligaments then become the primary restraint to anterior-posterior translation.[22] The CC ligaments, composed of the conoid and trapezoid ligaments, are responsible for superior-inferior stability of the distal clavicle with respect to the coracoid process.[21–24] The CC ligaments originate at the base of the coracoid process and insert on the inferior aspect of the distal clavicle. There is some variability in the attachment sites for the conoid and trapezoid ligaments as measured from the distal clavicle between individuals. The trapezoid ligament attaches to the distal clavicle approximately 2 to 3 cm from the AC joint.[20,25] The conoid ligament attaches approximately 4.5 cm from the AC joint.[20,25] On average, the distance between the coracoid process and undersurface of the clavicle, also known as the CC interspace, is approximately 1.1 to 1.3 cm.[26]

Apart from ligamentous anatomy, muscular anatomy surrounding the clavicle dictates many of the deforming forces after a fracture. Muscular attachments to the clavicle include the sternocleidomastoid, trapezius, pectoralis major and minor, and latissimus dorsi.[27] The anterior deltoid inserts on the anterior superior clavicle, whereas the trapezius inserts on the posterior superior clavicle. The subclavius muscle is found on the inferior surface or the subclavian groove of the clavicle. Anteriorly, the clavicular head of the pectoralis major originates on the medial clavicle. Posteriorly, the trapezius inserts posterosuperior while the clavicular head of the sternocleidomastoid inserts on the medial third of the clavicle.[27]

The 4 displacing forces on the distal clavicle, described by Neer[8] include the (1) trapezius, (2) weight of the arm, (3) trunk muscles attaching to the humerus and scapula, and (4) rotary displacement from scapula ligaments. The clavicular head of the trapezius attaches on the superior, outer third of the distal clavicle, and draws the clavicular shaft posteriorly.[8] The lateral fragment of the clavicle is pulled downward and anteriorly due to the weight of the arm.[8] The trunk muscles attaching to the humerus and scapula can displace the distal outer clavicular fragment medially toward the apex of the thorax.[8] Finally, the scapular ligaments can rotate the distal fragment as much as 40° with movement of the arm.[8]

The clavicle has an "S" shape in the coronal plane and cephalad-to-caudad bow. A cadaveric biomechanical study demonstrated that different regions of the distal clavicle have differences in bone mineral density and cortical thickness.[28] Length of screws inserted in the superior-inferior dimension can range from 14 to 16 mm in women and 16 to 18 mm in men.[27]

Concerning blood supply, the clavicle has periosteal contributions from the suprascapular artery, thoracoacromial artery, and internal thoracic or mammalian artery.[29]

Mechanism of Injury

The mechanism of injury for fractures of the distal clavicle fractures is typically from a medially directed force from either a fall or a traumatic event in which the lateral shoulder (tip of acromion) is driven into the ground or rigid surface.[30,31] In particular, when the arm is in an adducted position, this force can be transmitted through the AC joint to the distal clavicle and CC ligaments due to the robust stability of the sternoclavicular joint.[25] The bone fails superiorly with tension and inferiorly with compression.[32] These injuries are common in young active individuals who participate in sports or high-speed activities, such as after being tackled or falls from bicycles.[33] This is evidenced by the fact that the mean annual incidence is highest in men aged younger than 20 years.[34] Common sporting activities associated with clavicle injuries include American football, cycling, motocross, and horseback riding.[35]

Presentation and Physical Examination

Presentation is most common after a fall onto the lateral shoulder or from a direct, medially directed blow onto the distal clavicle.[30,31] On physical examination, patients typically present with tenderness to palpation about the distal clavicle and pain with both active and passive range of motion of the shoulder, in particular, cross-body adduction. If there is a significant soft tissue injury patients may present with ecchymosis and swelling, or if fracture displacement is significant enough, there may be tenting of the skin. A thorough examination of surrounding soft tissue should be undertaken. Although motor deficits from nerve injury are rare, paresthesias and numbness can be common, due to swelling, compression, or injury to the supraclavicular nerves.[33] Rarely, suprascapular nerve injuries can lead to weakness in external rotation with the arm adducted.[36]

Imaging

Imaging after the aforementioned presentation should include standard true anteroposterior (Grashey views) and axillary radiographs of the shoulder as well as dedicated clavicle XRs.[33] If a distal clavicle fracture has been identified, then imaging that includes the bilateral AC joints or a contralateral shoulder XR can be useful to compare fracture displacement with the uninjured side. This is particularly helpful for assessing fracture pattern and displacement when normalized to a patient's given anatomy.[33]

Additionally, a Zanca view, which is a shoulder XR with a 10° to 15° cephalic tilt, can be helpful for determining intra-articular involvement.[25]

Although not often included in diagnostic workup, if a fracture has significant comminution or intra-articular extension, or in cases of nonunion/malunion, a CT may also be considered to help better evaluate bony pattern. The authors recommend utilization of MRI if there is concern for concomitant soft tissue injury to the rotator cuff or intra-articular glenohumeral pathology is suspected, although this type of pathologic condition is rare.[37]

Classification

The Neer classification system, which is based on the fracture location in relation to the CC ligament on an anteroposterior radiograph, is widely used.[4,6,8] The original Neer classification[8] described in the 1963 described 3 fracture types in relation to the CC ligaments. In subsequent articles, addendums to include periosteal sleeve avulsion fractures in children and comminuted fractures with an inferior bony fragment were included.[4,8,27] Thus, the most commonly used classification today is a modification to the Neer classification, as follows[4,38] (**Fig. 1**).

Type I: extra-articular fracture lateral to the CC ligaments, with intact CC ligaments, and sparing the AC joint
Type II: fracture occurring medial to the CC ligament, with 2 subtypes
IIA: fracture occurs medial to the conoid ligament, both conoid and trapezoid ligaments remain intact
IIB: fracture occurs between the conoid and trapezoid ligaments with rupture of the conoid ligament
Type III: fracture lateral to the CC ligaments with extension into the AC joint
Type IV: fracture with disruption of the periosteal sleeve (in skeletally immature) and superior displacement of the medial fragment
Type V: fracture medial to the CC ligament, comminuted, and small inferior fragment attached to CC ligament

The modified Neer classification is helpful in determining management. In most cases, types I and III distal clavicle fractures are deemed stable and usually can be

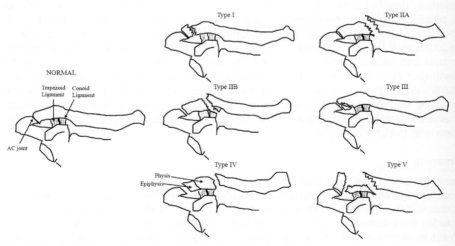

Fig. 1. Modified Neer classification for distal clavicle fractures.

managed conservatively, whereas types II and V are unstable patterns and can be managed either nonoperatively or operatively.

The AO classification[39] for distal clavicle fractures is below.

Type A: nondisplaced fracture with intact CC ligaments
    A1: extra-articular; A2: intra-articular
Type B: displaced fracture with intact CC ligaments
    B1: extra-articular; B2: comminuted
Type C: displaced with torn CC ligaments
    C1: extra-articular; C2: intra-articular

In more recent years, several studies have proposed new classification systems to improve interobserver and intraobserver reliability and utility of fracture classification. In 2018, Cho and colleagues[40] described a classification system utilizing anteroposterior and oblique views of the AC joint and axial shoulder radiographs. This classification system demonstrated moderate interobserver ($k = 0.434$) and substantial intraobserver ($k = 0.644$) reliability. This classification system describes.

Type I–stable: nondisplaced or minimally displaced (<5 mm) irrespective of location
Type II–unstable ($\geq$5 mm)
    IIA: medial to CC ligaments; conoid and trapezoid ligaments intact
    IIB: medial to CC ligaments; conoid ligament torn, trapezoid ligament intact
    IIC: lateral to CC ligaments; conoid and trapezoid ligaments torn
    IID: comminuted fracture with CC ligaments attached to inferior fragment

The authors' preferred classification system remains the Neer classification because this provides concise information that is clinically relevant to treatment algorithms (operative vs nonoperative) and allows for consistent communication, given its widely accepted utility.

Nonoperative Management

Determining whether to operate or not on distal clavicle fractures depends on many factors involving the patient, concomitant injuries, fracture characteristics, timing, and skin compromise. Many studies have attempted to elucidate prognostic factors for fracture healing without surgical intervention. Although some distal clavicle fracture patterns are more clearly defined, there are also fracture variations that may spark more controversy.

Absolute indications for surgical intervention include open fractures, skin tenting, neurovascular injury, or floating shoulder.[41] Indications for initial conservative management include stable fracture patterns such as Neer type I and III distal clavicle fractures. This is generally agreed upon as these fracture patterns do not disrupt the CC ligaments and are typically not significantly displaced.[33] Nondisplaced type II distal clavicle fractures can also typically be managed nonoperatively, although this is more controversial. Displaced type II and V fractures are more commonly treated operatively given their higher risk of nonunion, which can be symptomatic.[11,33,42,43] However, debate remains regarding the degree of dysfunction in patients who go on to develop nonunion, specifically older patients.[6,44]

Various nonoperative measures can be used. Most conservative treatment begins with sling immobilization for 2 weeks primarily for pain control, the authors recommend early initiation of passive range of motion, including pendulum exercises. The authors recommend repeating radiographs within 1 to 2 weeks of injury if any question of fracture stability remains following initial presentation. Although historically, figure-of-eight braces were used, no improvement in outcomes compared with sling immobilization has been demonstrated.[45] One randomized controlled trial demonstrated similar functional and cosmetic outcomes between sling immobilization and figure-of-eight bracing, while actually reducing short-term pain by wearing a simple shoulder sling.[46] Furthermore, figure-of-eight bandages may even lead to problems such as temporary neurovascular dysfunction and pseudoarthrosis.[45] As pain improves, gentle shoulder motion, including passive range of motion and active-assisted motion is initiated at 2 to 4 weeks.[33,35,41] At 6 weeks, the authors recommend repeat radiographs to be obtained to assess for fracture callus and maintenance of alignment. At that point, if pain has been managed well and there are radiographic signs of union, strengthening exercises are initiated,[33] with expected return to sport at 3 to 4 months[35] (**Fig. 2**A and B).

The bulk of the literature has focused on operative versus nonoperative treatment of type II distal clavicle fractures. Although good functional outcomes have largely been reported for conservatively managed type II fractures, nonunion rates after conservative management have been reported to range from 28% to 44%.[1,11,30,42,47–49] Important to note, however, is that only a fraction of patients who develop nonunion are symptomatic.[44] In one study, although 21% of patients with distal clavicle fractures went onto nonunion, only 14% required surgery for persistent symptoms.[30] Furthermore, many of these patients maintain their functionality despite radiographic nonunion.[30,44] In a large case series of 127 patients, there were no significant differences in Constant or Short Form-36 scores between patients with nonunion or those whose fractures had healed, or those who had nonunion and those who had undergone delayed surgery.[30] Conversely, a prospective, randomized controlled trial published in 2021[50] demonstrated that while functional outcomes were equivalent at 1 year between operatively and nonoperatively managed patients, 15% of patients in the nonoperative cohort needed surgery for symptomatic nonunion. In contrast, 44% of patients in the operative group underwent a second surgery—however all were for implant removal, which in contrast was a relatively benign procedure. The operative group also had a significantly higher percentage of patients return to work by 6 months (78% vs 44%) and all but one patient in the operative group achieved union.[50] More work must be done, in particular, likely randomized controlled trials, to elucidate which type II injuries should be managed operatively to avoid more symptomatic nonunions.[44]

Type I and Type III fractures are unique in that because the fracture is located lateral to the CC ligaments, they are inherently more stable and amenable to primary healing. To the authors' knowledge, there are no dedicated case series that report the rate of distal clavicle resection for these patients who go on to develop AC arthrosis following distal clavicle fracture union.

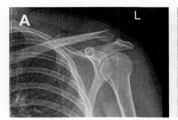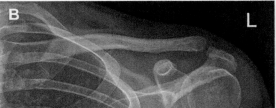

Fig. 2. (*A*) A 32-year-old man with left distal clavicle fracture sustained by fall directly onto lateral shoulder while playing soccer (*B*) Same individual after 4 months of nonoperative management, demonstrating excellent healing/remodeling.

CLINICS CARE POINTS

- Careful evaluation of radiographs to determine fracture pattern and stability at initial evaluation is essential for proper management.
- Shared decision-making[51] with discussion of risks and benefits of nonoperative and operative measures should be had with the patient regarding expectations and goals management of a distal clavicle fractures.
- If a patient with a Type II Neer distal clavicle fracture elects to pursue nonoperative treatment, they should understand that a malunion or nonunion can occur up to half of the time; however, full clarity of the clinical impact of this outcome is uncertain.

Summary

Most patients can expect good functional outcomes even with conservative management of distal clavicle fractures; however, in displaced type II and V fractures there is likely a benefit to operative management with regards to achieving reliable rates of union and returning to normal function at an earlier time point. Patients should understand that there may be residual cosmetic deformity if their fracture is displaced and they elect for nonoperative treatment. A sling is sufficient for nonoperative management for 2 weeks for pain control, at which point gentle range of motion exercises can be started. At 6 weeks, if signs of radiographic union are maintained, strengthening exercises can be incorporated in physical therapy.

DISCLOSURE

There are no relevant financial disclosures.

ACKNOWLEDGMENTS

The authors would like to thank Dr Lauren Crocco for assistance with figure contribution.

REFERENCES

1. Nordqvist A, Petersson C, Redlund-Johnell I. The natural course of lateral clavicle fracture: 15 (11–21) year follow-up of 110 cases. Acta Orthop Scand 1993;64(1): 87–91.
2. Postacchini F, Gumina S, De Santis P, et al. Epidemiology of clavicle fractures. J Shoulder Elbow Surg 2002;11(5):452–6.
3. TO M. Internal pin fixation for fracture of the clavicle. Am Surg 1951;17(7):580–3.
4. Charles SN. 5 Fractures of the distal third of the clavicle. Clin Orthop Relat Res 1968;58:43–50.
5. Nordqvist A, Petersson C. The incidence of fractures of the clavicle. Clin Orthop Relat Res 1994;300:127–32.
6. Bishop JY, Jones GL, Lewis B, et al. Intra- and interobserver agreement in the classification and treatment of distal third clavicle fractures. Am J Sports Med 2015;43(4):979–84.
7. Ockert B, Wiedemann E, Haasters F. Distal clavicle fractures. Classifications and management. Unfallchirurg 2015;118(5):397–406.
8. NEER CS 2nd. Fracture of the distal clavicle with detachment of the coracoclavicular ligaments in adults. J Trauma Acute Care Surg 1963;3(2):99–110.

9. Edwards D, Kavanagh T, Flannery M. Fractures of the distal clavicle: a case for fixation. Injury 1992;23(1):44–6.

10. Tsuei Y-C, Au M-K, Chu W. Comparison of clinical results of surgical treatment for unstable distal clavicle fractures by transacromial pins with and without tension band wire. J Chin Med Assoc 2010;73(12):638–43.

11. Yagnik GP, Porter DA, Jordan CJ. Distal Clavicle Fracture Repair Using Cortical Button Fixation With Coracoclavicular Ligament Reconstruction. Arthrosc Tech 2018;7(4):e411–5. https://doi.org/10.1016/j.eats.2017.10.012.

12. Quigley T. The management of simple fracture of the clavicle in adults. N Engl J Med 1950;243(8):286–90.

13. Neer CS. Nonunion of the clavicle. Journal of the American Medical Association 1960;172(10):1006–11.

14. McKee MD, Pedersen EM, Jones C, et al. Deficits following nonoperative treatment of displaced midshaft clavicular fractures. JBJS 2006;88(1):35–40.

15. McKee MD, Wild LM, Schemitsch EH. Midshaft malunions of the clavicle. JBJS 2003;85(5):790–7.

16. Nowak J, Holgersson M, Larsson S. Sequelae from clavicular fractures are common: a prospective study of 222 patients. Acta Orthop 2005;76(4):496–502.

17. Wick M, Müller E, Kollig E, et al. Midshaft fractures of the clavicle with a shortening of more than 2 cm predispose to nonunion. Arch Orthop Trauma Surg 2001;121(4):207–11.

18. Walley KC, Haghpanah B, Hingsammer A, et al. Influence of disruption of the acromioclavicular and coracoclavicular ligaments on glenohumeral motion: a kinematic evaluation. BMC Muscoskel Disord 2016;17(1):1–9.

19. Culham E, Peat M. Functional anatomy of the shoulder complex. J Orthop Sports Phys Ther 1993;18(1):342–50.

20. Renfree KJ, Riley MK, Wheeler D, et al. Ligamentous anatomy of the distal clavicle. J Shoulder Elbow Surg 2003;12(4):355–9.

21. Fukuda K, Craig E, An K, et al. Biomechanical study of the ligamentous system of the acromioclavicular joint. J Bone Jt Surg Am Vol 1986;68(3):434–40.

22. Debski RE, Parsons It, Woo SL, et al. Effect of capsular injury on acromioclavicular joint mechanics. JBJS 2001;83(9):1344–51.

23. Costic RS, Labriola JE, Rodosky MW, et al. Biomechanical rationale for development of anatomical reconstructions of coracoclavicular ligaments after complete acromioclavicular joint dislocations. Am J Sports Med 2004;32(8):1929–36.

24. Lee K-W, Debski RE, Chen C-H, et al. Functional evaluation of the ligaments at the acromioclavicular joint during anteroposterior and superoinferior translation. Am J Sports Med 1997;25(6):858–62.

25. Rios CG, Mazzocca AD. Acromioclavicular joint problems in athletes and new methods of management. Clin Sports Med 2008;27(4):763–88.

26. Bearden JM, Hughston JC, Whatley GS. Acromioclavicular dislocation: method of treatment. J Sports Med 1973;1(4):5–17.

27. Craig EV, Rockwood C, Green D, et al. Fractures in adults. Philadelphia: JB Lippincott Company; 1996. p. 928–90.

28. Chen RE, Soin SP, El-Shaar R, et al. What regions of the distal clavicle have the greatest bone mineral density and cortical thickness? A cadaveric study. Clin Orthop Relat Res 2019;477(12):2726.

29. Knudsen F, Andersen M, Krag C. The arterial supply of the clavicle. Surg Radiol Anat 1989;11(3):211–4.

30. Robinson CM, Cairns DA. Primary nonoperative treatment of displaced lateral fractures of the clavicle. JBJS 2004;86(4):778–82.

31. Stanley D, Trowbridge E, Norris S. The mechanism of clavicular fracture. A clinical and biomechanical analysis. Journal of bone and joint surgery British volume 1988;70(3):461–4.
32. Stenson J, Baker W. Classifications in brief: the modified NEER classification for distal-third clavicle fractures. Clin Orthop Relat Res 2021;479(1):205.
33. Banerjee R, Waterman B, Padalecki J, et al. Management of distal clavicle fractures. JAAOS-Journal of the American Academy of Orthopaedic Surgeons 2011; 19(7):392–401.
34. Robinson CM. Fractures of the clavicle in the adult: epidemiology and classification. Journal of bone and joint surgery British 1998;80(3):476–84.
35. Robertson GA, Wood AM. Return to sport following clavicle fractures: a systematic review. Br Med Bull 2016;119(1):111–28.
36. Huang K-C, Tu Y-K, Huang T-J, et al. Suprascapular neuropathy complicating a Neer type I distal clavicular fracture: a case report. J Orthop Trauma 2005; 19(5):343–5.
37. Anderson K. Evaluation and treatment of distal clavicle fractures. Clin Sports Med 2003;22(2):319–26.
38. Blaas LS, van Sterkenburg MN, de Planque AM, et al. New possibilities: the Lock-Down device for distal clavicle fractures. JSES international 2020;4(4):713–8.
39. Nambiar M, West LR, Bingham R. AO Surgery Reference: a comprehensive guide for management of fractures. Br J Sports Med 2017;51(6):545–6.
40. Cho C-H, Kim B-S, Kim D-H, et al. Distal clavicle fractures: a new classification system. J Orthop Traumatol: Surgery & Research 2018;104(8):1231–5.
41. Kim DW, Kim DH, Kim BS, et al. Current Concepts for Classification and Treatment of Distal Clavicle Fractures. Clin Orthop Surg 2020;12(2):135–44.
42. Robinson CM, McQueen MM, Wakefield AE. Estimating the risk of nonunion following nonoperative treatment of a clavicular fracture. JBJS 2004;86(7):1359–65.
43. Yagnik GP, Seiler JR, Vargas LA, et al. Outcomes of arthroscopic fixation of unstable distal clavicle fractures: a systematic review. Orthopaedic Journal of Sports Medicine 2021;9(5). 23259671211001773.
44. Kihlström C, Hailer NP, Wolf O. Surgical Versus Nonsurgical Treatment of Lateral Clavicle Fractures: A Short-Term Follow-Up of Treatment and Complications in 122 Patients. J Orthop Trauma 2021;35(12):667–72.
45. Andersen K, Jensen PØ, Lauritzen J. Treatment of clavicular fractures: Figure-of-elght bandage versus a slmple sling. Acta Orthop Scand 1987;58(1):71–4.
46. Ersen A, Atalar A, Birisik F, et al. Comparison of simple arm sling and figure of eight clavicular bandage for midshaft clavicular fractures: a randomised controlled study. Bone & Joint Journal 2015;97(11):1562–5.
47. Rokito AS, Zuckerman JD, Shaari JM, et al. A comparison of nonoperative and operative treatment of type II distal clavicle fractures. Bull Hosp Jt Dis 2002; 61(1–2):32–9.
48. Deafenbaugh M, Dugdale T, Staeheli J, et al. Nonoperative treatment of Neer type II distal clavicle fractures: a prospective study. Contemp Orthop 1990; 20(4):405–13.
49. Van der Meijden OA, Gaskill TR, Millett PJ. Treatment of clavicle fractures: current concepts review. J Shoulder Elbow Surg 2012;21(3):423–9.
50. Hall JA, Schemitsch CE, Vicente MR, et al. Operative Versus Nonoperative Treatment of Acute Displaced Distal Clavicle Fractures: A Multicenter Randomized Controlled Trial. J Orthop Trauma 2021;35(12):660–6.
51. Wilson CD, Probe RA. Shared Decision-making in Orthopaedic Surgery. J Am Acad Orthop Surg 2020;28(23):e1032–41.

Operative Management for Displaced Distal Clavicle Fractures

Mihir M. Sheth, MD[a], Theodore B. Shybut, MD[b],*

KEYWORDS

- Distal clavicle fracture • Lateral clavicle • Coracoclavicular ligaments
- Surgical fixation • Athlete

KEY POINTS

- Operative treatment is favored for fractures medial to the CC ligaments (Neer type 2A), with CC ligament injury (Neer types 2B and 5) and with concern for skin compromise. In addition, operative treatment is favored for displaced fractures in athletes.
- The most common fixation techniques currently include locked plating, CC fixation with a variety of devices, and combination locked plating with CC fixation. Hook plates may be useful for very lateral fractures, but surgeons should be aware of complications specific to this implant. Tension banding and K-wire constructs should not be considered a first choice.
- Arthroscopically assisted techniques allow the surgeon to address concomitant shoulder pathology.
- While the surgical outcomes of subacute or chronic injuries is inferior to acute injuries, they can be managed successfully through locking plates with CC fixation or salvage AC + CC reconstruction procedures if the lateral fragment is not amenable to fixation.
- The rate of symptomatic hardware requiring removal has been reported to be 50%, and surgeons should aim to use low-profile constructs when feasible.

INTRODUCTION

The previous section on the nonoperative management and classification of distal clavicle fractures has noted that many distal clavicle fractures are amenable to nonsurgical treatment. However, nonunion is estimated to occur in 31% of fractures treated nonoperatively, with the strongest predictors being a high degree of displacement (>100%) and advancing age.[1] These nonunions are estimated to be symptomatic in 50% of patients. A recent systematic review found 8% later undergo surgery.[2]

[a] Baylor College of Medicine, 7200 Cambridge Street, Suite 10A, Houston, TX 77030, USA;
[b] Southern California Orthopedic Institute, 6815 Noble Avenue, Van Nuys, CA 91405, USA
* Corresponding author.
E-mail address: tshybut@scoi.com

Clin Sports Med 42 (2023) 695–711
https://doi.org/10.1016/j.csm.2023.06.017
0278-5919/23/© 2023 Elsevier Inc. All rights reserved.
sportsmed.theclinics.com

While nonsurgical management is appropriate for many distal clavicle fractures, acute operative fixation of displaced fractures provides faster union and more predictable outcomes than nonoperative management. Hence surgery the treatment of choice in athletes for displaced fractures. A recently published prospective, randomized controlled trial of nonoperative versus operative treatment of displaced distal clavicle fractures found the nonoperative group to have a slower return to full activity and less satisfaction with their shoulder cosmesis than the surgery group. In addition, 63% of the nonoperative group developed a nonunion, of which 33% underwent a corrective surgery by 1 year; moreover, two of these patients required multiple procedures.[3] A separate study found that distal clavicle fixation at >4 weeks from injury resulted in lower function scores and a higher complication rate.[4] The literature lacks well-established predictors of which patients will not tolerate a nonunion. In light of inferior subacute outcomes, acute fixation is preferred for displaced fractures, particularly in athletes.

While surgeons may debate whether the frequency of symptomatic nonunion justifies fixation in general for these fractures, acute surgical fixation is the optimal strategy for displaced distal clavicle fractures in athletes because it facilitates return to play. Moreover, for other patient populations, acute surgical management reduces the risk of nonunion, avoids the surgeon having to guess if a patient will be symptomatic from a nonunion, and avoids the inferior results of subacute treatment. In this section, we review the operative management of displaced distal clavicle fractures, including relevant anatomy, indications for surgery, described techniques, and the current clinical outcomes literature.

RELEVANT ANATOMY AND BIOMECHANICS

The static stabilizers of lateral clavicle include the coracoclavicular (CC) and acromioclavicular (AC) ligaments (**Fig. 1**). The CC ligaments include the conoid ligament medially and the trapezoid ligament laterally, which originate from the coracoid and insert

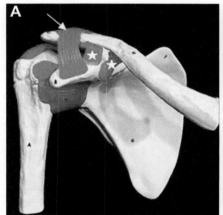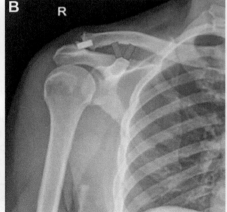

Fig. 1. Anatomy of distal clavicle and stabilizing ligaments. (*A*): Model shoulder including the acromioclavicular (AC) ligaments indicated by the white arrow and coracoclavicular (CC) ligaments indicated by white stars, with the conoid ligament being more medial. (*B*): A shoulder radiograph with a schematic representation of the AC ligaments in yellow and CC ligaments in blue.

approximately 45 and 25 mm from the lateral end of the clavicle.[5] The CC ligaments provide predominantly vertical stability to the lateral clavicle. The normal distance between the coracoid and clavicle at this level is 11-13 mm. This measurement can vary significantly based on radiographic projection, and a comparison to the contralateral side can be useful with < 5 mm of difference being considered uninjured.[6] The AC ligaments surround the AC joint capsule with thickenings anteroinferiorly and posterosuperiorly; the posterosuperior is the more robust bundle.[7] The AC ligaments provide predominantly horizontal stability.[7] These ligaments are rarely injured in lateral clavicle fractures, and an effort should be made to preserve the ligaments during surgery to avoid iatrogenic instability of the AC joint.

The dynamic stabilizers of the lateral clavicle include the anterior third of the deltoid and the trapezius, which originate on the anterior-inferior and posterior-superior surface of the lateral clavicle, respectively.

The clavicle serves as a lateral strut to the shoulder girdle and its length is essential to the complex mechanics of the scapulothoracic articulation. Shortened clavicle malunions have been shown to result in inferior, anterior, and medialized scapular position, and diminish tolerance for overhead activities.[8–11]

Evaluation and Imaging

The evaluation and imaging relevant to distal clavicle fractures are discussed in Lian and colleagues' article, "Classification of Distal Clavicle Fractures and Indications for Conservative Treatment," in this issue. The most important factor to evaluate on physical exam is the presence of an open fracture or impending skin compromise. Imaging should include radiographs with a 10 to 15° cephalic tilt, which will better assess the superior displacement compared to neutral tilt projections; this view is also known as a Zanca view. CC ligament injury can be inferred by the involvement of the inferior clavicle surface at their insertion. Computed tomography (CT) images can be obtained to assess lateral bone stock, but are generally not required.

Indications for Operative Management

There are not absolute evidence-based indications for the operative management of closed distal clavicle fractures, largely owing to the frequency of asymptomatic nonunions. In general certain fracture patterns are recognized to have a low rate of nonunion and may be treated nonoperatively:

Fractures lateral to intact CC ligaments and not involving the AC joint (Neer type 1).

Physeal fractures involving lateral clavicle tearing through the periosteal sleeve (Neer type 4).

Intra-articular fractures lateral to the intact CC ligaments have generally treated nonoperatively. Recently, some surgeons have advocated for operative repair of these injuries due to a higher than expected rate of nonunion, which they postulated was due to deforming forces of the deltoid and trapezius causing horizontal instability.[1,12] However, this is not yet a universally applied surgical indication.

Indications for operative management include.

- Displaced fractures medial to the CC ligaments (Neer type 2A)
- Displaced fractures involving partial (Neer type 2B) or complete CC ligament injury (Neer type 5)
- Open fractures or those with impending skin compromise.

As with all fractures, the patient's activity level and individual risk factors should be considered. Surgical fixation may be relatively indicated in physiologically younger and more active patients, although surgeons should be aware that advancing age is a risk factor for nonunion.[1] Smoking, malnutrition, and severe medical comorbidities have also been reported to increase the risk of nonunion,[1,13] but those factors are also relative contraindications to surgical treatment.

With regard to athletes, there are no studies directly comparing return to play for operative and nonoperative treatment to guide management. In general, non-displaced fractures can be treated non-operatively with return to play guided by signs of radiographic union. Surgical management is favored for displaced fractures. This preference relates to better predictability of fracture union and functional outcomes, and mitigating scapulothoracic dyskinesia related to loss of the clavicle strut. The trend towards surgical management in athletes is reflected in a recent systematic review that found 204 displaced lateral clavicle fractures in athletes were treated surgically compared to only 6 patients treated non-surgically.[14]

Surgical Techniques

Multiple techniques for operative fixation of distal clavicle fractures have been described. A comprehensive list can be found in **Table 1**. While successful outcomes have been reported with all of these techniques, the most common today are locking plates, CC repair with suture button implants or cerclage, combined plating with CC suture buttons or cerclage, and hook plates.

Locking plates

A 2021 survey found that the most common operative treatment was locking plates.[15]

Several commercially available anatomically contoured plates have lateral screw clusters to achieve fixation in even small fragments. For most of these cluster designs, obtaining three screws in the lateral fragment requires the fragment to be 10 to 15 mm in size. Some plates are designed with suture holes or to accommodate flush nesting of a suture button if the surgeon wishes to augment the construct with CC suspensory fixation. Drawbacks to locked plating include that lateral comminution can preclude adequate purchase and implant prominence. A retrospective review including 16 distal clavicle fractures treated with plates and screws (not including hook plates) found a 50% hardware removal rate,[16] although other studies have reported lower rates.[17–19] Successful outcomes have also been reported with non-locking "T" plates[20] and mini-fragment plates.[21]

Coracoclavicular suture fixation

CC suture fixation has been described using a suture anchor in the base of the coracoid, cortical button-based suspensory devices passed through the coracoid, and with cerclage sutures around the coracoid. CC screws, also referred to as Bosworth screws, are similar in concept but have fallen out of favor due to reports of migration, screw breakage, and loss of reduction. In addition, they require subsequent surgery for removal.

There are multiple descriptions of arthroscopically assisted techniques. The benefits of an arthroscopic approach include smaller incisions, less stripping of the clavicle's blood supply, and excellent visualization of the coracoid base. Arthroscopy also allows the identification and management of concomitant pathology, which is present in as high as 44% of patients.[22] This approach can be technically challenging (as reflected in longer operative times), and requires conversion to an open approach if scar tissue blocks CC reduction or in the event of coracoid injury. A systematic review on union rates and function following arthroscopically assisted CC fixation found similar results to open techniques.[22] Thus, surgeons may elect this approach based

Table 1
Operative techniques for distal clavicle fixation

Technique	Description	Variations	Pros and Cons
Locking plate	Osteosynthesis with locking fixation in small lateral fragment through a screw cluster	• Anatomic contoured plate • Locking mini-fragment plates • Volar distal radius locking plates	*Pros:* • Robust fixation in lateral fragment *Cons:* • Hardware prominence • Cannot use with lateral fragment < 10–15 mm
Coracoclavicular ligament suture/ suture button repair	Suture ± cortical button or anchor passed through or around clavicle and/or coracoid to stabilize conoid and trapezoid ligament attachments.	• Coracoid: anchor in base, button through coracoid, or sutures passed under coracoid • Clavicle: button on the superior clavicle, bone tunnels, or tied over top • Approach: open or arthroscopy assisted	*Pros:* • Low profile • More directly addresses vertical instability *Cons:* • Coracoid fracture • Clavicle fracture adjacent to tunnels (rare)
Locking plate with CC fixation	Anatomic plate augmented with CC fixation.	Various combinations of plate and CC fixation techniques.	*Pros:* Biomechanical strength *Cons:* Hardware prominence of plate
Hook plate	Cortical plate medially with a hook laterally that is positioned to sit beneath the acromion.	• 90° plate • 115° plate	*Pros:* Provides stable fixation for very small or comminuted lateral fragments. *Cons:* • Requires hardware removal • Acromial erosion or fracture • Subacromial impingement or rotator cuff tear • AC joint arthrosis

(continued on next page)

Table 1
(continued)

Technique	Description	Variations	Pros and Cons
Mini fragment plating	Osteosynthesis with mini fragment plates.	• Single "T" plate • Dual plating	*Pros:* Low profile *Cons:* Cannot use with lateral comminution
Trans-osseous suturing	2–3 high tensile strength sutures through drill tunnels in fragments.	With and without sutures around the coracoid.	*Pros:* Low profile *Cons:* Cannot use with lateral comminution
Coracoclavicular (Bosworth) screw	6.5 mm or 4.5 mm screw placed through clavicle and coracoid		*Con* • Requires hardware removal • Migration, screw breakage and loss of reduction
Kirschner wires/Knowles pin	Temporary pin fixation across fracture	• Trans-acromial pins • Tension band wiring • Intramedullary fixation	*Pros:* low cost *Cons:* • Skin irritation • Pin migration and higher rates of lost fixation

on their experience and comfort level. The potential to identify and address concurrent intra-articular pathology makes this an attractive option for the treatment of athletes.

Clinical outcomes of CC fixation have been reported to be similar to or better than anatomic plating. A retrospective cohort comparison of 15 CC fixations (augmented with K-wire fixation across the fragments) and 26 anatomic plates for type 2B at minimum 2-year follow-up found 100% union in both groups and no difference in function or pain scores (ASES and VAS pain). In addition, the CC fixation group had a better maintenance of coracoclavicular distance, shorter operative time and better cosmesis.[23] Moreover, CC fixation with suture buttons has been found to be cost-effective compared to locking and hook plates, due to lower reoperation rates and high rates of healing.[24]

There are limitations to isolated CC fixation. It is not well suited for fractures exiting medial to intact CC ligaments, or Neer type 2A injuries, because the fixation would have to be oblique towards the coracoid and the surgery may unnecessarily disrupt the intact native ligaments. Moreover, this technique would not be appropriate for fractures lateral to the trapezoid ligament that some authors have felt are horizontally unstable.[12] Other limitations include the risk of coracoid fracture with the use of fixation through the coracoid (suture buttons or anchors) or the risk of coracoid erosion due to the "sawing" effect of sutures passed under the coracoid.[25,26]

Locking plate with coracoclavicular suture reconstruction

Locking plate fixation can be augmented with combined CC fixation. Multiple implant systems are designed for this technique, but it can also be performed with any suture placed through or around a superior plate.

The combination of these techniques has been studied. Two biomechanical studies showed a higher load to failure with the addition of CC fixation compared to locking plates alone.[27,28] There are 2 retrospective clinical studies that have compared locking plates with and without CC fixation. In a series of 34 patients, Xu and colleagues[19] found a statistically significant faster union rate (mean 14 weeks vs 16 weeks) and 5 point advantage in mean Constant score at 1 year (95 vs 90) with the addition of CC fixation. There were no differences in complication and overall union rates. Salazar and colleagues[29] compared 16 patients treated with locking plates to 7 patients with the addition of CC fixation; they found no difference in union rates and function when CC fixation was added. While the number of comparative studies is limited, a recent systematic review found better Constant-Murley scores after locking plates when combined with CC fixation compared to without, but similar rates of union and complications.[2]

The decision to add CC fixation to a locking plate is also informed by studies on either fixation construct in isolation. Furuhata and colleagues[30] found that the use of a locking plate alone for fractures with CC ligament injury resulted in greater residual CC distance compared to fractures treated the same way without CC injury. This finding suggests that locking plates in isolation do not provide sufficient vertical stability in the setting of CC ligament. Therefore CC ligament injury may be an indication to add CC fixation. However, both this study and another similar study found no differences in function scores, union rate, and complications between the 2 groups.[30,31] Additionally, there are reports of favorable results with either technique in isolation for fractures with CC ligament injury.[2,32]

Overall the addition of CC fixation to locking plates improves the biomechanics of distal clavicle fracture repairs. Added CC fixation is warranted in fractures with partial or complete CC ligament injury (Neer 2B and 5), but may not be needed in many injuries with intact ligaments (Neer 2A). In the treatment of athletes, consideration should be given to their sport-specific demands, which may favor using the biomechanically strongest construct. If CC fixation is added to injuries with intact CC ligaments, we recommend cerclage fixation (around the coracoid) to avoid the disruption of the CC ligament origins on the coracoid, which might occur when drilling to place anchors or suture button suspensory devices.

Hook plate

Hook plates involve cortical screw fixation through the plate on the medial clavicle fragment, and fixation laterally via a hook placed underneath the acromion (**Fig. 2**). This construct provides a method for fixation in distal clavicle fractures with lateral fragments too small for locked plating. It also provides vertical stability and so can be utilized when there is a concurrent coracoid fracture that precludes CC fixation. For type 2B fractures it offers the advantage of achieving lateral fixation without requiring extensive dissection around the trapezoid ligament. A recent meta-analysis found a union rate of 98% and comparable function scores compared to other methods of fixation.[32]

Of concern, the hook can erode the undersurface of the acromion. Acromial erosion was reported in 27% of cases,[32] and some patients may sustain acromial fractures.[33–35] For this reason, implant removal is recommended after fracture union, which adds to the burden of treatment. Factors that increase the likelihood of acromion osteolysis include:

Hook position posterior to the ideal position of being just posterior to the AC joint and pointing anterior[36]

Mismatch of the hook with the slope of the acromion undersurface, that results in point loading rather than load sharing across the entire hook.[37]

Permitting shoulder abduction and flexion of >90° prior to plate removal.

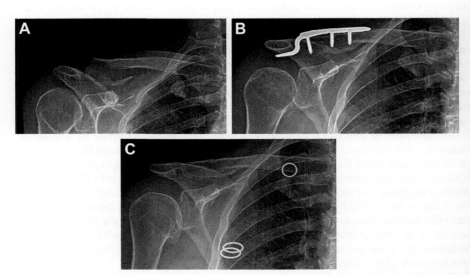

Fig. 2. Hook plate case example (A) Radiograph of an acute displaced distal clavicle fracture with lateral comminution. (B) Hook plate at 3 months post-operatively with radiographic healing. (C) Hook plate removed after radiographic healing. (Images courtesy of Peter S. Vezeridis, MD).

Delayed implant removal after fracture union (ie, noncompliance/loss to follow-up).

In addition, hook plates may be approached with caution when there is existing acromial erosion (such as in cuff tear arthropathy), osteoporosis, or an os acromiale.[38] The mismatch of the acromion slope and hook can be mitigated by manually contouring the plate or possibly by using newer plates with a 15° inferior angulation.[37,39] The anterior position can be ensured intra-operatively by using the posterior aspect of the AC joint capsule as a landmark for ideal hook position.

Other complications associated with hook plates include AC joint arthrosis (22%), clavicle fracture medial to the plate (22%), and painful stiffness or subacromial impingement (47%).[32,34] Rotator cuff tears have been reported, although an MRI study found no complete tears in 39 cases.[40] Lastly, one study found that 66% of athletes treated with a hook plate did not return to sports.[41] While this is a single study, these findings suggest primary distal clavicle fixation with a hook plate should be limited to narrow indications in athletes.

Trans-osseous suturing

Multiple authors have described interfragmentary suturing through anterior to posterior bone tunnels in each fragment with or without incorporating sutures passed under the coracoid.[42–44] Two retrospective reports of 20 and 12 patients showed union at a mean of less than 3 months in all but one patient.[42,43] This technique has the benefit of being low profile and inexpensive. Its limitations include not being possible for comminuted or small lateral fragments.

Other techniques (K-wires, tension band, knowles pinning)

K-wires, tension bands, and intramedullary Knowles pinning are inexpensive, now mostly historical techniques. They have been largely replaced by other methods. Two meta-analyses on the clinical outcomes and complication rates after various distal clavicle fixation techniques support abandoning Kirschner wires, Knowles pinning, and tension bands due to higher complication rates.[2,32]

TECHNIQUES FOR SUBACUTE AND CHRONIC INJURIES

The nonunion rates for displaced distal clavicle fractures suggest that surgeons who treat them initially without surgery will likely encounter symptomatic nonunions. Surgical fixation in these cases can be challenging due to the partial resorption of the lateral fragment. In addition, deformity in the clavicle for as short as 4 to 6 weeks can lead to scapular dyskinesis and affect final function.[8,45]

For cases with adequate bone quality in the lateral fragment, locking plates combined with CC fixation is the mainstay for treatment. A series of 38 nonunions treated with this technique showed a 100% union rate, alongside favorable functional outcomes and a 5% complication rate.[13] Some authors have added iliac crest or proximal humerus cancellous autograft to augment the biologic environment for healing.[46] When stable fixation of the lateral fragment cannot be achieved, we recommend fragment excision with the vertical stabilization of the medial fragment via CC ligament reconstruction using both tendon graft and suture and horizontal stabilization with acromioclavicular stabilization and/or graft reconstruction. Surgeons may elect other technique variations similar to those used for chronic AC joint separations.

The complication rates and functional outcomes of distal clavicle fracture fixation are inferior when surgery is performed at greater than 4 weeks from injury. Klein and colleagues[4] found a mean American Shoulder and Elbow Surgeons score of 78 and 36% complication rate in patients treated after 4 weeks compared to 65 and 7%, respectively, in patients treated before 4 weeks. As mentioned, surgeons should be aware of these inferior results when considering nonoperative treatment for displaced fractures. When considering the athlete's shoulder, these outcomes support acute surgical intervention for displaced fractures.

COMPARATIVE STUDIES ON FIXATION TECHNIQUES

Recent studies have directly compared the outcomes of fixation techniques, as summarized in **Table 2**.[3,18–20,23,47–50] In general, the majority of studies comparing locked plating or CC fixation to hook plates have found similar rates of union and final functional outcome, but inferior early function and more complications with hook plates (even when excluding planned hardware removals).[32] Studies comparing locked plating with and without CC fixation have found either similar results or favor the use of adding CC fixation.[19,29]

A recent systematic review and meta-analysis of 59 studies and 2284 patients compared the results of distal clavicle fixation techniques, including locked plating, CC fixation, hook plates, K-wires, and combinations of fixation constructs.[2] With regard to function, they found that hook plates showed lower Constant scores compared to CC fixation but were similar to locking plates and K-wire constructs. There was no significant difference in union rates across all fixation methods. K-wire constructs (including tension banding) had the highest rate of complications overall, as well as specifically for hardware failure, infection, and wound complications. Hook plates had the second highest rate of complications overall, with 1 of 5 patients experiencing a complication (excluding planned hardware removals); a separate systematic review found a higher rate of complications with hook plates compared to locked plating and CC fixation.[32] The authors concluded that the first choice of surgical fixation should be CC fixation alone, followed closely by a locking plate with CC fixation.

Overall, the recent literature has helped guide the selection of fixation techniques:

Low-profile techniques, such as isolated CC fixation and trans-osseous suturing, should be favored when possible due to the frequency of symptomatic hardware and similar union rates compared to plating techniques.

There is not currently strong evidence to support arthroscopic assisted CC fixation over an open technique.

There is no strong clinical evidence to support the addition of CC fixation to locked plating. Biomechanical studies support the combination construct, and thus it may be favorable in high-demand patients such as athletes.

K-wires and tension bands should not be considered a first choice because are associated with inferior results compared to multiple other techniques.

Hook plates should be reserved for fracture patterns in which adequate fixation of the lateral fragment cannot otherwise be achieved. The need for subsequent hardware removal, higher complication rate compared to other techniques (locking plates, CC fixation, trans-osseous suturing) and risk of particularly morbid complications (ie, acromial fractures) unique to hook plates preclude more routine use of these implants. Based on these data, we propose an algorithm for fixation techniques that are best suited for particular fracture patterns (**Fig. 3**). The main points to consider are whether the lateral fragment is large enough for fixation and if the CC ligaments are intact.

Return to Sport

Unlike mid-shift clavicle fractures, there is limited literature on return to sport after distal clavicle fractures. A systematic review[14] of 204 lateral clavicle fractures treated surgically attempted to analyze return to sport rates and times for various fixation

Table 2
Comparative studies of specific fixation techniques for distal clavicle fractures

Comparison (n)	Design	Union	Final Function	Complications
CCR (23) vs HP (49)[48]	Retrospective cohort	87% vs 92% [b]	CS: 95 vs 87.[a]	0% vs 25% [a]
HP (19) vs aCCR (21)[47]	Retrospective cohort	95% vs 95% [b]	CS: 89 vs 93 [b]	16% vs 10% [b]
LP (16) vs LP + CCR(18)[19]	Retrospective cohort	100% both groups	CS: 95 vs 90 [a]	17% vs 31% [b]
CCR (15) vs LP (26)[23]	Retrospective cohort	100% both groups	ASES: 92 vs 87 [b]	Higher rates of AC arthritis and cosmetic dissatisfaction with LP [a]
HP (13) vs **LP + CCR** (17)[18]	Prospective RCT	100% both groups	CS: 88 vs 88 [b]	Rate not specifically reported. All HP underwent HWR, compared to 1/17 LPs.
Non-op (30) vs LP/HP (27)[3]	Prospective RCT	64% vs 95% [a]	CS: 90 vs 90 [b]	13% vs 7% [b]
LP (20) vs **CCR (20)**[49]	Retrospective cohort, multicenter	100% both groups	UCLA: 35 vs 35 [b]	25% vs 10% [b]
aCCR (16) vs HP (32)[50]	Prospective cohort	100% both groups	ASES: 89 vs 84 [a]	0 vs 3% [b]
HP (30) vs non **locking T-plate** (30)[20]	Prospective cohort	100% both groups	CS: 92 vs 92 [b]	6% vs 3% [b]

Abbreviations: aCCR, arthroscopy-assisted coracoclavicular ligament suture reconstruction; CCR, coracoclavicular ligament suture reconstruction; HP, hook plate; HWR, hardware removal; LP, Locking plate; RCT, randomized controlled trial; CS, Constant Score.
Bold type denotes techniques this review finds preferable.
[a] Statistically significant difference.
[b] Not statistically significant difference.

techniques. The overall return to sport rate including all fixation techniques was 85% at a mean 19 weeks. The lowest return to sport rates were for hook plates (79%) and tension band wiring (40%). The mean time to return was reported only for transosseous sutures, Bosworth screws, and arthroscopic CC fixation, and were found to be 13, 36 and 17 weeks, respectively. Overall, this study was limited by the few studies reporting return to sport after these injuries, and further research in this area is needed to better prognosticate and optimize treatment for athletes.

CASE EXAMPLES
Case 1

29-year-old female recreational athlete presented the day of a fall onto her shoulder while running. She had no skin compromise and was neurovascularly intact. Radiographs (**Fig. 4**) showed a displaced lateral clavicle fracture that appeared to involve the conoid ligament insertion on the clavicle and a comminuted lateral fragment. This is classified as a Neer type 2B injury.

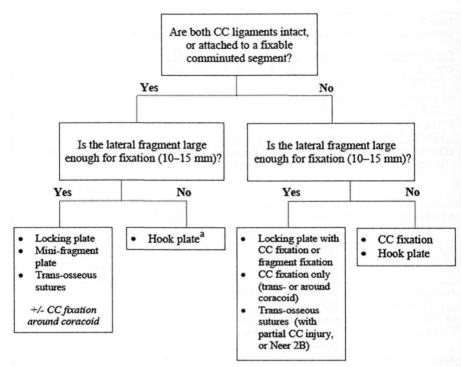

Fig. 3. Algorithm for recommended fixation techniques for acute displaced lateral clavicle fractures C ᵃ = this fracture pattern (lateral fragment too small for fixation with intact CC ligaments, Neer 1) is rare, and when it does occur, is typically nondisplaced. For all injury patterns, including ones with intact CC ligaments, CC fixation can be considered to augment the construct strength, but there is not strong clinical evidence to support its routine use. For injuries with intact CC ligaments, CC fixation around the coracoid is favored to avoid iatrogenic native CC ligament injury by fixation into the coracoid base.

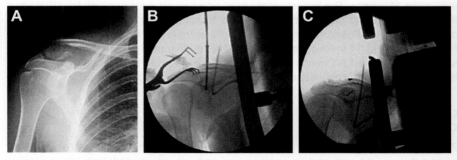

Fig. 4. Case example of a distal clavicle fracture treated with CC fixation only (A) Radiograph of an acute displaced distal clavicle fracture with CC ligament injury. Lateral fragment comminution is seen. (B) Intra-operative image shows coracoclavicular drilling. (C) Intraoperative image showing final reduction after suture button deployment and tensioning.

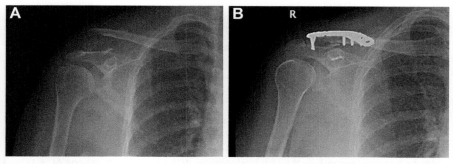

Fig. 5. Case example of displaced distal clavicle fracture treated with a locking plate and CC Fixation. (A) Radiograph of an acute distal clavicle fracture with > 100% displacement and a separate inferior clavicle fragment containing the CC ligament insertions. The lateral fragment measured 15 mm. (B) 3 month post-operative radiograph demonstrating fracture union.

Based displacement, desire to return to athletic activity, and cosmetic concerns, acute surgery consisting of CC fixation with a suture button was performed. Intraoperative fluoroscopy showing the button deployment and final reduction are shown (see **Fig. 4**B, C). At 2 months post-op she had near full active motion, the fracture was uniting, and she was progressing appropriately in physical therapy.

Case 2

59-year-old female housekeeper presented the day after a fall from standing onto the lateral aspect of her shoulder. She had no skin compromise and was neurovascularly intact. Radiographs (**Fig. 5**A) showed a displaced distal clavicle fracture with a comminuted segment involving the CC ligament insertions and a lateral fragment measuring 15 mm in length. This is classified as a Neer type 5 injury.

After a detailed discussion about treatment options, she elected acute surgical fixation. Locked plating in combination with suture button CC fixation was performed. Radiographic union was achieved at 3 months, as shown in **Fig. 5**B.

SUMMARY

Operative treatment of displaced lateral clavicle fractures is supported by a faster rate of recovery compared to nonoperative management, the risk with the nonsurgical treatment of symptomatic nonunion, and the inferior results of subacute operations. The fracture patterns at highest risk of nonunion that warrant fixation include fractures medial to the CC ligaments or involving CC ligament injury. Several techniques have been described with successful results, however an understanding of the injury pattern and clinical evidence can guide the surgeon to particular options. Surgeons should be aware of the high rates of symptomatic hardware with multiple techniques and the complication profile of hook plates when considering treatment options.

CLINICS CARE POINTS

- Operative treatment is favored for displaced distal clavicle fractures in athletes.
- More broadly, fracture patterns that favor operative treatment include those medial to the CC ligaments (Neer type 2A) or involving CC ligament injury (Neer types 2B and 5), and with concern for skin compromise.

- The most common fixation techniques currently include locked plating, CC fixation with a variety of devices, and combination locked plating with CC fixation.
- Arthroscopically assisted techniques allow the surgeon to address concomitant shoulder pathology.
- Hook plates may be useful for very lateral fractures, but careful attention to technique is critical to avoid complications specific to this implant, including subacromial erosion and fracture.
- Tension banding and other K-wire constructs are shown to provide inferior fixation and have higher complication rates, and should not be considered a first choice.
- While the surgical outcomes of subacute or chronic injuries is inferior to acute injuries, they can be managed successfully through locking plates with CC fixation or salvage AC + CC reconstruction procedures if the lateral fragment is not amenable to fixation.
- The rate of symptomatic hardware requiring removal has been reported to be 50%, and surgeons should aim to use low-profile constructs when feasible.

DISCLOSURE

The authors have nothing to disclose relevant to this topic.

REFERENCES

1. Robinson CM, Court-Brown CM, McQueen MM, et al. Estimating the risk of nonunion following nonoperative treatment of a clavicular fracture. J Bone Joint Surg Am 2004;86(7):1359–65.
2. Uittenbogaard SJ, van Es LJM, den Haan C, et al. Outcomes, union rate, and complications after operative and nonoperative treatments of neer type Ii distal clavicle fractures: a systematic review and meta-analysis of 2284 patients. Am J Sports Med 2021. https://doi.org/10.1177/03635465211053336. 3635465211053336.
3. Hall JA, Schemitsch CE, Vicente MR, et al. Operative versus nonoperative treatment of acute displaced distal clavicle fractures: a multicenter randomized controlled trial. J Orthop Trauma 2021;35(12):660–6.
4. Klein SM, Badman BL, Keating CJ, et al. Results of surgical treatment for unstable distal clavicular fractures. J Shoulder Elbow Surg 2010;19(7):1049–55.
5. Rios CG, Arciero RA, Mazzocca AD. Anatomy of the clavicle and coracoid process for reconstruction of the coracoclavicular ligaments. Am J Sports Med 2007;35(5):811–7.
6. Alyas F, Curtis M, Speed C, et al. MR imaging appearances of acromioclavicular joint dislocation. Radiographics 2008;28(2):463–79 [quiz: 619].
7. Nakazawa M, Nimura A, Mochizuki T, et al. The orientation and variation of the acromioclavicular ligament: an anatomic study. Am J Sports Med 2016;44(10): 2690–5.
8. McKee MD, Pedersen EM, Jones C, et al. Deficits following nonoperative treatment of displaced midshaft clavicular fractures. J Bone Joint Surg Am 2006; 88(1):35–40.
9. Ristevski B, Hall JA, Pearce D, et al. The radiographic quantification of scapular malalignment after malunion of displaced clavicular shaft fractures. J Shoulder Elbow Surg 2013;22(2):240–6.
10. Perskin CR, Egol KA. Conversion of Neer Type II Closed Distal Clavicle Fracture to an Open Fracture Following Surgery Delay: A Case Report. J Orthop Case Rep 2021;11(9):50–3.

11. Neer CS. Fractures of the distal third of the clavicle. Clin Orthop Relat Res 1968; 58:43–50.

12. Zhang Y, Yu P, Zhuang C, et al. Revising the modified Neer classification for distal clavicle fractures: Description and reliability. Injury 2021. https://doi.org/10.1016/j.injury.2021.11.018. S0020-1383(21)00927-X.

13. Robinson PG, Williamson TR, Yapp LZ, et al. Functional outcomes and complications following combined locking plate and tunneled suspensory device fixation of lateral-end clavicle nonunions. J Shoulder Elbow Surg 2021;30(11):2570–6.

14. Robertson GaJ, Wood AM. Return to sport following clavicle fractures: a systematic review. Br Med Bull 2016;119(1):111–28.

15. Sharma V, Modi A, Armstrong A, et al. The management of distal clavicle fractures – a survey of UK shoulder and elbow surgeons. Cureus 2021;13(8):e17305.

16. Davis BP, Shybut TB, Coleman MM, et al. Risk factors for hardware removal following operative treatment of middle- and distal-third clavicular fractures. J Shoulder Elbow Surg 2021;30(3):e103–13.

17. Gutman MJ, Joyce CD, Patel MS, et al. Outcomes following different fixation strategies of neer type IIB distal clavicle fractures. Arch Bone Jt Surg 2022;10(2): 160–5.

18. Orlandi TV, Rogers NS, Burger MC, et al. A prospective randomized controlled trial comparing plating augmented with coracoclavicular fixation and hook plate fixation of displaced distal-third clavicle fractures. J Shoulder Elbow Surg 2022; 31(5):906–13.

19. Xu H, Chen WJ, Zhi XC, et al. Comparison of the efficacy of a distal clavicular locking plate with and without a suture anchor in the treatment of Neer IIb distal clavicle fractures. BMC Musculoskelet Disord 2019;20(1):503.

20. Teimouri M, Ravanbod H, Farrokhzad A, et al. Comparison of hook plate versus T-plate in the treatment of Neer type II distal clavicle fractures: a prospective matched comparative cohort study. J Orthop Surg Res 2022;17(1):369.

21. Chen MJ, Salazar BP, Bishop JA, et al. Dual mini-fragment plate fixation for Neer type-II and -V distal clavicle fractures. OTA Int 2020;3(3):e078.

22. Yagnik GP, Seiler JR, Vargas LA, et al. Outcomes of arthroscopic fixation of unstable distal clavicle fractures: a systematic review. Orthop J Sports Med 2021;9(5). 23259671211001772.

23. Kim DJ, Lee YM, Yoon EJ, et al. Comparison of locking plate fixation and coracoclavicular ligament reconstruction for neer type 2B distal clavicle fractures. Orthop J Sports Med 2022;10(3). 23259671221086670.

24. Fox HM, Ramsey DC, Thompson AR, et al. Neer type-II distal clavicle fractures: a cost-effectiveness analysis of fixation techniques. J Bone Joint Surg Am 2020; 102(3):254–61.

25. Martetschläger F, Horan MP, Warth RJ, et al. Complications after anatomic fixation and reconstruction of the coracoclavicular ligaments. Am J Sports Med 2013; 41(12):2896–903.

26. Peng L, Zheng Y, Chen S, et al. Single tunnel technique versus coracoid sling technique for arthroscopic treatment of acute acromioclavicular joint dislocation. Sci Rep 2022;12(1):4244.

27. Madsen W, Yaseen Z, LaFrance R, et al. Addition of a suture anchor for coracoclavicular fixation to a superior locking plate improves stability of type IIB distal clavicle fractures. Arthroscopy 2013;29(6):998–1004.

28. Rieser GR, Edwards K, Gould GC, et al. Distal-third clavicle fracture fixation: a biomechanical evaluation of fixation. J Shoulder Elbow Surg 2013;22(6):848–55.

29. Salazar BP, Chen MJ, Bishop JA, et al. Outcomes after locking plate fixation of distal clavicle fractures with and without coracoclavicular ligament augmentation. Eur J Orthop Surg Traumatol 2021;31(3):473–9.

30. Furuhata R, Matsumura N, Udagawa K, et al. Residual coracoclavicular separation after plate fixation for distal clavicle fractures: comparison between fracture patterns. JSES Int 2021;5(5):840–5.

31. Shin SJ, Ko YW, Lee J, et al. Use of plate fixation without coracoclavicular ligament augmentation for unstable distal clavicle fractures. J Shoulder Elbow Surg 2016;25(6):942–8.

32. Asadollahi S, Bucknill A. Hook plate fixation for acute unstable distal clavicle fracture: a systematic review and meta-analysis. J Orthop Trauma 2019;33(8):417–22.

33. Chiang CL, Yang SW, Tsai MY, et al. Acromion osteolysis and fracture after hook plate fixation for acromioclavicular joint dislocation: a case report. J Shoulder Elbow Surg 2010;19(4):e13–5.

34. Lee SJ, Eom TW, Hyun YS. Complications and frequency of surgical treatment with AO-type hook plate in shoulder trauma: a retrospective study. J Clin Med 2022;11(4):1026.

35. Lopiz Y, Checa P, García-Fernández C, et al. Complications with the clavicle hook plate after fixation of Neer type II clavicle fractures. Int Orthop 2019;43(7):1701–8.

36. Shimpuku E, Uchiyama Y, Imai T, et al. Relationship between subacromial bone erosion and hook position of clavicular plate in distal clavicle fractures. J Orthop Trauma 2022;36(6):e243–9.

37. Kirsch JM, Blum L, Hake ME. Distal clavicle fractures: open reduction and internal fixation with a hook plate. J Orthop Trauma 2018;32(Suppl 1):S2–3.

38. Sun Q, Cai M, Wu X. Os acromiale may be a contraindication of the clavicle hook plate: case reports and literature review. BMC Musculoskelet Disord 2021;22(1):969.

39. Li G, Liu T, Shao X, et al. Fifteen-degree clavicular hook plate achieves better clinical outcomes in the treatment of acromioclavicular joint dislocation. J Int Med Res 2018;46(11):4547–59.

40. Schmidt J, Altmann T, Schmidt I, et al. The effects of hook plates on the subacromial space. A clinical and MRI study. Eur J Trauma Emerg Surg 2009;35(2):132–40.

41. Bhatia DN, Page RS. Surgical treatment of lateral clavicle fractures associated with complete coracoclavicular ligament disruption: Clinico-radiological outcomes of acromioclavicular joint sparing and spanning implants. Int J Shoulder Surg 2012;6(4):116–20.

42. Brereton DS, Robker JG, Gamez M, et al. Clinical and radiographic outcomes of a transosseous suture technique for displaced lateral clavicle fractures. J Shoulder Elbow Surg 2020;29(7S):S101–6.

43. Duralde XA, Pennington SD, Murray DH. Interfragmentary suture fixation for displaced acute type II distal clavicle fractures. J Orthop Trauma 2014;28(11):653–8.

44. Levy O. Simple, minimally invasive surgical technique for treatment of type 2 fractures of the distal clavicle. J Shoulder Elbow Surg 2003;12(1):24–8.

45. Jupiter JB, Leffert RD. Non-union of the clavicle. Associated complications and surgical management. J Bone Joint Surg Am 1987;69(5):753–60.

46. Tenpenny W, Caldwell PE, Rivera-Rosado E, et al. Arthroscopic-assisted bone graft harvest from the proximal humerus for distal third clavicle fracture nonunion. Arthrosc Tech 2020;9(12):e1937–42.
47. Flinkkilä T, Heikkilä A, Sirniö K, et al. TightRope versus clavicular hook plate fixation for unstable distal clavicular fractures. Eur J Orthop Surg Traumatol 2015; 25(3):465–9.
48. Hsu KH, Tzeng YH, Chang MC, et al. Comparing the coracoclavicular loop technique with a hook plate for the treatment of distal clavicle fractures. J Shoulder Elbow Surg 2018;27(2):224–30.
49. Katayama Y, Takegami Y, Tokutake K, et al. Comparison of functional outcome and complications of locking plate versus coracoclavicular fixation in the treatment of unstable distal clavicle fractures: the multicenter, propensity-matched TRON study. Eur J Orthop Surg Traumatol 2022. https://doi.org/10.1007/s00590-022-03358-0.
50. Nie S, Li HB, Hua L, et al. Comparative analysis of arthroscopic-assisted Tightrope technique and clavicular hook plate fixation in the treatment of Neer type IIB distal clavicle fractures. BMC Musculoskelet Disord 2022;23(1):756.

Traumatic Sternoclavicular Dislocations in Athletes

Diagnosis, Indications for Surgical Reconstruction, and Guide for Return to Play

Leah Brown, MD[a],*, Lisa M. Tamburini, MD[b]

KEYWORDS

- Sternoclavicular joint • SC dislocation • Figure-of-eight SC reconstruction
- SC plate stabilization • Closed reduction

KEY POINTS

- Instability of the sternoclavicular (SC) joint represents a rare but functionally limiting pathology for athletes.
- Computed tomography is an essential part of the diagnostic work up of SC injuries for visualization of direction of dislocation and associated retrosternal injuries.
- Closed reduction and/or surgical stabilization is superior to conservative therapy and delivers good functional results in the medium term.
- Graft-based stabilization in a figure-eight configuration is most commonly recommended as the surgical standard.
- Surgical treatment of chronic posterior SC joint dislocations should be reserved for centers with thoracic surgery.

INTRODUCTION

Shoulder injuries are common in sports, especially high-impact sports; however, much less frequent are injuries to the sternoclavicular (SC) joint. Traumatic SC injuries include sprain to the joint in which no instability is present, SC dislocations, and physeal disruption of the medial clavicle in skeletally immature athletes. Injuries to the SC joint represent only 3% to 5% of all injuries to the shoulder girdle with SC joint dislocations accounting for 1% to 3% of all injuries to the upper extremity. Eighty

[a] Banner Orthopaedic Sports Medicine, University of Arizona College of Medicine-Phoenix, 7400 North Dobson Road, Scottsdale, AZ 85256, USA; [b] Department of Orthopaedic Surgery, University of Connecticut, UConn Musculoskeletal Institute, 120 Dowling Way, Farmington, CT 06032, USA
* Corresponding author.
E-mail address: leah.brown2@bannerhealth.com

Clin Sports Med 42 (2023) 713–722
https://doi.org/10.1016/j.csm.2023.06.019
0278-5919/23/Published by Elsevier Inc.

percent of SC joint injuries are caused by either motor vehicle collisions (MVCs) or athletic injuries in contact and collision sports. Traumatic SC joint injuries are more common in male individuals. In patients aged 25 years and under, it is significant to distinguish SC joint dislocations from physeal fractures of the medial clavicle because physeal closure does not typically occur until 20 to 25 years of age.[1] Anterior SC joint dislocations are estimated to occur 9 times more frequently than posterior dislocations. In those posteriorly displaced, injury to the airway, vascular structures, and other mediastinal structures can occur that may be life-threatening. About 26% to 30% of patients with posterior SC dislocations sustain concurrent mediastinal injuries.[2–4]

There is currently a paucity of high-quality literature regarding SC joint injuries as these injuries are rare, which leads to difficulty in developing expertise in treatment. Published studies are primarily case reports and case series that are generally small and often include a mixture of atraumatic and traumatic SC joint dislocations, Salter-Harris type II fracture dislocations, and also include acute, chronic, or recurrent injuries. No level I evidence currently exists for these injuries, but several retrospective studies and surgical techniques have been described.[5]

ANATOMY/PATHOPHYSIOLOGY

The SC joint is the only articulation between the axial and appendicular skeleton of the upper limbs. Because only 50% of the medial clavicular surface articulates with the sternum, most of the stability is derived from the surrounding ligamentous structures. The ligamentous structures stabilizing the SC joint include the anterior capsule, posterior capsule, intra-articular disk ligament, inter-clavicular ligament, and costoclavicular ligament.

There are several critical anatomic structures that lie posterior to the SC joint. The innominate (also known as brachiocephalic) vein most often lies directly behind the SC joint. Other structures that one should be aware of due to their close proximity to the SC joint reconstruction drill holes include the common carotid arteries, subclavian veins, the superior vena cava, aortic arch, internal mammary arteries, and the trachea. These structures may be as close as 1 mm to the SC joint and are susceptible to becoming impinged or damaged in posterior SC joint dislocations and during surgical procedures.

CLASSIFICATION

Classification of SC joint instability is commonly described by a set of parameters that include acuity (acute or chronic), mechanism (atraumatic or traumatic), directionality (anterior or posterior), and degree (subluxation or dislocation) of instability.

In 1967, Allman and colleagues first described a system for classifying the severity of SC joint ligamentous disturbance and instability. A Type 1 SC joint instability reflects a sprain of the SC ligaments without subluxation or dislocation. Type 2 instability indicates anterior or posterior clavicle subluxation due to ligamentous injury. Type 3 SC instability indicates complete disruption of all ligamentous support with anterior or posterior clavicular dislocation.

MECHANISM OF INJURY

The most common mechanism of SC joint injury is an impact to the shoulder directed anteriorly or posteriorly. The costoclavicular ligament is suspected to act as a fulcrum, thus an anterior blow to the shoulder and lateral clavicle results in an anterior dislocation of the medial clavicle.[6] Similarly, a posterolateral blow, or a direct antero-medial blow, would result in a posteriorly dislocated SC joint. Injury to the posterior capsular apparatus of the SC joint requires 50% more force. In physeal injuries, the epiphysis remains attached to the sternum.

PRESENTATION/EVALUATION

Sports-related SC joint injuries are most commonly reported in rugby and football, but have also been described in basketball, hockey, wrestling, judo, ski racing, and in skatepark injuries.[1,7–13] Owing to the amount of energy required to cause SC joint instability, concomitant injury to the chest wall and surrounding structures must be considered.

Patients often believe a "pop" at the moment of impact, followed by immediate pain and swelling in the SC joint region. The prominence typically worsens with elevation and abduction of the arm, and the affected shoulder may seem shorter. Patients usually support the arm with the contralateral hand and tilt their head toward the injured side to relieve tension from the neck musculature. Pain may be relieved when the head is turned toward the affected shoulder.[14]

Posterior dislocations may present with a visible indentation; however, a hematoma will often mask this finding. If posterior instability is suspected a thorough history regarding dysphagia, stridor, retrosternal tightness, and dyspnea should be obtained and vascular congestion, paresthesias, and cardiac conduction abnormalities assessed. Thirty percent of patients who present with posterior dislocation of the SC joint sustained direct mediastinal injury from the posterior displacement of the clavicle.[11]

Radiological diagnostics include anterior-posterior (AP) and serendipity view radiographs. AP radiographs allow for the assessment of medial clavicle fracture. The serendipity view is obtained with the patient supine and the x-ray beam centered on the SC joint angled 40° cephalad (**Fig. 1**). In anterior dislocations, the affected clavicle will be visualized above the contralateral clavicle; in posterior dislocations, the opposite is true.

The gold standard is computed tomography (CT) for the exact depiction of the positional relationship providing a multiplanar evaluation of the joint space with three-dimensional reconstruction (**Fig. 2**).

In posterior dislocations, CT images can better visualize the mediastinal structures and assess for co-occurring injuries. In children, it is significant to distinguish SC joint dislocations from physeal fractures that are effectively visualized on CT. Angiography should be used if a vascular injury is suspected.

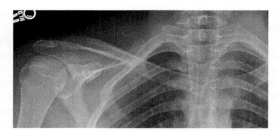

Fig. 1. Serendipity view radiograph demonstrating SC joint dislocation. (Image courtesy: Michael McKee, MD.)

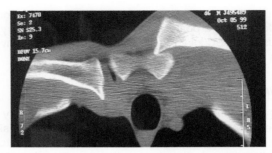

Fig. 2. Axial CT scan imaging showing anterior left SC joint dislocation. (Image courtesy Michael McKee, MD.)

TREATMENT

Differentiating between atraumatic spontaneous and acute traumatic SC dislocations is imperative as discussions around nonoperative treatment (including closed reduction) are primarily indicated for atraumatic spontaneous instability.

A limited role exists for nonsurgical management (without reduction or manipulation) in the setting of an acute SC joint dislocation. For many years treatment of SC joint dislocations has been a subject of controversy; however, scientific literature now describes and recommends conservative management with closed reduction and immobilization of the affected limb. For both anterior and posterior dislocations, initial management consists of a closed reduction attempt and subsequent percutaneous or open reduction with stabilization if unable to obtain a stable reduction with closed manipulation.

Several studies have recommended the immediate availability of a cardiothoracic surgeon when treating a posterior SC dislocation due to case reports of catastrophic complications.[15] In 2020, Leonard and colleagues[16] reported on the largest cohort of posterior SC joint dislocations and found that no vascular injuries occurred in the 140 patients treated in their cohort, and the authors called into question the necessity of this previous recommendation. The recommendation for cardiothoracic surgeon presence and availability remains controversial; hence, the treating physician must be aware of the possibility of catastrophic complications associated with critical mediastinal structures that is within 1 cm of the posterior SC joint.[17] Posterior injuries treated in a subacute and chronic manner may be particularly at risk because of the need for additional dissection to achieve reduction.[5]

Closed/Percutaneous Reduction

The preferred first line of management for patients with an acute anterior or posterior SC joint dislocation is closed reduction. In the acute setting, after reduction, internal stabilization is often not necessary.

Closed reduction can be attempted under sedation in some circumstances for acute anterior SC dislocations, but ideally, it is done under general anesthesia so that escalating reduction maneuvers including percutaneous and open techniques can be used if a closed reduction is unsuccessful. Patient should be placed in the supine position with a 3 to 4 in pad or rolled towel between the patient's scapulae. Closed reduction of an anterior dislocation is accomplished by continuous pressure in the posterior and lateral direction applied to the medial border of the clavicle where it meets the SC joint (**Fig. 3**). Closed reduction of a posterior dislocation is usually done under general anesthesia. The patient is placed in the supine position with a foam pad

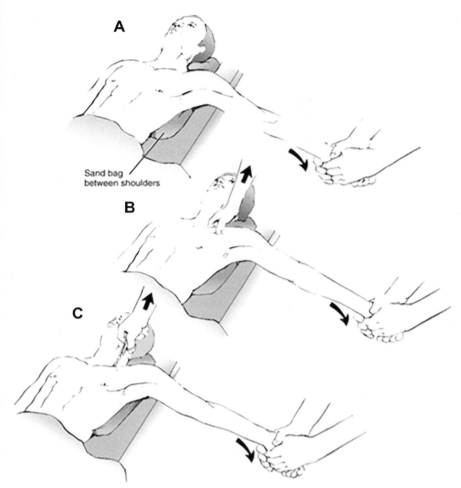

Fig. 3. Closed reduction maneuver for posterior SC joint dislocation. (Image courtesy Michael McKee, MD.)

or towel centered under their back to extend their shoulders. The arm is then abducted to 90° and the arm is pulled with constant pressure to gradually position the arm into full extension. The treating physician should consider a postoperative CT scan to evaluate the reduction. Immobilization of the affected extremity for 4 to 6 weeks is recommended.[18]

Surgical Indications

Surgical treatment of an SC joint injury is rare and carries substantial risks, including damage to surrounding structures, hardware migration, and poor cosmesis. Most treating surgeons refrain from surgery as the risks can heavily outweigh the benefits.

Operative treatment with open reduction and internal stabilization is indicated in the acute anterior or posterior dislocation that has failed closed reduction and has persistent instability, for chronic dislocations that are symptomatic, and posteriorly displaced medial physeal injuries. Urgent surgical management is mandated in individuals with a posterior dislocation and dysphagia, shortness of breath, an absent or asymmetric pulse, or vascular occlusion on angiography.

Surgical Techniques

Internal stabilization can be performed by ligament reconstruction, suture fixation, or plate and screw fixation. Owing to the rarity of injury, multiple techniques have been described, but few with long-term outcomes studied.

Open reduction internal fixation

During an open reduction internal fixation procedure, a locking compression plate, Balser plate, clavicular hook plate, or pre-contoured plate is used to provide fixation across the SC joint followed by sling immobilization for a minimum of 2 weeks[19] **(Fig. 4)**. Hardware removal is recommended to avoid the possible migration of the hook in the manubrial or posterior direction. Hardware removal before 3 months post-operation is avoided as it may lead to chronic SC joint instability.[11]

Ligament reconstruction

A variety of SC joint reconstruction techniques have been described in the literature including allograft or autograft figure-of-eight reconstruction, Roman numeral X reconstruction, intramedullary graft reconstruction, synthetic reconstruction using suture, and tenodesis using either the sternal head of the sternocleidomastoid or the subclavius. Tendon reconstruction is the most commonly used technique and has demonstrated the best outcomes. When comparing the most common tendinous reconstruction techniques, the figure-of-eight reconstruction demonstrates a load to failure almost three times greater in both anterior and posterior directions compared with other

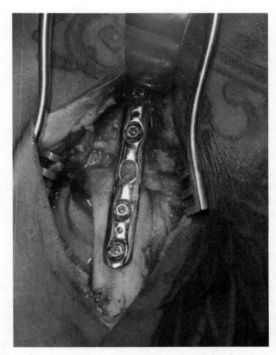

Fig. 4. Plate fixation of SC joint injury. (Image courtesy Michael McKee, MD.)

techniques.[20] The figure-of-eight technique has the benefit of providing multi-directional stability through a flexible construct.

In 2004, a biomechanical study compared 3 different types of ligament reconstruction techniques of the SC joint ligaments. The figure-of-eight technique had substantially higher mechanical strength in both the anterior and posterior directions when compared with the subclavius tendon technique and the intramedullary tendon technique. However, all 3 techniques were found to be biomechanically inferior to the native SC joint ligaments. Long-term outcomes of the figure-of-eight technique reveal significant improvement in functional outcomes and pain relief.[19] Lacheta and colleagues, published 5 years outcome data from their case series of 22 patients who underwent a figure-of-eight SC joint reconstruction using a hamstring autograft. They reported 90% construct survivorship with a minimum of 5 years follow-up. Of the patients that answered an optional sport questionnaire, 94% of them returned to their previous level of play.[21]

Other novel techniques are being used including sternal docking, internal bracing concept, and bone tunnels with permanent suture[22,23] (**Fig. 5**).

SC joint pain persists only in rare cases. The need for revision due to persistent, painful instability is estimated to be 5%. Revision procedures often include resection arthroplasty.[25–28]

Currently, no patient-reported outcome system specific to the SC joint exists. Studies have frequently used scores for glenohumeral joint function including the American Shoulder and Elbow Society Score, Subjective Shoulder Value, and Disability of the Arm, Shoulder, and Hand questionnaire. Better scoring systems specifically designed for the proximal shoulder girdle may have the potential to demonstrate subtle differences in outcomes between treatment groups.[5]

RETURN TO PLAY
Closed Reduction

Patients sustaining a posterior dislocation treated with closed reduction can be placed in a sling with gradual return to sport with appropriate rehabilitation. Athletes are usually able to return to full play without symptoms within a few weeks.[29]

Anterior dislocations are more likely to re-dislocate than posterior dislocations after closed reduction. Therefore, high-risk contact sports should be avoided for 3–4 months to prevent repeated injury and chronic instability of the SC joint.

Open Reduction Internal Fixation and Ligament Reconstruction

Rehabilitation protocols following SC joint reconstruction surgery vary according to the treatment intervention. Given the lack of data, there is significant variability among surgeons regarding post-operative protocols. Some surgeons recommend sling immobilization for 6 weeks with shoulder motion up to 90° of forward flexion and abduction beginning at 3 to 4 weeks and full motion allowed as early as 6 weeks. More conservative recommendations are to first place the patient in a figure-of-eight brace for 3 to 4, followed by sling immobilization for an additional 6 to 8 weeks. During this initial period following surgery, the patient is instructed to not elevate his or her arm more than 60° and heavily limit the use of the extremity. Following this protocol, at 12 weeks the patient can begin to use the extremity for daily activities and gradually return to strengthening and contact sports at his or her discretion.[30] Return to contact sports typically takes about 6 months. Hardware removal following plate stabilization should occur at approximately 6 months to avoid hardware complications.[31]

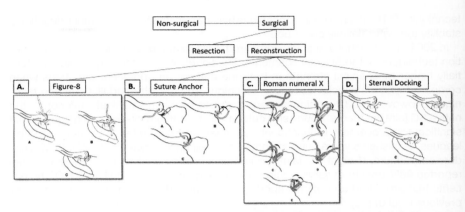

Fig. 5. Summary of the surgical techniques for SCJ instability management. (*A*) SCJ reconstruction using the figure-eight-surgical technique with grafted ligament or tendon. (*B*) SCJ reconstruction using the suture anchor technique described by Bak and colleagues (*C*) SCJ reconstruction using the Roman numeral X technique described by Guan and colleagues[24] (*D*) SCJ reconstruction using the Sternal Docking technique described by Sanchez-Sotelo et al. (*From* Garcia JA, Arguello AM, Momaya AM, Ponce BA. Sternoclavicular Joint Instability: Symptoms, Diagnosis and Management. Orthop Res Rev 2020;12:75-87. (In eng). https://doi.org/10.2147/orr.S170964.)

There are not enough data to provide an accurate assessment of the prognostic outcome for return to play for those athletes competing in collision sports who suffer this injury. Although this is a rare injury, future research efforts should be geared toward defining appropriate methods and criteria to determine the readiness of those athletes involved in collision sports before their return to play.

SUMMARY

SC injuries are rare injuries that occur following a significant amount of force. Collision and contact sports are second only to MVC as a cause for such trauma. Without a true gold standard treatment algorithm, the diagnosis and management of SC joint instability remain a challenge for orthopedic surgeons.

Establishing the correct diagnosis to allow for early intervention with closed reduction alone or with surgical stabilization is key to success in restoring joint stability, function, and ability to return to sport at the same level.

CLINICS CARE POINTS

- If an injury to the SC joint is suspected, prompt evaluation including thorough history regarding symptoms pertaining to mediastinal structures and radiographic evaluation with radiograph and CT scan are important.

- Patients sustaining anterior SC joint dislocations may have recurrent dislocations and therefore a slower more gradual return to play protocol must be followed.

- In individuals up to 25 years of age, SC joint dislocation must be differentiated from fracture through medial physis.

- Practitioners must be able to promptly identify patients with posterior SC joint dislocations and transfer them to a center with an available thoracic surgery team.

- Open reduction with surgical stabilization is indicated after failed closed reduction with persistent instability, symptomatic chronic dislocations, and posteriorly displaced medial physeal injuries.

DISCLOSURES

L. Brown has no disclosures. L.M. Tamburini has no disclosures.

REFERENCES

1. Quinn D. Skate park injury: a new mechanism of sternoclavicular joint dislocation. Emerg Med Australas 2014;26(3):316–7 (In eng).
2. Jaggard MK, Gupte CM, Gulati V, et al. A comprehensive review of trauma and disruption to the sternoclavicular joint with the proposal of a new classification system. J Trauma 2009;66(2):576–84 (In eng).
3. Mirza AH, Alam K, Ali A. Posterior sternoclavicular dislocation in a rugby player as a cause of silent vascular compromise: a case report. Br J Sports Med 2005;39(5):e28 (In eng).
4. Worman LW, Leagus C. Intrathoracic injury following retrosternal dislocation of the clavicle. J Trauma 1967;7(3):416–23 (In eng).
5. Obremskey WT, Rodriguez-Baron EB, Tatman LM, et al. Acute dislocations of the sternoclavicular joint: a review article. J Am Acad Orthop Surg 2022;30(4):148–54 (In eng).
6. Hellwinkel JE, McCarty EC, Khodaee M. Sports-related sternoclavicular joint injuries. Physician Sportsmed 2019;47(3):253–61 (In eng).
7. Asplund C, Pollard ME. Posterior sternoclavicular joint dislocation in a wrestler. Mil Med 2004;169(2):134–6 (In eng).
8. Baumann M, Vogel T, Weise K, et al. Bilateral posterior sternoclavicular dislocation. Orthopedics 2010;33(7):510 (In eng).
9. Carmichael KD, Longo A, Lick S, et al. Posterior sternoclavicular epiphyseal fracture-dislocation with delayed diagnosis. Skeletal Radiol 2006;35(8):608–12 (In eng).
10. Galanis N, Anastasiadis P, Grigoropoulou F, et al. Judo-related traumatic posterior sternoclavicular joint dislocation in a child. Clin J Sport Med 2014;24(3):271–3 (In eng).
11. Garcia JA, Arguello AM, Momaya AM, et al. Sternoclavicular joint instability: symptoms, diagnosis and management. Orthop Res Rev 2020;12:75–87 (In eng).
12. Lemire L, Rosman M. Sternoclavicular epiphyseal separation with adjacent clavicular fracture. J Pediatr Orthop 1984;4(1):118–20 (In eng).
13. Tompkins M, Bliss J, Villarreal R, et al. Posterior sternoclavicular disruption with ipsilateral clavicle fracture in a nine-year-old hockey player. J Orthop Trauma 2010;24(4):e36–9 (In eng).
14. Arner JW, Provencher MT, Bradley JP, et al. Evaluation and management of the contact athlete's shoulder. J Am Acad Orthop Surg 2022;30(6):e584–94 (In eng).
15. Jougon JB, Lepront DJ, Dromer CE. Posterior dislocation of the sternoclavicular joint leading to mediastinal compression. Ann Thorac Surg 1996;61(2):711–3 (In eng).
16. Leonard DA, Segovia NA, Kaur J, et al. Posterior sternoclavicular dislocation: do we need "cardiothoracic backup"? insights from a national sample. J Orthop Trauma 2020;34(2):e67–71 (In eng).
17. Ponce BA, Kundukulam JA, Pflugner R, et al. Sternoclavicular joint surgery: how far does danger lurk below? J Shoulder Elbow Surg 2013;22(7):993–9 (In eng).

18. Groh GI, Wirth MA. Management of traumatic sternoclavicular joint injuries. J Am Acad Orthop Surg 2011;19(1):1–7 (In eng).
19. Shuler FD, Pappas N. Treatment of posterior sternoclavicular dislocation with locking plate osteosynthesis. Orthopedics 2008;31(3):273 (In eng).
20. Spencer EE Jr, Kuhn JE. Biomechanical analysis of reconstructions for sternoclavicular joint instability. J Bone Joint Surg Am 2004;86(1):98–105 (In eng).
21. Lacheta L, Dekker TJ, Goldenberg BT, et al. Minimum 5-year clinical outcomes, survivorship, and return to sports after hamstring tendon autograft reconstruction for sternoclavicular joint instability. Am J Sports Med 2020;48(4):939–46 (In eng).
22. Fandridis E, Koutserimpas C, Raptis K, et al. Anterior dislocation of sternoclavicular joint: a novel surgical technique. Injury 2022;53(4):1562–7 (In eng).
23. Sanchez-Sotelo J, Baghdadi Y, Nguyen NTV. Sternoclavicular joint allograft reconstruction using the sternal docking technique. JSES Open Access 2018; 2(4):190–3 (In eng).
24. Guan JJ, Wolf BR. Reconstruction for anterior sternoclavicular joint dislocation and instability. J Shoulder Elbow Surg 2013;22(6):775–81 (In eng).
25. Bak K, Fogh K. Reconstruction of the chronic anterior unstable sternoclavicular joint using a tendon autograft: medium-term to long-term follow-up results. J Shoulder Elbow Surg 2014;23(2):245–50 (In eng).
26. Willinger L, Schanda J, Herbst E, et al. Outcomes and complications following graft reconstruction for anterior sternoclavicular joint instability. Knee Surg Sports Traumatol Arthrosc 2016;24(12):3863–9 (In eng).
27. Panzica M, Zeichen J, Hankemeier S, et al. Long-term outcome after joint reconstruction or medial resection arthroplasty for anterior SCJ instability. Arch Orthop Trauma Surg 2010;130(5):657–65 (In eng).
28. Martetschläger F, Imhoff AB. [Surgical stabilization of acute/chronic sternoclavicular instability with autologous gracilis tendon graft]. Oper Orthop Traumatol 2014;26(3):218–27 (In ger).
29. Yang JS, Bogunovic L, Brophy RH, et al. A case of posterior sternoclavicular dislocation in a professional american football player. Sports Health 2015;7(4): 318–25 (In eng).
30. Sanchez G, Frank RM, Sanchez A, et al. Sternoclavicular joint injuries in the contact athlete. Oper Tech Sports Med 2016;24(4):262–72.
31. Feng WL, Cai X, Li SH, et al. Balser plate stabilization for traumatic sternoclavicular instabilities or medial clavicle fractures: a case series and literature review. Orthop Surg 2020;12(6):1627–34 (In eng).

Atraumatic Sternoclavicular Joint Instability

Prevalence, Etiology, and Management

Wade Gobbell, MD, Christopher M. Edwards, BS,
Samuel R. Engel, MA, Katherine J. Coyner, MD, MBA*

KEYWORDS

- Sternoclavicular • Instability • Shoulder • Arthritis • Reconstruction

KEY POINTS

- The etiology of sternoclavicular joint instability may be posttraumatic, infectious, autoimmune, degenerative, or secondary to generalized laxity.
- Conservative treatment has been successful and encompasses activity modification, physical therapy, oral medications, and corticosteroid injections.
- Surgery is indicated for persistent symptoms despite conservative treatment and is broadly classified into resection and reconstruction, with generally successful results for both methods.

PREVALENCE

Sternoclavicular joint injuries rarely present in the orthopedic clinic. It is estimated that 3% of all injuries to the shoulder girdle involve the sternoclavicular (SC) joint.[1] Atraumatic etiologies leading to chronic instability and degeneration are even rarer. For this reason, there is a paucity of literature addressing the topic, particularly diagnosis and management. Numerous review articles cite small case reports, underpowered studies, and opinions.[1–3] Most SC joint injuries require high-energy trauma; therefore, the absence of history of trauma may contribute to missed diagnoses at the time of initial evaluation.[1] These undiagnosed conditions can progress to chronic problems with time. Even when acute SC joint dislocations are identified and treated nonoperatively, they can cause instability and/or degenerative changes that induce arthritis. Patients may return years after the initial injury with an uncertain chronology of symptoms. While the prevalence of SC symptoms is low, there are certainly patients suffering from chronic SC joint instability of atraumatic origin. This article is aimed

Department of Orthopedic Surgery, University of Connecticut School of Medicine, 263 Farmington Avenue, Farmington, CT 06030, USA
* Corresponding author.
E-mail address: coyner@uchc.edu

Clin Sports Med 42 (2023) 723–737
https://doi.org/10.1016/j.csm.2023.05.008
0278-5919/23/© 2023 Elsevier Inc. All rights reserved.

sportsmed.theclinics.com

at helping clinicians feel more comfortable addressing these problems by summarizing the relevant literature in the field.

ANATOMIC CONSIDERATIONS

The SC joint is a diarthrodial joint that serves as the primary articulation between the upper limb and axial skeleton. The articular surface of the clavicle is "saddle"-shaped, whereas the articular surface of the manubrium is convex. Less than half of the medial clavicle surface articulates with the sternum. Despite the inherent flaws of this configuration, the joint is extremely stable due to the strength of the costoclavicular, interclavicular, and capsular ligaments. There is extensive range of motion in the joint including 35° of elevation, 35° of anterior-posterior motion, and 50° of long-axis rotation.[1]

The costoclavicular or rhomboid ligament spans from the inferior margin of the medial clavicle to the synchondral junction between the manubrium and first rib (**Fig. 1**).[1] The anterior component prevents superior and lateral translation, whereas the posterior component prevents inferior and medial translation. The costoclavicular is notably the strongest of all SC ligaments.

The interclavicular ligament spans from the sternal aspect of one clavicle to the contralateral clavicle and attaches at the upper margin of the sternum. The primary function of this ligament is to resist superior translation of the medial clavicle.

The capsular ligament comprises anterosuperior and posterior capsular thickenings and inserts on the medial clavicular epiphysis. The medial clavicle physis is in fact the last physis to close. Because this structure does not appear until late adolescence and does not ossify until the middle of the third decade or later, apparent injuries to the SC joint in adolescents are typically physeal separations.[2]

The capsular ligaments are the most important structures for resisting superior displacement of the clavicle. Bearn demonstrated that isolated division of the capsular ligaments caused inferior-anterior translation of the clavicle in biomechanical studies.[4]

The SC joint itself contains a durable fibrocartilaginous intra-articular disc that attaches to the anterior and posterior sternoclavicular ligaments and capsule. The disc divides the SC joint into two synovial lined cavities. Degeneration of the disc increases with age, and cadaveric studies have shown that the disc is incomplete in individuals over the age of 70 years.[5]

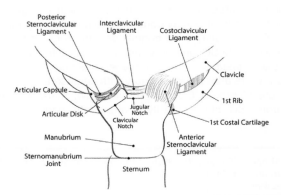

Fig. 1. Sternoclavicular joint anatomy. (*Data from* Stahel PF, Barlow B, Tepolt F, Mangan K, Mauffrey C. Safe surgical technique: reconstruction of the sternoclavicular joint for posttraumatic arthritis after posterior sternoclavicular dislocation. *Patient Saf Surg.* 2013;7(1):38. Published 2013 Dec 31. doi:10.1186/1754-9493-7-38.)

ETIOLOGY

There are numerous sources of SC joint instability. Structural bone or ligament abnormalities can disrupt the normal articulation of the joint. Arthritic changes to the joint can lead to chronic or persistent instability. Friedrich's disease, an aseptic osteonecrosis of the medial clavicle of idiopathic origin, can cause arthritic changes in young patients. Nonstructural (muscular) causes of instability from injury to any of the five muscles inserting on the clavicle (sternocleidomastoid, pectoralis major, deltoid, trapezius, and subclavius muscles) can affect stability of the joint. SC joint instability can also be post-traumatic, neurological, or a combination of these factors. Damage to the nerves innervating the SC joint (medial supraclavicular nerve and the nerve to subclavius) can also contribute to instability.

Instability of the SC joint is classified in several different ways. As previously described, instability can be classified by direction (anterior or posterior), cause (traumatic or atraumatic), severity (sprain, subluxation, or dislocation), and onset (acute or chronic). Historically, Allman classified SC joint injuries into three categories based on the degree of ligament disruption (**Table 1**). Type 1 constitutes a sprain of the SC ligaments without subluxation or dislocation. Type 2 involves SC ligaments and capsular disruption with subluxation of the medial clavicle. Type 3 represents total rupture of ligaments with dislocation anteriorly and posteriorly.[6]

Lewis and colleagues reported the utility of using the Stanmore triangle system for instability of the SC joint (**Fig. 2**).[7] This system was originally designed for classifying instability of the glenohumeral joint. Sewell and colleagues also reported on the utility of the model for the SC joint, citing the ability to track changing pathology with time and monitor response to treatment.[3] The dynamic model is represented by a triangle with each group assigned to a vertex: type I traumatic structural, type II atraumatic structural, and type III muscle patterning nonstructural pathology. Patients can be placed at one of the vertices, along any of the edges, or within the triangle itself to reflect the nature of instability. Clinicians can use this as a baseline and follow the patient's progression with time due to successful/unsuccessful management, further degeneration of the joint, and so on. The advantage of this model is that it is fluid and allows for multifactorial causes of instability.

PATIENT EVALUATION

Because the SC joint is a synovial joint, it is prone to various forms of arthritis as well as inflammatory disorders.[2] When assessing patients for disorders of the SC joint, it is important to start with a thorough medical history including history of present illness

Table 1
The Allman classification of traumatic sternoclavicular joint injuries*

Grade	Description
I	Sprain of the sternoclavicular joint without laxity and minimal pain
II	Rupture of the sternoclavicular ligaments without rupture of the costoclavicular ligaments
III	Complete rupture of the sternoclavicular and costoclavicular ligaments with anterior or posterior displacement

From Kendal JK, Thomas K, Lo IKY, Bois AJ. Clinical Outcomes and Complications Following Surgical Management of Traumatic Posterior Sternoclavicular Joint Dislocations: A Systematic Review. *JBJS Rev.* 2018;6(11):e2. doi:10.2106/JBJS.RVW.17.00157; with permission.

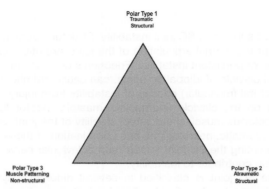

Polar Type 1
Traumatic
Structural

Polar Type 3
Muscle Patterning
Non-structural

Polar Type 2
Atraumatic
Structural

Fig. 2. The Stanmore triangle system for classifying sternoclavicular instability. A patient may move fluidly within the triangle over time based on pathophysiologic adaptations. (*Data from* Farrar NG, Malal JJ, Fischer J, Waseem M. An overview of shoulder instability and its management. *Open Orthop J.* 2013;7:338-346. Published 2013 Sep 6. doi:10.2174/1874325001307010338.)

with information about the nature and chronology of symptoms. SC joint disorders can present acutely, insidiously, or progressively, and patients may complain of localized pain and/or swelling. Past medical histories should document history of systemic illnesses, arthritis, and recent infections, as well as any familial arthritis and inflammatory disorders. Important conditions to ask about include osteoarthritis (OA), rheumatoid arthritis (RA), seronegative spondyloarthropathies, infection, and gout.

Physical Examination

Physical examination is essential for developing a differential diagnosis around sternoclavicular instability. Examiners should begin by observing the joint for noticeable joint hypertrophy, symmetry/asymmetry, and erythema. The patient should move his or her shoulder through the range of abduction-adduction and into forward flexion so the examiner can observe the articulation of the joint and document specific movements that elicit pain. Abduction and forward elevation tend to accentuate joint deformity. Movements of the SC joint include elevation-depression, protraction-retraction, and axial rotation. Palpation of the joint will reveal any localized pain or tenderness, as well as warmth and swelling.

Imaging

Imaging workup should start with conventional AP radiographs. From this modality, subchondral sclerosis, osteophytes, joint space narrowing, hyperostosis, and calcification may be identified.[8] Due to the oblique orientation of the joint, AP views of the affected SC joint are limited in their ability to identify subtle asymmetry or subluxation. Serendipity views, with the beam positioned 40° cephalad, allow bilateral comparison. Other imaging to consider based on individual patient factors includes computed tomography (CT), magnetic resonance imaging (MRI), and isotype scanning. CT can reveal both bony destruction and ossifying lesions. It is also the most sensitive modality for detecting the direction (ie, anterior or posterior) of subluxation or dislocation. MRI is used for identifying soft-tissue abnormalities due to inflammation (**Fig. 3**), as well as osteonecrosis that may be seen with Friedrich's disease. Isotope scanning would be reserved for concerns about malignancy or inflammation.

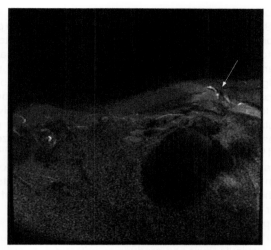

Fig. 3. MRI showing hyperintensity in the sternoclavicular joint on T2-weighted axial MRI.

With proper training in the technique, clinicians may implement ultrasound in the clinic setting for an efficient, economical, and less-invasive alternative to CT or MRI. Ultrasound has been demonstrated to be appropriately sensitive for diagnosing pathology of the SC joint. In a study of 103 age- and sex-matched individuals with RA, blinded ultrasound and clinical examinations of 412 SC joints identified 89 arthritic SC joints compared with 36 in the control group.[9] Features assessed include osteophytes, synovitis, erosions, and intraarticular power Doppler, which can determine the density of synovial vasculature in patients with RA. In addition to demonstrating that the prevalence of SC joint pathology in RA patients is higher than that previously reported, the study confirmed the utility and reliability of the technique.

Laboratory tests for consideration primarily include inflammatory markers. Complete blood count (CBC) with differential, erythrocyte sedimentation rate (ESR), C-reactive protein (CRP) rheumatoid factor, antinuclear antibodies, and antigen tests for HLA-B27 (autoimmune disease specific) should be included in the patient workup. Joint aspiration or arthrocentesis also has a diagnostic value. The procedure should be performed under ultrasound guidance to avoid damaging underlying mediastinal structures. The aspirated joint fluid should be analyzed with Gram staining and cultured for bacteria. Infection can be identified from increased leukocyte count or known pathogens. Crystalline-induced arthritis may be recognized by observing crystals in the joint aspirate on microscopy.

DIFFERENTIAL DIAGNOSIS

Narrowing the differential for atraumatic SC joint instability requires ruling out several conditions that may present with similar symptoms. OA is considered the most common cause of pain and swelling at the SC joint and may be asymptomatic for some patients.[2] The prevalence of OA of the SC joint is estimated to be 90% in individuals older than 60 years in some studies[10] while others have reported moderate to severe degenerative joint changes in 53% of individuals older than 60 years.[11] The patient profile at the highest risk of this disorder includes men and women older than 40 years, in particular, postmenopausal women, manual laborers, and individuals who have had a radical neck dissection.[2] Medical history for patients with SC joint OA may or may not include a history of trauma.[1] Patients will complain of pain with abduction or forward flexion past 90°. The pain may be severe for some patients and can radiate to the shoulder, neck, or breast. Physical examination may demonstrate medial clavicle prominence due to the presence of osteophytes, as well as pain and crepitus with movement.[1,2] Maneuvers that should be performed include the push-down test, cross-shoulder sign (**Fig. 4**), and resisted arm abduction.[1] Radiographic imaging may be positive for joint space narrowing, osteophytes, sclerosis, or cysts.[11]

In patients with known RA with SC joint involvement, approximately one-third report asymmetry, crepitus, hypertrophy, tenderness, or restriction and pain with movement.[2] SC joint instability in patients with RA is not well characterized. Studies have reported 1% to 41% of patients with RA have SC joint involvement.[10,12] In a study using ultrasound as a diagnostic tool, 19% of patients with RA had SC joint involvement.[9] RA affects women more frequently than men and may affect patients of any age. Radiographs may show arthritic features. Labs may be positive for rheumatoid factor and/or antinuclear antibodies.[2]

Seronegative spondyloarthropathies include conditions such as ankylosing spondylitis, psoriatic arthritis, Reiter's syndrome, and colitic arthritis. These disorders can involve the sternoclavicular joint and produce an inflammatory arthritis targeting the large peripheral joints. Emery and colleagues identified acute inflammatory arthropathy involving the SC joint in 4% of patients with ankylosing spondylitis.[13] Taccari and colleagues found SC joint involvement in 9 out of 10 patients with psoriatic arthritis using CT imaging.[14] Interestingly, only 50% of patients were symptomatic.[14] Kumar Digge and colleagues describe a case of atraumatic posterior SC dislocation in a 26 year-old male with Reiter's syndrome,[15] although arthritis symptoms are more common. Men younger than 40 years are more commonly affected by seronegative spondyloarthropathies. Radiographs may be normal or show arthritic changes. Labs may be positive for HLA-B27 and negative for autoantibodies, which is diagnostic.[2]

Tophaceous gouty arthritis can occasionally affect the SC joint although literature is limited to a few case reports.[16–18] Gout and pseudogout can be diagnosed by aspiration of joint fluid followed by examination under polarized microscopy. Gout displays negative birefringent, whereas pseudogout displays positive birefringent crystals. Both conditions are known to affect the SC joint. Crystalline arthropathies occur more frequently in older men. In addition to joint fluid analysis, an elevated ESR can

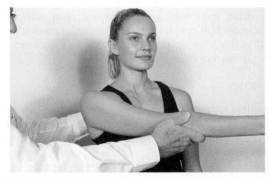

Fig. 4. The cross-shoulder sign demonstrates adduction, which accentuates pain and deformity at the SC joint. (*From* Pillemer R. Examination for Specific Conditions of the Shoulder. In: Pillemer, R. *Handbook of Upper Extremity Examination*. Springer Nature; 2021: 187-210; with permission.)

support diagnosis during an acute attack. Radiographs may or may not show arthritic changes. Soft-tissue calcification may be present as well.

Among the arthritic mimickers of atraumatic SC instability, including OA, RA, sero-negative spondyloarthropathies, and gout, it is important to note that pain and swelling are the cardinal features rather than gross instability. The potential for erosive changes and ligament attenuation in arthritic pathologies should not be minimized, however.

Infectious sources of SC joint pathology consist of septic arthritis and osteomyelitis. Infection is an important diagnostic consideration for patients presenting with unilateral SC joint arthritis. It has been reported that the SC joint was involved in as many as 9% of patients with septic arthritis.[12] This condition can occur in patients of any age but is most commonly present in patients with risk factors such as immunocompromise or intravenous drug use. Clinicians should recognize acute presentations of pain and swelling accompanied by systemic signs of sepsis. Note that elderly and immunocompromised patients may not present with these features. Labs should check for infection markers. Ultrasound aspiration of the joint is also indicated. Purulent aspirate requires workup with Gram staining and bacterial culture with sensitivity. Imaging may show evidence of swelling and sclerosis. In existing literature, there is little mention of instability as sequela of septic arthritis of the SC joint. The authors of a recently published case report performed simultaneous debridement and allograft stabilization to prevent iatrogenic instability after medial clavicle and manubrium resection.[19]

Osteomyelitis and SAPHO syndrome (synovitis, acne, pustulosis, hyperostosis, osteitis) share common features and are characterized by culture-negative osteomyelitis. However, chronic recurrent multifocal osteomyelitis is an idiopathic inflammatory disorder primarily affecting children and adolescents, whereas SAPHO syndrome is a spectrum of chronic skin and osteo-articular conditions (synovitis, acne, pustulosis, hyperostosis, and osteitis) typically affecting middle-aged adults (**Fig. 5**). Patients with chronic recurrent multifocal osteomyelitis will present with localized pain and swelling bilaterally. Labs may show elevated ESR. Lesions do not usually cross the SC joint and primarily affect the medial end of the clavicle. When the disease is active, isotope scanning will show activity, and MRI will show edema in the soft tissues and abnormalities within the clavicle. Despite resolution of the disease, patients will have sclerosis and expansion of the medial clavicle.[2] Symptoms can persist for years. Similarly, patients with SAPHO will have localized pain, swelling, and limited mobility. Skin lesions are

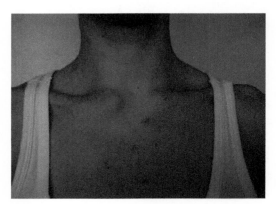

Fig. 5. This patient with SAPHO syndrome demonstrates bilateral sternoclavicular edema due to osteitis and hyperostosis, as well as acne of the anterior chest. (*Data from* Rukavina I. SA-PHO syndrome: a review. *J Child Orthop.* 2015;9(1):19-27. doi:10.1007/s11832-014-0627-7.)

usually pustular and are present in most cases. Labs may show elevated ESR and CRP. CT imaging will show 3 stages of progression.[2] Stage 1 includes involvement from the costoclavicular ligament with a soft-tissue mass and new bone formation. Stage 2 shows SC joint arthropathy and sclerosis of the clavicle, first rib, sternum, and costal cartilage. In stage 3, there is evidence of clavicular and sternal sclerosis, hyperostosis, and hypertrophy that also affects the upper ribs. There are adjacent arthritic changes as well. MRI shows edema of the soft tissue and bone. Isotype scanning reveals a "bull's head" pattern, a classic finding for the condition (**Fig. 6**).[2] Histological findings include infiltrates, edema, and inflammation of the periosteum. This can progress to sclerosis and fibrosis. Patients may experience a few symptomatic attacks with resolution or more frequently encounter a chronic disease that can move to other locations.

Friedrich's disease or aseptic osteonecrosis of the medial clavicle has unknown pathophysiology. It presents with discomfort, swelling, and crepitus of the SC joint, and in some cases, loss of shoulder mobility. Osteonecrosis of the medial clavicle is usually accompanied by cystic changes. Lab values will be normal including serum leukocyte count and ESR. Radiographs will show osteolysis of the medial clavicle, and MRI will display necrotic bone within the metaphysis.[20] Histology will usually demonstrate necrotic bone fragments with cystic changes accompanied by normal intact bone. The clinical course of this disease is not well understood or characterized.

MANAGEMENT

Surgical treatment for atraumatic SC joint pathology is reserved for cases refractory to conservative management. Nonoperative treatment options include rest, activity

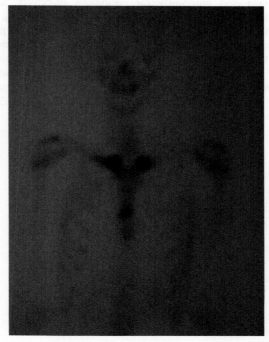

Fig. 6. Increased Tc-99m uptake at the SC joints demonstrates the described "bull's head" pattern in SAPHO syndrome. (*Data from* Rukavina I. SAPHO syndrome: a review. *J Child Orthop*. 2015;9(1):19-27. doi:10.1007/s11832-014-0627-7.)

modification, anti-inflammatory medications, intra-articular corticosteroid injections, and local cryotherapy.[1] Physical therapy may also be prescribed for both acute instability and atraumatic structural instability.[1,3] A muscle compensatory component should be recognized and addressed in therapy at the risk of persistent pain and instability.

Chronic instability often results from a failure of reduction of traumatic dislocation. A survey of practicing orthopedic surgeons revealed that 52% first attempted closed reduction, but 80% reported that the reduction was not maintained in more than half of their treated patients.[5] While traumatic dislocations are often recognized and stabilized acutely, attempted closed reduction of subacute or chronic atraumatic instability is of uncertain benefit. Recurrent subluxation and/or dislocation may lead to chronic, painful instability ultimately requiring surgical intervention. Indications for surgical management include instability that has become symptomatic or functionally limiting. Surgical options are broadly categorized into two categories: reconstruction of the costoclavicular ligaments and resection of the medial clavicle.

The costoclavicular ligaments are usually torn or attenuated. A subperiosteal incision may be made parallel to the orientation of the clavicle to expose the medial clavicle. The decision whether to remove or preserve the medial clavicle is influenced by the presence of ligamentous attachments to the clavicle. If the ligaments are disrupted, resection of approximately 2 cm of medial clavicle can result in pain relief. If this is done, the anterosuperior corner of the clavicle may be feathered to prevent prominence. Regardless, when resection arthroplasty is selected as the treatment of choice, outcomes are improved if the costoclavicular ligaments are preserved.[21] Patients should be counseled regarding postsurgical cosmesis and potential functional limitations at their preoperative visit. Specifically, patients may expect some degree of limitation in overhead function and sport activities.[21] For this reason, medial clavicle resection may be preferred for lower-demand individuals; although Dekker and colleagues demonstrated high rates of patient satisfaction and return to sport after medial clavicle resection, this study was performed in patients undergoing treatment for OA and not for SC instability.[22]

Reconstruction of the sternoclavicular joint has been described by a variety of techniques. Graft may be autograft or allograft, with gracilis or semitendinosus tendons frequently chosen.[23–25] Reconstruction using synthetic weave ligament grafts has also been described in the literature.[26] A figure-of-eight configuration (**Fig. 7**) has shown superior biomechanical strength[27] to other reconstruction techniques, but alternative methods have been implemented due to lower rates of neurovascular injury. Fixation may be performed using suture, anchors, or cannulated screws.[24]

Treatment implications for chronic instability vary based on the presence of anterior- or posterior-directed instability just as they do for acute dislocations. Anterior dislocations are typically better tolerated than posterior due to effects on the surrounding anatomy. Severe complications of nonoperative treatment of posterior instability include neurovascular compromise, (subclavian artery compression), thoracic outlet syndrome, intrathoracic injury, and erosion of the medical clavicle into the posteriorly-situated hilar structures. Indications for surgical management of post-traumatic posterior instability include failed closed reduction with symptoms or recurrent posterior dislocations. A CT of the chest should be performed before surgical intervention, and arteriography may be added in any case with signs or symptoms suspicious for vascular compression. A thoracic surgery consultation and availability during surgery should be strongly considered. An open reduction may be attempted. Many chronic dislocations are unable to be successfully reduced, or the reduction remains unstable. In this case, a medial clavicle resection can be performed without substantial risk of functional deficit.

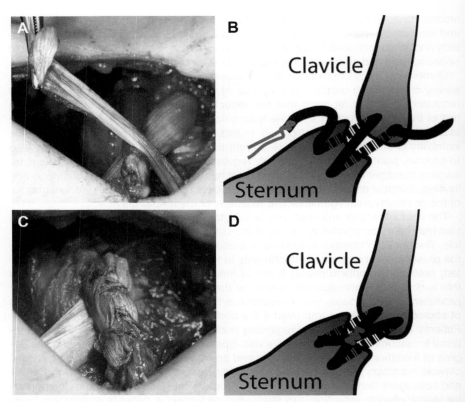

Fig. 7. Intraoperative photo demonstrates hamstring graft passage (*A*) with an associated schematic illustration (*B*) for SC joint stabilization. Intraoperative photo (*C*) depicts the final construct of stabilization using the figure-of-8 configuration, as also shown in the schematic illustration (*D*). (*From* Singer G, Ferlic P, Kraus T, Eberl R. Reconstruction of the sternoclavicular joint in active patients with the figure-of-eight technique using hamstrings. *J Shoulder Elbow Surg.* 2013;22(1):64-69. doi:10.1016/j.jse.2012.02.009; with permission.)

Postoperative care should involve the use of a shoulder immobilizer for a total of 3 to 6 weeks. A progressive shoulder range of motion and strengthening program may be initiated thereafter.

TREATMENT OUTCOMES

Treatment of chronic SC instability is associated with inferior outcomes compared with those of acute SC dislocation. A systematic review of 16 case studies including 151 patients reported the delay in treatment from symptom onset to definitive treatment.[28] In this study, 87.5% of acute dislocations were treated with excellent/good results, whereas 73% of chronic dislocations had excellent/good results. Patients treated for acute dislocations achieved better functional outcomes than patients treated for chronic dislocations. Chronic anterior dislocations treated by open reduction achieved functional outcomes that were not significantly different from those of dislocations treated nonoperatively.

Rockwood and Odor reported no limitation of activity or restriction of lifestyle in 29 patients at mean 8-year follow-up with atraumatic anterior dislocations treated nonoperatively.[29] These were compared to 8 patients who were treated with resection arthroplasty or SC joint reconstruction by other surgeons. All patients treated surgically reported limitations of activity and lifestyle, and surgical complications included persistent pain, instability, and dissatisfaction with the appearance of their scars. Of the entire cohort, 90% experienced persistent subluxation. Similarly, Eskola and colleagues reported on 12 patients with chronic SC instability treated with reconstruction, fascial stabilization, or medial clavicle resection.[30] Of the eight patients treated with reconstruction or fascial stabilization, four were judged to have good results while four were fair. However, all four patients treated with resection arthroplasty had results classified as poor. It is important to note that the surgical procedures performed in these two cohorts have been supplanted by a number of newer techniques.

Despite this historical evidence suggesting superiority of nonsurgical treatment, more recent surgical techniques have shown positive short-term clinical and patient-reported outcomes. Sabatini and colleagues demonstrated an increase in American Society of Elbow Surgeons (ASES) score from 35.3 to 84.7 after figure-of-eight SC joint reconstruction, and visual analog scale (VAS) scores decreased from 7 to 1.2.[31] Bak and Fogh described a technique that involves drilling holes and anchor placement at an angle of 20° oblique to the horizontal on the lateral manubrium to avoid the risk of anterior-to-posterior drilling.[32] Obliquely-oriented screws are placed in the medial articular facet exiting the anterior aspect of the medial clavicle. This study showed an improvement in the Western Ontario Shoulder Instability Index (WOSI) score from 44% to 75%.[32] Another alternative to the figure-of-8 graft pattern is the Roman numeral X. This method incorporates unicortical drilling and placement of inferior and superior drill holes through which the graft is passed to provide communicating inferior and superior transverse support (**Fig. 8**).[33] This technique resulted in significant improvement in VAS scores compared to the preoperative condition. Sanchez-Sotelo et al. described a method for sternal docking of semitendinosus allograft, which involved passing the graft through anteroinferior and anterosuperior drill holes in the medial clavicle, through superior and inferior holes in the sternum connected by an oblong tunnel, and suturing the ends of the graft together anteriorly. These patients demonstrated significant improvement in VAS and Disabilities of

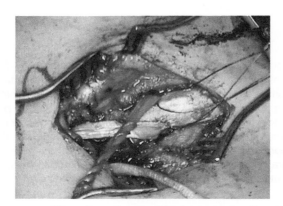

Fig. 8. The Roman numeral X configuration for SC joint reconstruction. The graft is passed diagonally over the SC joint both anteriorly and posteriorly, and the limbs are sutured together at each crossing point. (*From* Guan JJ, Wolf BR. Reconstruction for anterior sternoclavicular joint dislocation and instability.*J Shoulder Elbow Surg.* 2013;22(6):775-781. doi:10.1016/j.jse.2012.07.009;with permission.)

Arm, Shoulder, and Hand (DASH) scores.[34] Tashjian and colleagues described single-loop reconstruction using a semitendinosus allograft and demonstrated satisfactory VAS, ASES, and Simple Shoulder Test scores.[35] There was no residual instability in any patient and 8 of 9 patients reported satisfaction with the procedure.

Treatment of atraumatic SC instability in athletes has shown mixed outcomes. Open SC resection arthroplasty with capsulorrhaphy to treat pain from OA resulted in significant improvement in clinical outcomes, patient satisfaction, return to sports, and pain reduction at a minimum of 5 years in follow-up.[22] In this study, 21 sternoclavicular joints in 19 patients were treated with resection of the medial clavicle and intra-articular disc and capsulorrhaphy for SC joint OA in 19 patients with a mean age of 39.4 years. Nineteen SC joints in 16 patients were treated with resection of the medial clavicle and intra-articular disc with capsulorrhaphy for OA. At a mean follow-up of 6.7 years, outcome scores improved significantly from preoperative to postoperative assessments for the ASES, SANE, QuickDASH, and SF-12 PCS. Median satisfaction with surgical outcomes was 9 out of 10. Pain levels improved from a score of 8/10 to 3/10. Twelve of 14 athletes (86%) successfully returned to sports although the level of participation was not specified. Pain at its worst and with competition significantly decreased preoperatively to postoperatively. Three patients (15%) had recurrent SC joint pain and were treated with revision surgery.

SC joint reconstruction with figure-of-eight technique using hamstring tendon autograft resulted in significantly improved clinical outcomes compared to the preoperative condition, with high patient satisfaction and 90% survivorship at midterm follow-up.[23] Of this patient population, 94% returned to their previous level of sports participation. With regard to the concern for advanced postinstability arthritis, patients maintained a significant decrease in pain at minimum 5-year follow-up, suggesting a longer latency period before the development of clinically evident OA.

Fifteen pediatric patients treated for chronic anterior sternoclavicular joint instability using either ligamentous reconstruction or resection arthroplasty were reviewed by Bae and colleagues at a mean of 4 years in follow-up, the mean ASES score was 85, and 60% of patients reported a pain-free, stable shoulder, but 87% of patients had limitation in recreational sports and activities.[36]

In an athletic population, synthetic reconstruction using an artificial weave ligament showed improvement at 29 months in follow-up with 100% return to sport.[26]

SUMMARY

Atraumatic sternoclavicular joint instability is a rare condition with a myriad of etiologies. If a history of significant trauma has been eliminated, diagnostic workup should include radiographs, serum lab studies (CBC, ESR, CRP, rheumatologic panel), and advanced imaging. Initial treatment is conservative and focused on physical therapy, oral anti-inflammatory medications, and corticosteroid injections. For refractory cases, surgery is indicated and involves either medial clavicle resection arthroplasty or SC joint reconstruction. A number of reconstruction techniques have been described using both autograft and allograft and with various fixation methods. These generally show favorable outcomes but wide variety in return to sport metrics.

CLINICS CARE POINTS

- The etiology of sternoclavicular joint instability may be post-traumatic, infectious, autoimmune, degenerative, or secondary to generalized laxity.

- Conservative treatment has been successful and encompasses activity modification, physical therapy, oral NSAIDs, and corticosteroid injections.
- Surgery is indicated for persistent symptoms after failed conservative treatment and is broadly classified into resection and reconstruction, with generally successful results for both methods.
- Figure-of-eight reconstruction techniques provide the greatest biomechanical strength but are associated with risk of neurovascular injury.
- A number of alternative reconstruction methods have been described to mitigate risk of neurovascular injury with favorable short-term outcomes.

DISCLOSURE

K.J. Coyner reports speaking fees from Arthrex, Inc., and Smith & Nephew and research support from Arthrex and Food and Drug Administration (FDA) outside the submitted work. The other authors have no disclosures.

REFERENCES

1. Martetschläger F, Warth RJ, Millett PJ. Instability and degenerative arthritis of the sternoclavicular joint: a current concepts review. Am J Sports Med 2014;42(4): 999–1007.
2. Robinson CM, Jenkins PJ, Markham PE, et al. Disorders of the sternoclavicular joint. J Bone Joint Surg Br 2008;90(6):685–96.
3. Sewell MD, Al-Hadithy N, Le Leu A, et al. Instability of the sternoclavicular joint: current concepts in classification, treatment and outcomes. Bone Joint Lett J 2013;95-B(6):721–31.
4. Bearn JG. Direct observations on the function of the capsule of the sternoclavicular joint in clavicular support. J Anat 1967;101(Pt 1):159–70.
5. Van Tongel A, McRae S, Gilhen A, et al. Management of anterior sternoclavicular dislocation: a survey of orthopaedic surgeons. Acta Orthop Belg 2012;78(2): 164–9.
6. Allman FL Jr. Fractures and ligamentous injuries of the clavicle and its articulation. J Bone Joint Surg Am 1967;49(4):774–84.
7. Lewis A, Kitamura T, Bayley JIL. The classification of shoulder instability: new light through old windows. Curr Orthop 2004;18(2):97–108.
8. Arlet J, Ficat P. Osteo-arthritis of the sterno-clavicular joint. Ann Rheum Dis 1958; 17(1):97–100.
9. Higginbotham TO, Kuhn JE. Atraumatic disorders of the sternoclavicular joint. J Am Acad Orthop Surg 2005;13(2):138–45.
10. Thongngarm T, McMurray RW. Osteoarthritis of the sternoclavicular joint. J Clin Rheumatol 2000;6(5):269–71.
11. Kier R, Wain SL, Apple J, et al. Osteoarthritis of the sternoclavicular joint. Radiographic features and pathologic correlation. Invest Radiol 1986;21(3):227–33.
12. Yood RA, Goldenberg DL. Sternoclavicular joint arthritis. Arthritis Rheum 1980; 23(2):232–9.
13. Emery RJ, Ho EK, Leong JC. The shoulder girdle in ankylosing spondylitis. J Bone Joint Surg Am 1991;73(10):1526–31.
14. Taccari E, Spadaro A, Riccieri V, et al. Sternoclavicular joint disease in psoriatic arthritis. Ann Rheum Dis 1992;51(3):372–4.

15. Kumar Digge V, Meena S, Khan SA, et al. Spontaneous atraumatic dislocation of sternoclavicular joint in Reiter syndrome. Chin J Traumatol 2012;15(4):251–3.

16. Sant GR, Dias E. Primary gout affecting the sternoclavicular joint. Br Med J 1976; 1(6004):262.

17. Sahdev N, Smelt J, Avila Z, et al. Tophaceous gout in the sternoclavicular joint. J Surg Case Rep 2020;2020(10):rjaa398.

18. Fedeli MM, Vecchi M, Rodoni Cassis P. A Patient with Complex Gout with an Auto-inflammatory Syndrome and a Sternoclavicular Joint Arthritis as Presenting Symptoms. Case Rep Rheumatol 2020;2020:5026490.

19. Hanhoff M, Jensen G, Dey Hazra RO, et al. Innovative Surgical Concept for Septic Sternoclavicular Arthritis: Case Presentation of a Simultaneous Joint Resection and Stabilization with Gracilis Tendon Graft Including Literature Review. Z Orthop Unfall 2022;160(1):64–73 [published correction appears in Z Orthop Unfall. 2022 Feb;160(1):e4]. Innovatives OP-Konzept bei septischer Arthritis des Sternoklavi-kulargelenks: Falldarstellung einer simultanen Gelenkresektion und Stabilisierung mit Gracilissehnengraft inklusive Literaturübersicht [published correction appears in Z Orthop Unfall. 2022 Feb;160(1):e4].

20. Fischel RE, Bernstein D. Friedrich's disease. Br J Radiol 1975;48(568):318–9.

21. Rockwood CA Jr, Groh GI, Wirth MA, et al. Resection arthroplasty of the sterno-clavicular joint. J Bone Joint Surg Am 1997;79(3):387–93.

22. Dekker TJ, Lacheta L, Goldenberg BT, et al. Minimum 5-Year Outcomes and Return to Sports After Resection Arthroplasty for the Treatment of Sternoclavicular Osteoarthritis. Am J Sports Med 2020;48(3):715–22.

23. Lacheta L, Dekker TJ, Goldenberg BT, et al. Minimum 5-Year Clinical Outcomes, Survivorship, and Return to Sports After Hamstring Tendon Autograft Reconstruction for Sternoclavicular Joint Instability. Am J Sports Med 2020;48(4):939–46.

24. Kawaguchi K, Tanaka S, Yoshitomi H, et al. Double figure-of-eight reconstruction technique for chronic anterior sternoclavicular joint dislocation. Knee Surg Sports Traumatol Arthrosc 2015;23(5):1559–62.

25. Wang D, Camp CL, Werner BC, et al. Figure-of-8 Reconstruction Technique for Chronic Posterior Sternoclavicular Joint Dislocation. Arthrosc Tech 2017;6(5): e1749–53.

26. Quayle JM, Arnander MW, Pennington RG, et al. Artificial ligament reconstruction of sternoclavicular joint instability: report of a novel surgical technique with early results. Tech Hand Up Extrem Surg 2014;18(1):31–5.

27. Spencer EE Jr, Kuhn JE. Biomechanical analysis of reconstructions for sternocla-vicular joint instability. J Bone Joint Surg Am 2004;86(1):98–105.

28. Glass ER, Thompson JD, Cole PA, et al. Treatment of sternoclavicular joint dislocations: a systematic review of 251 dislocations in 24 case series. J Trauma 2011; 70(5):1294–8.

29. Rockwood CA Jr, Odor JM. Spontaneous atraumatic anterior subluxation of the sternoclavicular joint. J Bone Joint Surg Am 1989;71(9):1280–8.

30. Eskola A, Vainionpää S, Vastamäki M, et al. Operation for old sternoclavicular dislocation. Results in 12 cases. J Bone Joint Surg Br 1989;71(1):63–5.

31. Sabatini JB, Shung JR, Clay TB, et al. Outcomes of augmented allograft figure-of-eight sternoclavicular joint reconstruction. J Shoulder Elbow Surg 2015;24(6): 902–7.

32. Bak K, Fogh K. Reconstruction of the chronic anterior unstable sternoclavicular joint using a tendon autograft: medium-term to long-term follow-up results. J Shoulder Elbow Surg 2014;23(2):245–50.

33. Guan JJ, Wolf BR. Reconstruction for anterior sternoclavicular joint dislocation and instability. J Shoulder Elbow Surg 2013;22(6):775–81.
34. Sanchez-Sotelo J, Baghdadi Y, Nguyen NTV. Sternoclavicular joint allograft reconstruction using the sternal docking technique. JSES Open Access 2018; 2(4):190–3.
35. Tashjian RZ, Ross H, Granger E, et al. Single loop allograft reconstruction for sternoclavicular joint instability. JSES Int 2020;4(4):719–23.
36. Bae DS, Kocher MS, Waters PM, et al. Chronic recurrent anterior sternoclavicular joint instability: results of surgical management. J Pediatr Orthop 2006;26(1):71–4.

UNITED STATES POSTAL SERVICE® Statement of Ownership, Management, and Circulation
(All Periodicals Publications Except Requester Publications)

1. Publication Title
CLINICS IN SPORTS MEDICINE

2. Publication Number
000 – 702

3. Filing Date
9/18/2023

4. Issue Frequency
JAN, APR, JUL, OCT

5. Number of Issues Published Annually
4

6. Annual Subscription Price
$379.00

7. Complete Mailing Address of Known Office of Publication *(Not printer) (Street, city, county, state, and ZIP+4®)*
ELSEVIER INC.
230 Park Avenue, Suite 800
New York, NY 10169

Contact Person
Malathi Samayan

Telephone *(Include area code)*
91-44-4299-4507

8. Complete Mailing Address of Headquarters or General Business Office of Publisher *(Not printer)*
ELSEVIER INC.
230 Park Avenue, Suite 800
New York, NY 10169

9. Full Names and Complete Mailing Addresses of Publisher, Editor, and Managing Editor *(Do not leave blank)*

Publisher *(Name and complete mailing address)*
Dolores Meloni, ELSEVIER INC.
1600 JOHN F KENNEDY BLVD. SUITE 1600
PHILADELPHIA, PA 19103-2899

Editor *(Name and complete mailing address)*
Megan Ashdown, ELSEVIER INC.
1600 JOHN F KENNEDY BLVD. SUITE 1600
PHILADELPHIA, PA 19103-2899

Managing Editor *(Name and complete mailing address)*
PATRICK MANLEY, ELSEVIER INC.
1600 JOHN F KENNEDY BLVD. SUITE 1600
PHILADELPHIA, PA 19103-2899

10. Owner *(Do not leave blank. If the publication is owned by a corporation, give the name and address of the corporation immediately followed by the names and addresses of all stockholders owning or holding 1 percent or more of the total amount of stock. If not owned by a corporation, give the names and addresses of the individual owners. If owned by a partnership or other unincorporated firm, give its name and address as well as those of each individual owner. If the publication is published by a nonprofit organization, give its name and address.)*

Full Name	Complete Mailing Address
WHOLLY OWNED SUBSIDIARY OF REED/ELSEVIER US HOLDINGS	1600 JOHN F KENNEDY BLVD. SUITE 1600 PHILADELPHIA, PA 19103-2899

11. Known Bondholders, Mortgagees, and Other Security Holders Owning or Holding 1 Percent or More of Total Amount of Bonds, Mortgages, or Other Securities. If none, check box ▶ ☐ None

Full Name	Complete Mailing Address
N/A	

12. Tax Status *(For completion by nonprofit organizations authorized to mail at nonprofit rates) (Check one)*
The purpose, function, and nonprofit status of this organization and the exempt status for federal income tax purposes:
☒ Has Not Changed During Preceding 12 Months
☐ Has Changed During Preceding 12 Months *(Publisher must submit explanation of change with this statement)*

PS Form **3526**, July 2014 *[Page 1 of 4 (see instructions page 4)]* PSN: 7530-01-000-9931 PRIVACY NOTICE: See our privacy policy on www.usps.com

---

13. Publication Title
CLINICS IN SPORTS MEDICINE

14. Issue Date for Circulation Data Below
JULY 2023

15. Extent and Nature of Circulation

		Average No. Copies Each Issue During Preceding 12 Months	No. Copies of Single Issue Published Nearest to Filing Date
a. Total Number of Copies *(Net press run)*		142	137
b. Paid Circulation *(By Mail and Outside the Mail)*	(1) Mailed Outside-County Paid Subscriptions Stated on PS Form 3541 (Include paid distribution above nominal rate, advertiser's proof copies, and exchange copies)	99	69
	(2) Mailed In-County Paid Subscriptions Stated on PS Form 3541 (Include paid distribution above nominal rate, advertiser's proof copies, and exchange copies)	0	0
	(3) Paid Distribution Outside the Mails Including Sales Through Dealers and Carriers, Street Vendors, Counter Sales, and Other Paid Distribution Outside USPS®	23	23
	(4) Paid Distribution by Other Classes of Mail Through the USPS (e.g., First-Class Mail®)	13	18
c. Total Paid Distribution *(Sum of 15b (1), (2), (3), and (4))* ▶		135	130
d. Free or Nominal Rate Distribution *(By Mail and Outside the Mail)*	(1) Free or Nominal Rate Outside-County Copies included on PS Form 3541	6	6
	(2) Free or Nominal Rate In-County Copies Included on PS Form 3541	0	0
	(3) Free or Nominal Rate Copies Mailed at Other Classes Through the USPS (e.g., First-Class Mail)	0	0
	(4) Free or Nominal Rate Distribution Outside the Mail (Carriers or other means)	1	1
e. Total Free or Nominal Rate Distribution *(Sum of 15d (1), (2), (3) and (4))* ▶		7	7
f. Total Distribution *(Sum of 15c and 15e)* ▶		142	137
g. Copies not Distributed *(See Instructions to Publishers #4 (page #3))* ▶		0	0
h. Total *(Sum of 15f and g)* ▶		142	137
i. Percent Paid *(15c divided by 15f times 100)* ▶		95.07%	94.89%

* If you are claiming electronic copies, go to line 16 on page 3. If you are not claiming electronic copies, skip to line 17 on page 3.

16. Electronic Copy Circulation

	Average No. Copies Each Issue During Preceding 12 Months	No. Copies of Single Issue Published Nearest to Filing Date
a. Paid Electronic Copies ▶		
b. Total Paid Print Copies (Line 15c) + Paid Electronic Copies (Line 16a) ▶		
c. Total Print Distribution (Line 15f) + Paid Electronic Copies (Line 16a) ▶		
d. Percent Paid (Both Print & Electronic Copies) (16b divided by 16c × 100) ▶		

☒ I certify that 60% of all my distributed copies (electronic and print) are paid above a nominal price.

17. Publication of Statement of Ownership
☒ If the publication is a general publication, publication of this statement is required. Will be printed in the OCTOBER 2023 issue of this publication. ☐ Publication not required.

18. Signature and Title of Editor, Publisher, Business Manager, or Owner

Malathi Samayan — Distribution Controller

Date 9/18/2023

Malathi Samayan - Distribution Controller

I certify that all information furnished on this form is true and complete. I understand that anyone who furnishes false or misleading information on this form or who omits material or information requested on the form may be subject to criminal sanctions (including fines and imprisonment) and/or civil sanctions (including civil penalties).

PS Form **3526**, July 2014 *(Page 3 of 4)* PRIVACY NOTICE: See our privacy policy on www.usps.com

Moving?

Make sure your subscription moves with you!

To notify us of your new address, find your **Clinics Account Number** (located on your mailing label above your name), and contact customer service at:

Email: journalscustomerservice-usa@elsevier.com

800-654-2452 (subscribers in the U.S. & Canada)
314-447-8871 (subscribers outside of the U.S. & Canada)

Fax number: 314-447-8029

Elsevier Health Sciences Division
Subscription Customer Service
3251 Riverport Lane
Maryland Heights, MO 63043

*To ensure uninterrupted delivery of your subscription, please notify us at least 4 weeks in advance of move.

Printed and bound by CPI Group (UK) Ltd, Croydon, CR0 4YY

08/05/2025

01864750-0001